THE NURSE AS THERAPIST: A Behavioural Model

The Nurse as Therapist
A Behavioural Model

Edited by Philip J. Barker and Douglas Fraser

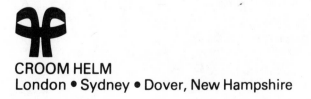

CROOM HELM
London • Sydney • Dover, New Hampshire

© 1985 Philip J. Barker and Douglas Fraser
Croom Helm Ltd, Provident House, Burrell Row,
Beckenham, Kent BR3 1AT
Croom Helm Australia Pty Ltd, Suite 4, 6th Floor,
64–76 Kippax Street, Surry Hills, NSW 2010, Australia

British Library Cataloguing in Publication Data

The Nurse as therapist: a behavioural model.
  1. Behaviour therapy   2. Psychiatric nursing
  I. Barker, Philip J.   II. Fraser, Douglas
  616.89′142′024613   RC489.B4

  ISBN 0-7099-3253-7

Croom Helm, 51 Washington Street, Dover,
New Hampshire 03820, USA

Library of Congress Cataloging in Publication Data
Main entry under title:

The Nurse as therapist.

  Includes index.
  1. Nursing. 2. Behavior therapy. I. Barker,
Philip J. II. Fraser, Douglas, 1949–
[DNLM: 1. Behavior Therapy—Nurses' instruction.
2. Nursing Care—methods. 3. Psychiatric Nursing—
methods. WY 160 N9723]
RT41.N84   1985   616.89′142′024613   85-10935
ISBN 0-7099-3253-7 (pbk.)

Phototypeset by Words & Pictures Ltd,
Thornton Heath, Surrey

Printed and bound in Great Britain by
Biddles Ltd, Guildford and King's Lynn

CONTENTS

Foreword
F.M. McPherson
List of Contributors

Part One: General Issues

1. Introduction   3
    Annie T. Altschul
2. The Development of Behaviour Therapy   16
    Philip J. Barker and Douglas Fraser
3. Rehabilitation in Psychiatric and Mental Handicap   47
    Hospitals
    Philip J. Barker and Douglas Fraser
4. The Nurse Therapist in a Primary Care Setting   92
    Philip J. Barker and Douglas Fraser
5. Creating Therapeutic Environments   115
    Robert C. Durham

Part Two: Case Studies

6. The Treatment of Bathing and Eating Problems in   147
    a Mentally Handicapped Woman
    Peggy Griffiths
7. A Time-limited Treatment Programme for   168
    Phobic Avoidance Behaviour
    Ilse Ablett
8. Increasing the Speech Output of a Mentally   186
    Handicapped Man
    Lydia M. Stephenson
9. A Time-limited Therapy in Late Pregnancy   208
    Jean Kirby
10. Reducing the Weight and Increasing the Work   226
    Output and Social Activity of a Long-stay Patient
    Christopher Portues
11. The Management of Chronic Pain   265
    William Harkin
Author Index   295
Subject Index   300

FOREWORD

This book has grown out of the course in behaviour therapy nursing which is organised by Tayside Area Clinical Psychology Department in conjunction with Dundee College of Nursing, the authors all being, or having been, closely associated with the course: Philip Barker as course leader; Douglas Fraser and Rob Durham as teachers and clinical supervisors; Annie Altschul as external examiner; and the case-study contributors as students on the course.

When this course was started in 1975, the aim was not to produce 'behaviour therapists', far less assistant or cut-price psychologists. Rather it was hoped to make a significant contribution to *nursing*, by providing nurses with knowledge and skills that would enable them to do their existing jobs, in ward, community or management, more effectively, or to develop new nursing roles, e.g. as clinical nurse specialists. The intention was that nurses should return from the course to serve as examples of good practice, and as 'prime movers', encouraging the development of behaviour therapy nursing in its various forms in their parent hospitals and services. For this reason, the course has always emphasised the teaching of behavioural *principles* as well as techniques, has encouraged the integration of the behavioural approach with more traditional nursing practice, and has tried to prepare the students for the practical difficulties of implementing new approaches within normal National Health Service settings.

These interactions and concerns are reflected in the various chapters of this book. The first two, by Professor Altschul and by Douglas Fraser and Philip Barker, show how behaviour therapy nursing is as much a product of processes within nursing as it is of external influences, e.g. from behavioural psychology. Many of the other chapters provide examples of how, by combining the approaches and methods of nursing with those of behavioural psychology, behaviour therapy nurses can make a contribution to treatment and care which is quite distinct from that made either by conventionally trained psychiatric nurses, or by clinical psychologists; in particular, they show how behaviour therapy nurses and psychologists can provide complementary, rather than alternative, services.

When behavioural programmes fail, it is often because the

organisational problems associated with the introduction of new modes of working have been underestimated, or recognised but not resolved. Rob Durham's chapter takes up these issues, and in particular the role-confusion and conflict which can be caused in multidisciplinary teams when nurses acquire and employ therapeutic expertise. The chapters of case studies which make up Part Two provide ample evidence of the scope of behaviour therapy nursing: of the wide range of problems with which appropriately trained nurses can deal, and the very different settings in which they function. These chapters also testify to the very high levels of theoretical and practical expertise which behaviour therapy nurses are capable of achieving.

Although the 10 years since the course began have seen dramatic developments in the scope, methods and expertise of behaviour therapy nurses, their numbers remain very small. The few courses, at Tayside, the Maudsley Hospital, Graylingwell, and elsewhere, produce a mere handful annually, and the majority of psychiatric and mental handicap hospitals and services in the UK have no nurses who have had formal training in behavioural methods. One reason for this slow development has been that many nursing managers have been unaware of the full scope and potential of behaviour therapy nursing, as indeed have many psychiatrists and clinical psychologists. What has been written has tended to appear in specialist journals, and no overview of the whole field has been available. This book fills this gap most impressively; no one reading it can doubt that, appropriately encouraged and organised, behaviour therapy nursing can make a significant, almost revolutionary, contribution not only to psychiatric nursing but to the health services in general.

F.M. McPherson

LIST OF CONTRIBUTORS

Ilse Ablett, Nurse Behaviour Therapist, North Tees District General Hospital, Stockton-on-Tees, Cleveland TS19 8PE, UK.

Annie T. Altschul, Emeritus Professor of Nursing, University of Edinburgh, Adam Ferguson Building, George Square, Edinburgh EH8 9LL, UK.

Philip J. Barker, Clinical Nurse Consultant in Behaviour Therapy, Royal Dundee Liff Hospital, Dundee DD2 5NF, UK.

Robert C. Durham, Principal Psychologist, Tayside Area Clinical Psychology Department, Royal Dundee Liff Hospital, Dundee DD2 5NF, UK.

Douglas Fraser, Principal Psychologist, Tayside Area Clinical Psychology Department, Royal Dundee Liff Hospital, Dundee DD2 5NF, UK and Sunnyside Royal Hospital, Montrose DD10 9JP.

Peggy Griffiths, Charge Nurse, Dingleton Hospital, Melrose, Roxburghshire TD6 9HN, UK.

William Harkin, Charge Nurse, Ravenscraig Hospital, Greenock PA16 9HY, UK.

Jean Kirby, Nurse Therapist, Community Psychiatric Nursing Service, St. Luke's Hospital, Marton Road, Middlesbrough, Cleveland TS4 3AF, UK.

F.M. McPherson, Director, Tayside Area Clinical Psychology Department, Royal Dundee Liff Hospital, Dundee DD2 5NF, UK.

Christopher Portues, Charge Nurse, The Westbury Centre, Winterton Hospital, Sedgefield, Near Stockton-on-Tees, Cleveland TS21 3EJ, UK.

Lydia M. Stephenson, Nurse Behaviour Therapist, Gogarburn Hospital, Corstorphine, Edinburgh EH12 9BJ, UK.

PART ONE: GENERAL ISSUES

1 INTRODUCTION

Annie T. Altschul

Mentally disordered people exist in all cultures and in all societies. There have always been unhappy, maladjusted, or ineffective people, or those whose behaviour seems strange to others. In different societies and at different periods of time, what is done about such people varies. How such people are described, classified and labelled determines to some extent whose responsibility it is to do something about them. Description, classification and labelling in turn are the expression, on the one hand, of the beliefs and values which members of society share, and, on the other hand, the result of the professional socialisation of those to whom society has assigned responsibility for such people.

Books on the history of psychiatry remind us of the tortures of the Middle Ages, of the way in which the Renaissance period sanctioned witch hunts and of the deplorable conditions of the madhouses of the seventeenth and eighteenth centuries (see Walk, 1961). 'Humane treatment arrived', according to Ackner (1964), in 1792 when Pinel removed the chains from patients at the Bicetre Hospital in Paris. We are not naive enough today to believe that enlightenment simply 'arrived' or that it was coincidence that such humane and enlightened doctors as Pinel in France and Tuke in England should simultaneously decide to liberate the mentally disordered from the degrading restraints which had been placed on them. Tuke and Pinel were representatives of the educated classes of their society, reading contemporary literature, discussing modern philosophical and psychological ideas, studying recent scientific and medical writings. Lewis (1967) provides a masterly sketch of the background against which the work of these pioneers should be viewed.

One point which we should perhaps remember is that in the dark period of the Middle Ages 'community care' was practised. People who were mad were at large, and fools had a place at court; it was later, at the height of the 'age of reason', that institutions were created to house all those no longer acceptable to society. The mad, the criminal and the poor were housed in the same institutions.

The achievement of the pioneers of psychiatry was to separate the

3

mentally ill from all the others who were confined to institutions: on moral grounds, because it seemed wrong to judge the insane whose own ability to make moral judgements was diminished, and on pragmatic grounds, because the insane were considered to be a danger to other prisoners and in danger from them.

It is interesting to note that in order to separate the mentally ill for treatment from others whose wrongdoings were to be punished, medical skills and judgement were believed to be necessary. One of the by-products of the achievement of these early efforts to liberate the mentally disordered was probably to delay reforms for prisoners; another, now regarded as unfortunate by some people, was to lodge responsibility for the care of the insane firmly in the orbit of the medical profession. Medical skills included careful observation, rigorous categorisation of the phenomena called symptoms, and documentation of the circumstances in which these phenomena occurred. The repeated coexistence of certain phenomena led to speculation about their explanation, to a process of naming the syndromes, i.e. 'diagnosing' the disease, and to the planning of appropriate treatment. Pinel was among the earliest doctors who also advocated the practice of carrying out a statistical analysis of the incidence of the observed phenomena in order to help in understanding and evaluating the outcome of the prescribed treatment.

The usefulness of careful observation and accurate documentation has become increasingly evident to all who care for the mentally ill. Though nurses were slow to incorporate these in their practice, those nurses who have become interested in behavioural therapy were quickest off the mark. All nurses who have committed themselves to any form of systematic nursing care now base the process of their action on reliable and valid observation and documentation. The usefulness of statistical treatment of observations has also now become generally accepted among nurses.

The interesting stage, that of grouping symptoms into syndromes and of labelling these, was necessary to ensure that statistical analysis compared like with like. However, the effort to classify mental disorder by symptom group has, in the opinion of some people (including nurses and doctors), had unfortunate effects. It has emphasised description, paying less attention to the dynamics or to the aetiology of the disorder. It has resulted in the study of disorder rather than the human being behind the classificatory frame. It has led to an attitude in which one sees symptoms as belonging to the patient rather than concentrating on disordered interaction between the patient and others. A description of a patient as aggressive, hostile, combative, which is still sometimes to be found in textbooks, is the outcome of such an attitude. It leads people to ask how to treat a 'combative patient', instead of asking what behaviour of others has caused the patient to fight.

In spite of this, however, it was clear to the early psychiatrists that historical events in the patient's life and environmental circumstances had an influence on the manifestation of symptoms.

Tuke believed that, in the calm surroundings of a country retreat, mental disorder had the best chance of subsiding. Pinel believed in a more positive influence of the hospital environment as a place where temperance and other moral values could overcome the patient's wildness and wickedness. It took nearly another 50 years before these ideas found widespread application in psychiatric hospitals. It was Conolly in 1839 who appears first to have realised that the right kind of environment for the mentally disordered had to be carefully created and that staff had to be specially selected and trained for the purpose. Conolly is quoted by Lewis (1967) as saying:

It appears to me that only after the abolition of mechanical restraint could the proper study of insanity begin, the removal of restraint and of all violent and irritating methods of control, thus permitting the student to contemplate disorders of the mind in their simplicity, no longer modified by exasperating treatment.

Conolly at Hanwell and later Browne at the Crichton Royal Hospital considered in detail the role of the 'attendants of the insane'. Their lectures from 1837 onwards and their later *Handbook for Attendants of the Insane*, published in 1885 by the Royal Medico-Psychological Association, gave a clear indication that the predecessors of psychiatric nurses were taught how to control and modify behaviour.

Psychiatric nurses in the United Kingdom have been controlling and influencing patients' behaviour without mechanical restraint since at least the late nineteenth century. The Lunacy Acts of 1890 specifically prohibited their use. Though seclusion (locking up a patient in a room by himself) was permitted under medical orders, if strictly controlled and reported to the Board of Control, this was generally believed to be non-therapeutic and only to be resorted to when it became necessary to protect staff in emergencies until more help could be obtained.

It would be of interest to find out why the 'enlightenment' which had such a profound effect on the care of the mentally ill in France and in the United Kingdom did not affect their treatment in the rest of Europe. In the United States, where Dorothea Dix campaigned against the conditions in poorhouses early in the nineteenth century and where several small private asylums were created as early as 1818–25, humane treatment of the insane did not become established practice for a long time.

It is a paradox that the psychodynamic theory of Freud and the psycho-biological theory of Adolf Mayer of the late nineteenth and early twentieth centuries should have had as much or even more influence on American psychiatry as they have in the United Kingdom; and nevertheless the care of the mentally ill in institutions remained restrictively custodial there for much longer than in the United Kingdom. Until quite recently, nursing textbooks published in the USA, for example, described the use of cold wet packs to control combative behaviour of patients.

Conditions described by Goffman (1961) in 'total institutions' continued to exist in the USA for much longer than they did in the United Kingdom. It was only in 1960 that a committee on psychiatric nursing of the Group for the Advancement of Psychiatry began to explore how nursing care could be improved. On the other hand, American nurses identified their therapeutic role in work with individual patients long before British psychiatric nurses did so.

We may obtain a clue to the different approaches by looking at the way nursing education has developed on the two sides of the Atlantic.

In the United Kingdom, mental-nurse training has an uninterrupted history from the time when the Royal Medico-Psychological Association began to interest itself in the preparation of those to whom they delegated the task of managing institutions. Medical Superintendents felt responsible for all aspects of the life of their 'patients' and consequently for the quality of the 'attendants' and, later the 'nurses' who were employed. They ensured that every institution for the insane became a training school for staff, taught and examined the nurses and, through their professional organisations, issued certificates to successful candidates. In 1871, Maudsley proposed that the RMPA set up a register of 'good attendants' to raise the standards of care. General nurse training, under the model introduced by Florence Nightingale, had no part to play in the training of asylum staff and they did not organise their qualifications on a national basis until 1919 when a registration of nurses was achieved (against the ideas put forward by Florence Nightingale).

In America, it was a nurse trained on the Nightingale model, Linda Richards, who first decided that the mentally ill needed care from trained personnel. McLean Hospital, Massachusetts, established a training school in 1882. By the end of the century there were about twenty American 'asylums' providing programmes of training. However, in the majority of institutions the mentally ill continued to be cared for by untrained attendants.

Early in the twentieth century, schools of nursing in American general hospitals were, however, beginning to seek a period of affiliation to a psychiatric hospital for their students, and by 1952 some psychiatric nursing experience was a requirement for registration. In the United Kingdom, even optional experience in psychiatric nursing only became available in the 1960s, and a compulsory psychiatric component of general nursing had to await the directives of the European Economic Community late in the 1970s.

In America, the objective of the psychiatric experience was to help nursing students to improve their interpersonal skills, to learn to study their own psychological make-up and to establish control over their own behaviour in interaction with their patients. Nursing students were encouraged to develop the ability to use themselves as a therapeutic tool in their dealings with patients.

It was not envisaged that nurses, after only a few weeks of psychiatric nursing experience, would have a role in in-patient settings. A number of nurses educated in the growing academic setting in America found their psychiatric experience of sufficient interest to want to progress beyond the elementary level of the Bachelor's course. Masters and Doctorate programmes developed rapidly, preparing nurses for intensive therapeutic work with individual patients. Different theoretical frameworks are used as a basis in different schools of nursing. Peplau (1952), the originator of the 'therapeutic use of self', based her work on the interpersonal theory of Sullivan (1953). The nurse, according to Peplau, helps the patient to improve his competence in interpersonal relationships or learns new ways of developing these. The nurse, in the process, must assess her own interpersonal behaviour and its effect on the patient.

Mellow (1966), who encouraged her students to work with severely disturbed schizophrenic patients, based her work on Freudian and Neo-Freudian explanations of emotional development. The role of the psychiatric nurse, according to Mellow, is to share with the patient highly charged emotional experiences, hoping to achieve resolution of the acute phase of the illness.

More recently (ANA, 1976) the role of psychiatric nurses came to be seen to encompass the use of group skills, milieu therapy and learning theory, but still only in the individual treatment of the patient, not in the day-to-day management of the treatment setting.

Meanwhile, mental-nurse training in the United Kingdom, having remained entirely separate from general nurse training even after the General Nursing Councils had accepted responsibility for training, examinations and registration, continued to emphasise the importance of environmental factors in the control of mental disorder and in the management of the patient.

Nurses (and psychiatrists) in the United Kingdom have always been more eclectic than their American colleagues. They have incorporated a variety of theoretical frameworks into their practice, without ever finding it necessary to base their work entirely on any one of them.

The goal of all therapy is to change some unsatisfactory aspect of a patient's experience or personality or behaviour, but generally nurses have managed to work for change without attempting to clarify the theoretical assumptions they hold about the nature of such experience, or the development of personality, or the causes of certain kinds of behaviour. The principles underlying the introduction of change did not concern them very much either.

What was at times described as 'moral treatment' seems to have suited nursing staff who were recruited for their kindly, tolerant and humane behaviour towards patients. The effectiveness of moral treatment depends on the contract in the ordinary activities of everyday living between patients and staff. The creation of a cohesive ward and hospital community where standards of living for patients were relatively high, and one small enough for the establishment of easy personal relationships, seemed to be the essence of moral treatment (Rees, 1958).

It was recognised that the ordinary activities of daily living should resemble the normal circumstances of the patients as much as possible. Opportunity for work, sports and recreation, for example, were provided. Nursing staff were recruited at least partly because of their interest in football or in theatrical performance, or their ability to instruct patients in crafts or farming. Patients and staff worked side by side in the hospital laundry, bakery, clothing store, kitchens and gardens, and on the cricket pitch. It was only when hospitals had become too big and impersonal that the social distance between staff and patients increased, that the patients' ability to work became exploited and the conditions described by Barton (1976) developed, and that life in the institution became antitherapeutic.

Although there have been ups and downs over the years in the levels of humanising ideology among nursing staff of psychiatric hospitals, the shift from 'moral treatment' towards 'milieu therapy' and the introduction of 'therapeutic community' ideologies seemed a natural progression. The 'therapeutic' community' approach views the hospital or the psychiatric ward as a social system within which the attitudes and actions of each person affect the quality of life, the behaviour and the relationships of staff and patients. One of the underlying assumptions is that patients' difficulties become manifest in their participation in ward life and that these difficulties must be examined in regular open discussion with all concerned, i.e. fellow patients, staff and possibly significant others such as the patients' family and friends. Free discussion of the problems as they arise can only happen if continuous effort is made to resolve conflicts between staff and to create an atmosphere in which staff respect each other and are willing to examine their own motives. A democratic egalitarian ideology which facilitates a breaking down of the distinction between patient and staff roles and between the doctors' and other staff members' roles is a necessary condition if patients are to use the ward effectively as a learning environment.

The theoretical bases for the practice of milieu therapy or therapeutic community approaches are to be found, on the one hand, in the psychodynamic interpretation of interpersonal behaviour and, on the other hand, in social psychology and the concept of 'social learning'. Without necessarily examining these theoretical stand-points, nurses have been able to adapt to the role expectations which are implied, namely to provide the patients with a safe environment which offers the opportunity to gain insight and to learn alternative modes of operating. No specific approach to individual patients is required, but it is necessary that the nurse should see herself as a facilitator of patients' growth and learning rather than as an active agent who administers nursing care. Parsons and Bales (1965) have described this as the 'expressive function' in contrast to the instrumental function which doctors assume in some treatment settings.

How psychiatric nurses can learn and adapt to this role is described by Towell (1975). The transition from moral treatment to the therapeutic community approach has not been entirely without interruption in the history of psychiatric nursing.

The phase of predominantly 'custodial' care may perhaps be put down to the effect of the increased size of the hospitals, and the difficulties in a period of full employment of finding high-quality staff, especially as financial incentives for work in mental hospitals were lacking. However, Lader and Allderidge (1973) put it down to the fact that once moral treatment has been accepted, it usurped any attempt at medical treatment. Several hundred patients in the 'care' of a single medical officer who was mainly concerned with the management of moral treatment may have been the cause for medical pessimism, and the cause of the increase in the numbers of chronic patients and the overcrowding of hospitals where nothing could be done beyond the provision of basic care and supervision.

A renewed wave of interest by the medical profession had its origin in Europe: in Germany, with the introduction of malarial treatment for general paralysis of the insane; in Vienna with the use of insulin coma therapy for schizophrenia; in Hungary with the induction of epileptic fits, first in patients suffering from schizophrenia, later to reduce depression; and, in Portugal, with operations to divide the pathways between the frontal lobes of the brain and the thalamus to reduce the intensity of emotions which had disrupted the behaviour of severely disturbed patients.

A renewed interest in the relationship between brain disease and mental disorder and, more generally, between physical and mental disorder resulted in much progress, but as far as nursing was concerned, also in considerable setbacks.

All physical forms of treatment in the first instance rendered patients more ill and dependent, and it was therefore necessary to introduce into psychiatric hospitals nurses with experience in general nursing. That the introduction of general nurses depressed the status of the mental nurse had been pointed out even before the advent of physical treatment (Walk, 1961), but became even more obvious later when the General Nursing Councils introduced a syllabus for training patterned on that for general nurse training and largely irrelevant to work with psychiatric patients, and when Health Authorities began to regard general nursing qualifications as prerequisites for promotion.

One might think that under the influence of general nurses, psychiatric nursing would have shifted from moral treatment to patient-centred care, but this was not the case. It became task centred and management orientated, not only in practice but also in its ethos. Fitting in with hospital life appeared to become a goal by which patient progress could be measured, and a system of 'progressive care' was introduced in many hospitals in which patients moved 'up' and 'down' a series of wards according to whether they appeared more or less able to adapt to the expectations of the ward. This system is not entirely without merit if one views the psychiatric hospital as a learning laboratory, but it does not encourage planning of care for individual patients or provide any continuity of relationships either with staff or with other patients.

All the varieties of psychiatric nursing practice discussed so far are based on the underlying assumption that behaviour, irrespective of the patients' diagnosis or of the likely aetiology of their disorder, is capable of changing and that nurses can, by some ill-defined method, act as change agents. How, specifically, any one individual patient might be helped to change his behaviour did not appear to be considered by either doctors or nurses. It was psychologists who first addressed themselves to this question.

Psychologists originally found their way into the psychiatric field as people whose training might enable them to observe and describe behaviour, record conditions under which it occurred, and thus assist the psychiatrist in diagnosis. They were fulfilling a similar function in education, in helping to classify children for the purpose of providing suitable schooling or corrective treatment if they were delinquent. However, in their training, psychologists had also learned to produce abnormal behaviour, for example in rats, and had developed theories of learning which explained how desirable behavioural responses could be increased and undesirable ones decreased. Psychologists began to make their influence felt in the early 1960s (Eysenck, 1959), and the history of behaviour therapy from then will be discussed in a later chapter. Here it is only intended to touch briefly on the way the psychologists' perspective affected psychiatric nurses. No systematic analysis is attempted.

Where the psychologists' new approach was most easily acceptable was in the area of habit training, especially with children, because, in spite of the nurses' general ideology which decreed that all patients should be treated alike, those who wetted the bed or whose toilet training had been delayed demanded personal attention and had to be given extra care. The pad-and-bell method for waking sufferers from nocturnal enuresis, for example, found quick acceptance.

Nurses also agreed readily that it could be their function to assess the self-help skills required by mentally handicapped patients. Although they found it easy to give approval whenever patients gained any success, they found it difficult to withhold attention when patients behaved inappropriately, as all their nursing training and the personality characteristics which brought them into nursing in the first place dictated that the more ill and helpless a patient is, the more attention he should command. That they might actually be reinforcing inappropriate behaviour by their attention to the patient was difficult to accept. Psychologists who themselves introduced behaviour-modification schemes successfully found that staff behaviour was not maintained when their research was completed.

Another group of patients who obtained early attention from psychologists was that of austistic children. The profound distress which a psychotic child so frequently manifests, the restlessness and withdrawal from other children, seemed to call for undivided attention from a single person for long periods of time. It was not easy for nurses to realise that they might be reinforcing the child's abnormal pattern of behaviour.

Other problems arose for nurses when psychologists attempted to design programmes for individual patients (Shapiro, 1961). The nurses' unwillingness or inability to adopt tailormade programmes for one patient, for example not to urge the patient to come to the dining room while doing so for the other patients, or to accompany one patient alone on the way to another department whereas they escorted others in groups, resulted partly from their general approach of concerning themselves with the ward as a whole, and partly from their traditional position in the relationship pattern of the mental hospital. It was usual for nurses to take instructions from doctors but not from other staff, such as psychologists. It was also usual for them to be consulted by doctors. Psychologists did not always consult nurses, even though at times nurses would have been the most appropriate people to help identify suitable reinforcers or to provide relevant baseline observational data. Nurses were generally unenthusiastic about behavioural therapy until relatively recently.

From psychiatrists they adopted the belief that behaviour modification programmes were able only to relieve symptoms and that they ignored underlying psychodynamic or personality problems. It is of note that psychiatric textbooks on the whole tend to deal with behavioural therapy only very briefly, dismissing it as of very limited importance or highlighting the possible dangers of other symptoms emerging as substitutes.

Some of the earliest behaviour modification techniques were particularly distasteful to nurses (as indeed to others), for example the aversion therapies applied to the consumption of alcohol or to overeating or gambling.

Token economy programmes did, at first, appear acceptable to nurses. It was self-evident to psychologists and to psychiatrists that these could only be initiated with the wholehearted co-operation of nursing staff, as it was they who had to deliver the tokens whenever appropriate behaviour occurred, so the principles of behaviour modification had to be taught to nurses. Their relationships with patients played an important part in the functional analysis of behaviour, in target setting and in negotiating schedules of rein-forcers. But ethical problems troubled nurses a good deal. First, they felt guilty about ignoring some of the behaviour which it was hoped would not be repeated because it was ignored. They had misgivings about their right to control other people's behaviour, they disliked using tokens, which they often regarded as bribes, and they disliked the artificial value assigned to those activities which patients were expected to pay for with tokens they had earned.

There has been a marked change in recent years and nurses have enthusiastically adopted behavioural therapy as their proper role. How and why this change has come about is well documented by Barker (1982). Perhaps one of the reasons lies in the demonstration by Marks, Hallam, Philpott and Connolly (1977) that nurses can carry out behaviour therapy as effectively as other professionals. From Mark's point of view, it is an advantage that they do so more cheaply, though this argument is not likely to be attractive to nurses. Another reason may be that behavioural therapy was recognised by the Joint Board of Clinical Nursing Studies and the Committee for Clinical Nursing Studies for Scotland, and that each developed a syllabus and approved advanced training schemes now operated under the aegis of the respective National Boards for Nursing, Midwifery and Health Visiting.

The post-registration qualifications that are awarded designate behavioural therapy nursing as a speciality, outside the mainstream of psychiatric nursing or of the nursing of the mentally handicapped. To call nurses who have gained such a qualification 'therapists' deliberately sets them aside, a trend deplored by many. Tierney (1976), for example, as a result of her work with mentally handicapped children, strongly advocated that the skills of behaviour modification should be acquired by all nurses.

It would seem that the main reason for the acceptance by nurses of the principles and practice of behaviour modification is that nursing generally has moved in that direction. No longer do nurses mainly want to care for wards; they want to deliver individualised nursing care under whatever name — nursing process, holistic nursing or behavioural therapy.

All nurses have accepted the need for assessment for recording and for evaluation. Behavioural therapists are showing them how this can be done. Psychiatric nurses have recognised that the purpose of all nursing care is to help people to increase their ability to exercise their own judgement and their ability to cope. Behavioural therapy is no exception. It does not imply that the therapist decides what behaviour is desirable or undesirable; it is designed to help the patient in the task of identifying for himself satisfactory and unsatisfactory ways of coping. Psychiatric nurses have come to realise that the goals of behaviour change must be related to the needs and well-being of the patient, not the institution. They have accepted that they cannot opt out of the business of controlling the behaviour of their patients. To do so by behavioural techniques is not incompatible with their mandate of creating a special environment in which the patient can learn. The nurses' therapeutic orientation must accommodate simultaneously a model of illness and of social learning. Nurses do not necessarily have to decide between social deviation and illness, but they must understand the theoretical assumptions about human nature which guide their actions in their professional role.

References

Ackner, B. (1964) *Handbook for Psychiatric Nurses*, 9th edition, Baillière, Tindall and Cox, London

ANA (1976) Division on Psychiatric and Mental Health Nursing Practice. *Statement on Psychiatric and Mental Health Practice*, ANA, Kansas City

Barker, P. (1982) *Behaviour Therapy Nursing*, Croom Helm, London

Barton, R. (1976) *Institutional Neurosis*, 3rd edition, Wright, Bristol

Eysenck, H. (1959) 'Learning Theory and Behaviour Therapy', *Journal of Mental Science*, *105*, 61–75

Goffman, E. (1961) *Asylums*, Doubleday, New York

Lader, M. and Allderidge, P. (1973) *The SK & F History of British Psychiatry*, Smith, Kline and French Laboratories, Welwyn Garden City

Lewis, A. (1967) 'The Story of Unreason (1961) and Phillippe Pinel and the English (1955)', in *The State of Psychiatry: Essays and Addresses*, Routledge and Kegan Paul, London

Marks, I.M., Hallam, R.S., Philpott, R. and Connolly, J. (1977) *Nursing in*

Behavioural Psychotherapy, Royal College of Nursing, London
Mayer, A. (1957) *Psychobiology: A Science of Man*, Charles Thomas Publishers, Springfield, Ill.
Mellow, J. (1966) 'Nursing Therapy as a Treatment and Clinical Investigation. Approach to Emotional Illness', *Nursing Forum*, 5 (3), 64
Parsons, T. and Bales, R. (1965) *Family, Socialisation and Interaction Process*, The Free Press, Clencoe, Illinois
Peplau, H. (1952) *Interpersonal Relations — Nursing*, Pitman, New York
Rees, T.P. (1957) 'Back to Moral Treatment', *Journal of Mental Science, 103*, 303–25
Shapiro, M.B. (1961) 'A Method of Measuring Psychological Changes Specific to the Individual Psychiatric Patient', *British Journal of Medical Psychology, 34*, 151–5
Sullivan, H. (1953) *The Interpersonal Theory of Psychiatry*, Norton, New York
Tierney, A. (1976) 'Behaviour Modification in Mental Deficiency Nursing', PhD Thesis, University of Edinburgh
Towell, D. (1975) *Understanding Psychiatric Nursing*, Royal College of Nursing, London
Walk, A. (1961) 'The History of Mental Nursing', *Journal of Mental Science* (monograph), *107*, 446

2 THE DEVELOPMENT OF BEHAVIOUR THERAPY

Philip J. Barker and Douglas Fraser

Introduction

Every historical account of significant developments in politics, science or the arts is a personal history which tells us a great deal about the author in addition to providing us with fresh insights into his subject matter. The decisions which the historian takes in selecting, condensing and editing material for his work reflect his personal as well as his professional attitude towards the events that he is trying to portray. There is little doubt, therefore, that the historian is irredeemably biased in his reporting of the 'facts'. With this in mind, you should be aware from the outset that our account of the integration of behaviour therapy into nursing practice is, likewise a biased account. What follows is no more than our interpretation of the way in which two entirely separate disciplines established a relationship, and of the advances which were promoted by this union. In tracing the most significant developments in the theory and practice of the behavioural model of nursing which issued from this relationship, we are relating a story with a beginning and a middle but, as yet, with no foreseeable ending.

The Roots of the Therapeutic Model

In order to examine the roots of this behavioural model of nursing practice, we need to trace the developments of the significant 'learning theories' that provide the backcloth to this story. In particular we need to distinguish clearly between 'instrumental learning' theory and 'classical conditioning' theory. (See Figure 2.1.) These two fundamental theories help us to understand, and to distinguish between, behaviour which is shown 'voluntarily', and that which is involuntary or appearing to be beyond the control of the individual. Instrumental learning theory is concerned with the effects of the 'environment' upon patterns of behaviour which the person shows 'voluntarily'. Classical conditioning theory focuses on the mechanism by which 'reflex' behaviour is produced and maintained.

16

Figure 2.1: Major Contributors to the Development of Behaviour Therapy

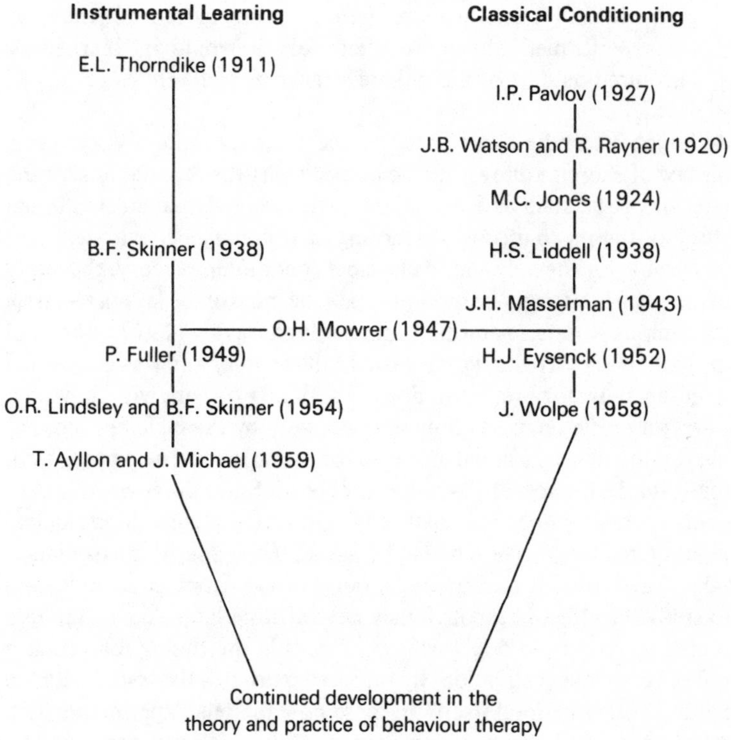

Instrumental Learning

E.L. Thorndike (1911)

B.F. Skinner (1938)

————— O.H. Mowrer (1947) —————

P. Fuller (1949)

O.R. Lindsley and B.F. Skinner (1954)

T. Ayllon and J. Michael (1959)

Classical Conditioning

I.P. Pavlov (1927)

J.B. Watson and R. Rayner (1920)

M.C. Jones (1924)

H.S. Liddell (1938)

J.H. Masserman (1943)

H.J. Eysenck (1952)

J. Wolpe (1958)

Continued development in the
theory and practice of behaviour therapy

One of the earliest instrumental learning theorists was the American, Edward Thorndike. In 1911 he published a book describing 'animal intelligence'. In the course of his research into this subject, Thorndike formulated two important 'laws of learning'. These were related to his famous trial-and-error learning experiments in which he studied the way cats learned how to escape from 'puzzle boxes': special cages with a range of complex 'release' mechanisms. Thorndike's two laws were as follows:

(1) The law of effect: here he proposed that if the animals' attempts to escape from the puzzle box were closely followed by some form of 'satisfaction', then the animal would tend to repeat this successful pattern of escape behaviour when placed again in the same situation. Conversely, any action on the part of the animal

which was closely followed by 'discomfort' would be less likely to occur again in the future.

(2) The law of exercise: here he proposed that the more *often*, the more recently, and the more *vigorously*, any pattern of behaviour was performed, the more effectively it would be learned or acquired as part of the animal's repertoire of behaviour.

Although Thorndike later modified these laws, eventually retracting his law of exercise altogether, he helped to lay the foundations for the later theorists, such as B.F. Skinner, who were also interested in the study of the mechanisms of learning in voluntary behaviour.

Turning for the moment to classical conditioning theory, this body of research is strongly linked — even in the mind of the layman — with the famous Russian neurophysiologist Ivan Pavlov (1927). Much of his work was carried out at the turn of the century and was concerned with the salivatory reflex in dogs. As all dog owners will know, the salivatory reflex can be stimulated not only by the taste of food, but also by the sight, the smell and even the sound of food being prepared; for example, the sound of a tin being opened. Since the sound of a can-opener working does not 'naturally' produce a change in biological functioning, the question had to be asked: 'How does this association take place?' Pavlov constructed a range of sophisticated experiments to study the effect of an obviously neutral stimulus — the sound of a tuning fork — on a dog's behaviour. Could the tuning fork elicit a reflex behaviour (salivation) by repeated pairing of the sound with the natural stimulus, food itself? In these now famous experiments with Alsatian dogs he showed how a tuning fork which was sounded just before the presentation of food would ultimately produce the salivatory response even when the food was absent. As the salivatory reflex was produced by a previously 'neutral' stimulus, the response was now called a 'conditional reflex' — it had been acquired through learning — and the neutral stimulus was now referred to as a 'conditioned stimulus'. (See Figure 2.2).

Other processes of 'learning' and 'unlearning' were also observed by Pavlov. Of prime importance were the concepts of extinction and generalisation. *Extinction* refers to the process by which the conditioned stimulus loses its power to produced the conditioned reflex. Pavlov found that by repeatedly sounding the tuning fork in the absence of food presentation, the conditioned salivatory reflex gradually disappeared: it was extinguished. As we shall show later, this process was thought to be crucial to the understanding of how

Figure 2.2: The Process of Classical Conditioning

Stage 1

Presentation of a neutral stimulus	⟶	closely followed by presentation of an unconditioned stimulus	⟶	elicits a reflex response
(e.g. sounding a tuning fork)		(e.g. food)		(salivation)

Stage 2

After repeated pairings of the neutral stimulus and the unconditioned stimulus, the following is observed:

Presentation of ⟶ elicits the conditioned response
the conditioned
stimulus
(formerly the
neutral stimulus)

i.e. sounding of the tuning fork ⟶ elicits salivation

phobias could be overcome, or unlearned. *Generalisation* refers to the way in which the reflex behaviour can be produced by stimuli which are similar to, but not identical to, the original conditioned stimulus. For example, Pavlov noted that when the dog was conditioned to salivate in response to the sound of a middle C tuning fork, it would also salivate to a range of other tuning forks up and down the scale from middle C. However, it would be likely to produce less saliva the further away from middle C the note was sounded. It was clear that the same response would occur under different conditions, but would become weaker and weaker as the nature of the stimulus changed from the original. This generalisation process has been used to explain the way in which fears acquired under one set of conditions may spread over time to situations which appear to bear little resemblance to the one in which the fear was first experienced. For instance, a person who experiences a panic attack in a supermarket may, some weeks or months later, feel fearful of entering a small corner shop; or a child who is frightened by a dog barking at him may 'generalise' his fear to dogs on television, in pictures or even in toy form.

Development of a Practical Model

Having established the role of influential figures such as Thorndike and Pavlov as founding fathers of instrumental learning and classical conditioning, we will now chart the development of these theories separately. We shall begin with the instrumental learning model, or, as it later became known, operant conditioning.

Thorndike's law of effect was taken a significant stage further through the work of an American psychologist, Burrhus Frederick Skinner (1938). He was unhappy with the definition of what Thorndike had called 'a satisfying event' since this referred to an internal state. Skinner noted that this state was not observable, and therefore was not amenable to scientific investigation. He subsequently developed a theory of 'reinforcement', which referred only to the *observable events* that preceded and resulted from the animal's behaviour. A 'reinforcer' was defined, therefore, as any consequence of the animal's behaviour which made the future occurrence of that behaviour more probable. Conversely, a punisher was defined as any consequence of behaviour which reduced the future probability of occurrence of that behaviour.

Skinner also developed an 'extinction' model. He discovered that when 'reinforcing events' were removed, the newly acquired behaviour would soon stop — or be extinguished. However, he also noted that this did not happen right away. The frequency of performance of the behaviour usually *increased* first, before gradually dropping off: usually at a dramatic rate until it ceased altogether. He also pointed out that the animal could learn how to 'escape' from punishing events; and later use 'avoidance' to make sure that it was not punished. He argued that these specific 'escape and avoidance' behaviours would be strengthened — or reinforced — in a negative way: by ensuring that they prevented the presentation of punishing events. The basic features of this *operant conditioning* theory are shown in Table 2.1. As the table shows, when a positive consequence is presented, this is called reinforcement. When a negative consequence is presented, this is punishment. Alternatively, when the positive consequences are removed, extinction takes place; and when negative consequences are removed — by the animal escaping from or avoiding the situation, escape or avoidance learning takes place.

These principles of operant conditioning stemmed from laboratory work with rats and pigeons which Skinner studied under highly controlled conditions: the 'Skinner box'. This was a soundproof box

Table 2.1: Basic Features of Operant Conditioning Theory

Type of consequence	Presenting	Removing
Positive	Reinforcement	(By experimenter) Extinction
Negative	Punishment	(By organism) Escape/avoidance

which carried a lever on one wall, when rats were the subject of this experiment, or a disc, when pigeons were involved. After being placed in the box, the animal, which had been deprived of food for some time, gradually learned to press the lever or to peck the disc, in order to gain food pellets, which were delivered automatically down a chute into the box. The food pellets represented a positive consequence of the pressing or pecking behaviour, and food delivery was observed to increase the frequency of these responses. A grid was frequently incorporated into the floor of the box to allow the delivery of electric shocks to the animal's feet, in order to study the effects of the delivery of punishing consequences.

Skinner's work was first reported in the late 1930s but was not applied to the study of learning in people until much later. The first recorded attempt to use the principles of operant conditioning in this way was made by Paul Fuller (1949). In this report, to which he gave the unfortunate title of 'Operant Conditioning of a Vegetative Human Organism', he described how he translated some of Skinner's principles with a male, profoundly handicapped patient. The patient was first of all deprived of food for several hours, in the same way as Skinner had starved his laboratory animals. Then Fuller 'reinforced' slight movements of the arm, made by the man, by injecting warm sugared milk into his mouth. Since the frequency of arm movements increased significantly during this experiment, Fuller argued that this very simple experiment showed the potential of operant conditioning in the case of someone who previously had been thought to be incapable of any kind of learning.

However, we had to wait a further 10 years to see any development of this simple application of operant principles. In 1959 Teodoro Ayllon and Jack Michael published an article entitled 'The Psychiatric Nurse as a Behavioural Engineer'. In this report of a study in a large American state hospital they described how the reinforcement, extinction, escape and avoidance procedures, described by Skinner some 20 years previously, could be used to modify the behaviour of long-term psychiatric patients. Most of the patients involved in the study were classified as schizophrenic, but a proportion of the group were also thought to be mentally handicapped. The real significance of this study was that it was carried out by nursing staff working under the direction of clinical psychologists. Also, a very wide range of clinical problems were tackled, including delusional speech, aggressive behaviour, eating difficulties and the hoarding of rubbish. We are of the opinion that this study represents the starting point of a major therapeutic movement: the nurse as behaviour therapist. Consequently, we believe that the report should be read in its original form, rather than summarised or paraphrased by others. We draw your attention, therefore, to the reference section at the end of this chapter, where the original source of the article is cited.

We have described the early developments of therapeutic methods based on operant conditioning, but what use was made of the theory of classical conditioning? It is intereresting to note that Pavlov's theories of reflex conditioning were adopted, and developed, much more quickly than Thorndike's laws of instrumental learning. In particular, a number of people began to show an interest in how animals and people acquired various fears or 'neuroses'. Could such fears be conditioned through Pavlov's classical learning model? In 1920 John B. Watson and Rosalie Rayner reported the now infamous experiment in which they tried to condition a specific phobia in an 11-month-old child named Albert. 'Little Albert' — as he was subsequently referred to — was observed playing happily with a variety of small animals, including a white rat. It was also noted that this happy state could be disrupted, and an intense startle reaction produced, when, unobserved by Albert but in close proximity to him, the experimenter clashed a hammer against an iron bar. Watson and Rayner decided to find out if they could 'condition' little Albert to show this startle reaction in response to some innocuous stimulus for which purpose they chose the white rat. In their experiment, each time they presented little Albert with the rat, one of the experimenters would strike the iron bar loudly behind him, just as the child began to play with the animal. This was repeated a number of times. It was then noted that Albert became very distressed whenever the experimenters tried to give him the rat to play with. Watson and Rayner blithely concluded that they had succeeded in establishing a conditioned 'fear response' in the child. Later, when Albert was presented with similar stimuli — a white rabbit, a dog, a fur coat, cotton wool — he showed the same sort of 'fear response' which he had acquired in the white-rat experiment. The experimenters concluded that this was a demonstration of *generalisation* of the conditioned fear response similar to the generalisation effect described by Pavlov. It is sad to report that Albert was allowed to leave the hospital before his recently acquired fears could be deconditioned.

The process of treating conditioned fear reactions was amply demonstrated only a few years later. Mary Cover Jones (1924), working under Watson's direction, tried to resolve the phobic problems of young children using the principles of classical conditioning. One of the most widely reported examples is that of little Peter, a young boy who showed severe anxiety towards animals and a host of 'furry' objects, including fur coats, cotton wool, fur rugs and feathers. The boy showed the greatest degree of fear towards a rabbit, and this was selected as the 'target' stimulus for the treatment programme. The 'counter-conditioning' was achieved by feeding the child in the presence of stimuli which produced only a little anxiety and by gradually increasing the strength of the stimuli. While Peter was eating his favourite food, a rabbit in a cage was placed some distance away from him. Each day the cage was brought gradually closer, and the rabbit was eventually released from the cage. At the end of the treatment, not only was he unafraid of the rabbit when it was placed on his lap, but he spontaneously expressed a fondness for the animal which once he feared. Tests later showed that the extinction of his fear of the rabbit had generalised to other fur-like objects. Cover Jones used a variety of techniques, which she called 'verbal and direct conditioning'. Some of these techniques are recognisable under different titles in contemporary behaviour therapy. However, although this study is regarded as highly influential, it took another 34 years before the principles of classic conditioning were to be used as the theoretical basis of behaviour therapy techniques (Wolpe, 1958).

The experimental work with animals which began with Pavlov at the turn of the century continued into the 1930s with Liddell's (1938) conditioning of fears in sheep; and into the 1940s with Masserman's (1943) experiments with cats. With hindsight, it seems apparent that the behavioural movement was slow to make use of the principles of learning which had been expressed in the conditioning experiments of Pavlov and Thorndike. Indeed, those academic psychologists who did pick up the trail continued to restrict their studies to the microcosmic world of the animal laboratory. It should be apparent from our historical sketch that the pioneering work of people like Watson, Rayner and Cover Jones made little impact on the prevailing attitudes towards the treatment of the mentally disordered. Indeed, it was not until the early 1950s that the movement which we now know as behaviour therapy surfaced and in the operant-conditioning field it emerged as a by-product of 'pure' research. In the USA, Skinner, along with one of his disciples, Ogden Lindsley, set up a laboratory in the Metropolitan State Hospital in Massachusetts in 1953. Their intention was not to 'treat' patients but to study the behaviour of psychotic patients in an attempt to produce medically useful, objective, laboratory measures of the psychoses (Lindsley and Skinner, 1954). They studied the behaviour of chronic and acute 'psychotic' patients as well as a range of 'normal' people, using a small, six-foot-square, room which contained a reinforcement machine, complete with lever and a stimulus panel. When the patients pulled the lever, a range of small objects was delivered as reinforcement. In a series of experiments, sweets, cigarettes and projected pictures were used. The experimenters were able to record the frequency and sequence of lever-pulling; noting how the performance of this action was interrupted by long pauses during which the patient engaged in 'psychotic' behaviour. Some of these patients were studied in daily sessions for nearly 5 years: the reinforcement schedules (or predetermined criteria for reinforcer delivery) becoming more complex and the reinforcement list growing to include food, money, male and female nude pictures, music, tokens and the opportunity to give milk to kittens. Although these studies were concerned only with producing detailed measures of 'psychotic behaviour' — in terms of how it interfered with lever-pulling — the findings had obvious implications for the design of treatment programmes. It was noted that for some patients, as the frequency of lever-pulling was increased through reinforcement, the frequency of 'psychotic behaviour' decreased. For some patients the reduction in psychotic behaviour during the sessions appeared to generalise to the environment outside of the room. These and other findings gave impetus to the development of the use of operant principles in the treatment of chronic psychiatric patients. Of special note is the fact that Skinner and Lindsley were the first to use the term 'behaviour therapy', meaning the use of operant conditioning to change behaviour.

At around the same time as Skinner and Lindsley were experimenting in Massachusetts, Joseph Wolpe, a South African doctor who had become disenchanted with psychodynamic therapy, began to publish detailed descriptions of specific treatment techniques that he had developed in clinical practice. Wolpe's methods were strongly influenced by the animal experiments of Pavlov and Masserman, and he began his own series of experiments into the development of neurosis in cats. In these experiments Wolpe found that his cats refused to eat in the cages where they had been experimentally 'shocked': this food refusal was apparent after several days of food deprivation. Wolpe was interested in the way in which this experimentally induced anxiety inhibited feeding and in the possibility that, under different circumstances, feeding might inhibit anxiety. This led him to formulate his concept of *reciprocal inhibition*: one reaction, anxiety, inhibited the other, feeding, and vice versa. Using a 'graded' process which was very similar to Cover Jones' treatment of little Peter, Wolpe *desensitised* his cats by feeding them in situations which became more and more like the cage setting in which they had been shocked. By using this graded approach, in conjunction with the anxiety-inhibiting feeding response, the cats were eventually able to eat in the 'shock cage' with no apparent anxiety. Wolpe applied this line of research to his own patients' problems by using progressive relaxation training as a mechanism that inhibits anxiety. His patients were taught to imagine scenes that usually induced fear or anxiety: they were then taught to relax — thereby inhibiting the anxiety usually associated with the scene. These scenes were graded on a hierarchy representing the anxiety-arousing power of different situations. Their presentation to the patient was ordered from the least anxiety-arousing, gradually ascending to the most frightening. His most significant contribution to behaviour therapy was his description of *systematic desensitisation*, an approach which used this combination of hierarchies with the inhibition of anxiety through progressive relaxation. Details of his approach were published in 1958 in a textbook to which we have referred earlier in this chapter.

In Britain, Hans Eysenck emerged in the early 1950s as the leader of what became known as the Maudsley Group: a group of psychologists who were anxious to promote the development of clinical psychology which would be involved in both the objective assessment and treatment of psychiatric patients. They saw a means of achieving this goal through the development of a learning-based therapy, founded on experimental research with animals and on clinical research. As we have noted earlier, 'behaviourism' —

although historically as old as psychoanalysis — had made little progress as a clinical activity by the end of the Second World War. By contrast, psychoanalysis had staked its claim on the field of mental disorder: as the accepted way of explaining mental illness and as the exclusive means of relieving it. However, in 1952, Eysenck published his oft-cited critique of psychoanalytic therapy, in which he asserted that psychotherapy, of an analytic nature, was no more effective than no treatment at all. That is to say that the spontaneous remission rates of untreated patients were equivalent to the recovery rates of patients undergoing psychoanalysis. This publication led to a change in the attitude towards traditional forms of psychotherapy. Interest in the application and evaluation of behaviour therapy began to grow, and faith in the value of traditional psychotherapy began to weaken. Eysenck then went on to publish accounts of behaviour therapy methods in clinical practice (Eysenck, 1960), and in 1963 he established *Behaviour Research and Therapy*, the first journal devoted solely to developing the theory and practice of behaviour therapy. London then became a key centre for the training of psychologists and psychiatrists in behaviour therapy and, 10 years later, was to provide the base for the first training course for nurses in this approach.

Bridging the Models

The developments described above reflect two, seemingly incompatible, models of learning. Classical conditioning restricted itself to reflex behaviour and autonomic functioning, whereas operant learning was concerned with voluntarily emitted behaviour. By the 1960s these two approaches (behaviour therapy, commonly associated with the use of classical learning, and behaviour modification, emphasising operant conditioning) ran in parallel but were seen as two distinct methods of therapy with vastly differing ranges of applicability. However, much earlier (in 1947) O. Hobart Mowrer tried to link the operant and classical traditions in an effort to explain the process of fear acquisition more fully. Mowrer believed that neither model could, by itself, provide a comprehensive description of such a complex process. In particular he was interested in the *avoidance* behaviour shown by people expressing fear of certain situations or objects. How did people, or animals, develop this avoidance response: Mowrer did not believe that Pavlovian conditioning alone could account for this. Consequently he developed what has become known as his 'two-factor' theory. In very simple terms, this model suggested that people *acquired* a fear response through classical conditioning. The person then learned how to 'solve' this problem through operant learning: by escaping from the situation the anxiety or fear is reduced. Subsequently the person *avoids* the feared situation because he has experienced the 'reinforcement' of anxiety reduction, brought about by his escape methods. It should be apparent that Mowrer was using Thorndike's earlier experiments with cats as the basis for this model. In those studies cats 'escaped' from cages: this was described by Thorndike as leading to 'satisfaction' — a concept later redefined by Skinner to mean reinforcement. Consequently Mowrer's two-factor theory asserts that a fear response which is acquired by classical learning is maintained by operant reinforcement: which is gained through performing escape and, later, avoidance behaviour. This theory represented an important advance in behavioural theory and is frequently echoed by contemporary psychological theorists. (An illustration of Mowrer's two-factor theory is shown in Figure 2.3.)

Figure 2.3: A Two-factor Theory Concerning the Acquisition and Maintenance of Fears

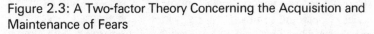

Neutral Stimulus   Reflex Response   Reinforcement

Unconditioned Stimulus   Operant Response

For example, the following sequence of events:

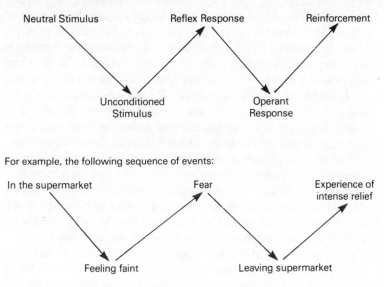

In the supermarket   Fear   Experience of intense relief

Feeling faint   Leaving supermarket

New Directions

The publication of the social learning theory of Albert Bandura and his colleagues in the late 1950s and early 1960s heralded further advances in behavioural theory and practice. Bandura (1969) was critical of the operant model because of its strict reliance upon external or environmental determinants of behaviour. His research suggested that the behaviour of the individual can affect the environment as well as vice versa. Bandura was the first of a long line of 'dissenting' voices that called for a change in the prevailing theoretical standpoint. In particular he wanted to replace environmental determinism, which assumed a one-way process of influence, with the concept of *reciprocal determinism* — a two-way process of influence.

One of the key features of Bandura's model was his argument that behaviour was *largely* learned through vicarious rather than direct experience. By vicarious he meant through others. Rosenthal (1982) argues that a wide range of complex behaviours, acquired throughout a person's lifespan, are in fact learned in this way through indirect experience. For instance, 'grammar patterns and language labels, strategies for solving conceptual problems; expressive and assertive styles of personal conduct; criteria to steer such abstract judgements as ethical decisions; and the approach to subjectively threatening events — all have been amenable to teaching through demonstration' (page 343). Rosenthal goes on to list a number of studies in which behaviour patterns have been developed by the use of these methods involving such complex 'behaviours' as standards for personal achievement, generosity, persistence, and tolerance of pain. Not only did Bandura question the assertion of all earlier theorists that learning had to be direct, but he also introduced the concept of the role of certain functions of the central nervous system as *mediators* of the learning experience: these became known as the *mediational processes*.

One of the important contributions made by social learning theory is to our understanding of *cognition*. Although the picture is by no means complete, the work of Bandura and his colleagues suggests that at least four cognitive processes are at work in bridging the gap between events that happen in the outside world and the eventual performance of 'response behaviour'. These are as follows.

Attention: We need not only to be able to 'focus' our attention upon stimuli coming from our environment, but we need also to be able to 'process' this information. This information-processing function appears to involve the use of memory as well as other decision-making functions. In a matter, literally, of a few microseconds we pick up, identify, label and in general 'recognise' the sounds and sights that we call environmental stimuli. If we do this incorrectly, we may be 'attending' to the *wrong* stimuli. This will influence the rest of the information-processing action.

Retention: A further stage in the process involves analysis of the stimuli. Here we begin to categorise the stimuli; allocating different stimuli, if you like, to different pigeon-holes in our memory bank. Here the information is stored for further use.

Reproduction: Here we give ourselves specific instructions to aid us in the performance of some pattern of overt behaviour. The information which has been processed in the two stages above is now retrieved, and used to help us to perform some pattern of motor behaviour.

Motivation: In the last stage a cognitive judgement is made about where and when it would be appropriate to show specific patterns of overt behaviour. This motivational judgement will also draw upon information stored in our memory: information which will help us to decide upon appropriate ways of behaving under different conditions.

Bandura and his colleagues have integrated much of the pure research on cognition with their experimental approaches towards the learning of overt patterns of behaviour. The summary given above is a necessarily crude representation of their social learning theory. However, it serves as a good illustration of the difference between the conditioning models of learning described earlier, and the mediational model described by Bandura. In the former it is assumed that learning takes place primarily as the result of the effect of 'external' variables. Bandura took a different viewpoint. He acknowledged that these external factors were important. However, he argued that it was the way in which the individual 'processed' this information coming from the outside world which determined whether or not he learned a specific behaviour. In a series of clever experiments Bandura and his colleagues showed that children could learn through *imitation* — i.e. through studying the behaviour of other children. They could store this behaviour — on a cognitive level — only showing it when the conditions were appropriate. From these experiments Bandura sought to show that most of our behaviour was learned *through* manipulation of these cognitive processes and that any technology of learning should take due note of this fact.

These imitative-learning experiments are very important since it was already clear that people acquired patterns of behaviour — both adaptive and maladaptive — through indirect experience, as well as by direct learning. One need not have had a bad experience with a snake to become a snake phobic. Similarly people can learn to tie shoelaces simply by watching someone else perform this complex motor task. Many of the techniques of behavioural change that were developing within the operant and classical learning traditions at this time were using *modelling* methods: where, with the patient as observer, the therapist performed a required behaviour, such as approaching a feared object, or demonstrating a skill. Clearly, learning under these conditions could not be explained completely by recourse to the operant or classical conditioning models. Bandura's social-learning model — which acknowledged the role of operant and classical learning — within an 'information-processing' paradigm seemed to offer a better explanation of the facts.

The Cognitive Therapies

The late 1960s and early 1970s saw a flourishing of interest in this mediational model. Several psychologists, such as Mike Mahoney (1974) and Donald Meichenbaum (1977), began to develop specific therapeutic techniques which were directed at the 'hidden behaviours' of thinking, memory, etc., referred to by Bandura. These techniques showed how *thinking* — which is an umbrella term for a wide range of 'mental processes' — could be used to assist in the performance of overt patterns of behaviour. Of particular significance at this time were Meichenbaum's experiments in which he first of all helped psychotic patients to control their 'thought disorder' and then helped children to reduce their impulsive acting-out behaviour. Both of these experiments used a technique that he called 'self-instructional training', and which relied heavily upon the manipulation of certain cognitive processes.

At around the same time, psychotherapists Albert Ellis (1962) and Aaron Beck (1976), were developing their own brands of psycho-therapy as alternatives to traditional psychoanalysis. Both therapies — 'rational emotive therapy' and 'cognitive therapy' — shared a similar assumption: that patients' disturbed patterns of behaviour were a function of certain thinking errors, which in turn were a function of some dysfunctional belief system. The cognitive therapy of Beck has shown the greatest potential to date, and involves a highly structured therapeutic process through which the patient is taught to recognise dysfunctional patterns of thinking and is then taught how to *challenge* these — through rational deduction. This focus upon the thinking patterns of the patient is linked to more overt patterns of behaviour. The patient learns to plan and execute 'behavioural experiments', each of which is designed to test out his thinking errors and to demonstrate the maladaptive nature of his belief system.

Cognitive therapy is an important advance since it provides a further, practical extension of the model articulated by Bandura. Beck's therapy helps the patient to learn about the relationship between his patterns of thinking, his emotions and his outward patterns of behaviour. A vast body of data has already been presented on the use of the approach with specific disorders — such as some forms of depression — and Beck (1976) argues that it is only a matter of time before the cognitive model of the 'emotional disorders' is shown to be of value with other types of psychiatric disorder.

The Applicability of Behaviour Therapy

It should be apparent that what we have described as 'behaviour therapy' is a very broad therapeutic system indeed. Some might argue that some practices — such as the 'cognitive therapies' — do not even fall within the scope of the behavioural model. However, Kazdin and Wilson (1978) have recently argued that all of these approaches are united by the following features:

(1) They present 'a psychological model of human behaviour that differs fundamentally from the traditional intrapsychic, psycho-dynamic, or quasi-disease model of mental illness'.
(2) They share 'a commitment to scientific method, measurement and evaluation' (page 7).

There is, however, a wide divergence of opinion concerning the range of applicability of behaviour therapy. For example, Marks, writing in 1979, suggests that 'in perhaps 12% of all psychiatric out-patients, which means 25% of neurotic out-patients, behavioural psychotherapy can be regarded as the approach of choice' (page 629). Marks is quite cautious in defining the boundaries of the province of behaviour therapy. He outlines the 'usefulness' of behaviour therapy as follows:

'Treatment of choice':
  phobic disorders
  social anxiety
  compulsive rituals
  sexual deviation and dysfunction
  nocturnal enuresis
  learning problems in children

'Probably useful':
  social skills deficits
  obsessive thoughts
  impulse control and habit disorders
  eating disorders
  morbid grief
  marital dysfunction
  nightmares
  child abuse
  conversion hysteria
  rehabilitation of chronic disorders
  conduct disorders in children

'Not useful':
  acute schizophrenia
  severe depression
  hypomania

Writing around the same time, Kazdin and Wilson (1978) considered that the following problems fell within the province of behaviour therapy:

'Neurotic disorders':
  generalised anxiety
  social anxiety
  phobic reactions (including agoraphobia)
  insomnia
  sexual deviation and dysfunction
  marital discord
  compulsive disorders
  obesity
  alcoholism

'Psychotic disorders' (focusing upon behaviours that may have contributed to the diagnosis, or may be a product of hospitalisation, rather than on psychosis as such):
  self-care behaviours
  participation in activities
  job performance
  social interaction
  delusional speech
  ritualistic behaviour

'Other applications':
  childhood disorders
  the mentally handicapped
  the elderly

Although we are in agreement with Marks' contention that behaviour therapy is 'not useful' with a certain, small, proportion of psychiatric disorders, we are much more in agreement with the broad-spectrum approach of Kazdin and Wilson: a wide range of 'problems of living' are amenable to remediation via an extensive repertoire of behaviour-change procedures. Hopefully, an indication of this range of applicability will become apparent in subsequent chapters of this book.

The Integration of Behaviour Therapy into Nursing Practice

As our review illustrates, the experimental and theoretical base of behaviour therapy is as old as Freudian 'ego psychology'. However, whereas Freud and his followers translated their theories very quickly into psychotherapy practice, there was a significant time-lag between the development of the early learning theories and the resultant therapeutic procedures. It is also clear that the behavioural model of mental disorder has grown more complex and sophisticated with the passage of time. Although the history of behaviour therapy spans less than three decades, in that time practitioners have progressed from dealing with discrete psychological problems to the manipulation of a complex range of factors associated with the patient's dysfunctional state. Therapists have progressed from using what now appear to be rather mechanical techniques of behaviour change, to using techniques which can involve the manipulation of imagery, thought processes, fantasy and memory as well as more overt patterns of behaviour. In the last decade behaviour therapists have shown their willingness to tackle such complex areas of psychological distress as depression, interpersonal relationship problems and psychological disorders associated with physical illness. The demonstrated effectiveness of these therapeutic innovations indicates that the behavioural model has much to offer patients whose problems involve more than simple phobic anxiety or learning deficits.

When we turn to consider the development of the nurse's role in behaviour therapy, we must study this within the historical development of psychiatric nursing itself. As the introductory chapter shows, nursing has evolved from a largely custodial, or caretaking, function into something resembling a true profession. Although nurses are now more sophisticated in their care of patients, their role is still described largely in terms of 'looking after people', 'preserving patients from harm or 'meeting individual patient needs'. The continued use of such vague concepts of care suggests that, in principle, psychiatric and mental-handicap nursing has not changed since the days of the great reformers like Tuke in the nineteenth century. In recent years, however, more emphasis has been placed on the nurse's role in changing the patient's behaviour. The influence of various intra-psychic and interpersonal theories of human behaviour led many nurses to experiment with forms of nursing care which involved a direct manipulation of the patient's social environment. This kind of 'milieu therapy' is associated traditionally with the work of innovators like Maxwell Jones (1952) and in the United States led to the development of a role for nurses as 'group therapists' or 'individual counsellors'.

To a large extent this role is still seen by many psychiatric nurses as the very basis of their art, especially since it can be traced back to the early psychodynamic theories from which modern psychiatry has evolved. However, as Hauser (1978) has commented, although psychiatric nurses were frustrated with their custodial role, and clamoured to learn and to utilise the theories of psychodynamic counselling and group work, this kind of care has never been properly evaluated. Indeed the key characteristics of such roles — which eschew the use of any systematic, tried-and-tested methods of effecting change — is the almost *magical* nature of the therapeutic effort: trying to effect change by means which are not clearly apparent to nurse or patient, if indeed they exist at all. You may wonder why we are stressing this point. What is the significance of this traditional psychotherapeutic role as far as the development of the nurse as behaviour therapist is concerned? We believe that it is important to stress the differences between the model of behaviour therapy and the psychotherapeutic model which nurses were beginning to develop from the early 1950s onwards. This model was derived from a range of psychodynamic theories which were, and indeed still are, largely unscientific in orientation. Such 'therapies' emphasised the manipulation of ill-defined social, interpersonal and intrapersonal processes as a way of helping patients. The developing model of behaviour therapy which we have described stands out in stark contrast. Drawing on the early laboratory experiments of Pavlov and Skinner, psychologists like Bandura began to develop a more 'scientific' framework for understanding how psychological problems could be acquired and remediated. This framework, originally drawn from studies with animals, later began to emphasise the complexity of human functioning and this has led to the development of therapeutic systems which are capable of meeting the challenge of the complexity of human behaviour. Developments like 'cognitive behaviour therapy' are beginning to embrace populations as diverse as mentally handicapped children (Borkowski and Cavanaugh, 1979) and depressed elderly patients. The therapy, although fundamentally practical in its application, acknowledges the complexity of the person behind the patient label. In this sense at least, such developments constitute radical departures within behaviourism, if not within psychiatry as a whole.

Early Experiments in Collaboration

It is worth noting that at the same time as nurses in Britain and the USA were developing their 'psychotherapeutic role', the experiment with the nurse as 'behaviour change agent' was also beginning. As we noted earlier, Teodoro Ayllon and Jack Michael were the first to investigate seriously the role of nurses as behaviour therapists. Although the role described was a limited one — the nurses worked under the direction of two psychologists all the time — this was the first clear example of how nurses could translate their traditional 'caring' role into one involving therapeutic change. As we discussed earlier, these nurses were successful in helping highly disturbed and institutionalised patients to become more independent and more 'self-controlled'. More importantly, the experiment showed the potential of various therapeutic procedures which could be learned by almost any nurse and which might help almost any institutionalised patient. It was also clear that the patients who were the focus of this experiment were not the kind of patients who might benefit from individual counselling or group therapy. It was also true that some of the staff who were given a chance to become 'therapists' would have otherwise been relegated to implementing the obscure ethos of the 'milieu therapy' setting. However, of paramount importance in our view was the illustration of the way in which nurses and psychologists might work together in a therapeutic partnership. The possibility was raised here that nurses might be willing to relinquish their largely subservient role relationship with doctors in favour of a more equal partnership with the ward psychologist.

The relationship between nurse and psychologist was not, however, purely a marriage of convenience. A number of researchers had shown that nurses (or rather nursing care) often made patients more disturbed or dependent. Instead of promoting 'health', nurses often were antitherapeutic.

This sort of finding was graphically described by Gelfand and her colleagues (1967). Studying the interaction of nurses and patients in a hospital setting, they found that nurses tended to ignore patients who showed acceptable or 'non-problematic' behaviour. Instead, they gave most of their attention to patients who were manifestly 'sick' or showing unacceptable patterns of behaviour. These nurses were influenced by the kind of psychodynamic theories which spawned the counselling/milieu therapy revolution. They took the view that, for example, very withdrawn patients were crippled by negative self-evaluations. The nurse's role was to provide the patient with sympathy and comfort, in order to re-establish his self-esteem. Gelfand noted that this view was promoted by a number of nursing textbooks which recommended that, for example, a mute patient should be handled by 'sitting with him for long periods and doing little things for him, like combing his hair or getting him a drink'. Gelfand took the view that such tender loving care only made 'sick' or maladaptive behaviour more likely, since only very withdrawn or disturbed patients received such intimate and specialised care.

This caring orientation was evident in nursing with other populations. In mental handicap, nurses tended to be supportive or custodial, acting on the assumption that most of their patients were ineducable or untrainable. Consequently attention focused upon providing 'total care': feeding, dressing and caring for personal hygiene. Ironically, this 'caring' approach also had negative side-effects. Studies conducted in large institutions in the mid 1960s showed that mentally handicapped people who lived in states of 'high dependence' were more likely to show highly disturbed patterns of behaviour, especially in the form of aggression, destruction or self-mutilation (Klaber and Butterfield, 1965). Most nurses viewed these problems as another facet of the condition of handicap itself, rather than as an unnecessary outcome of a restrictive care system. It should be noted, however, that many doctors were of a similar mind, many maintaining such myths of mental handicap well into the 1980s. Gradually the realisation began to dawn. Experiments such as that of Ayllon and Michael with psychotic patients were followed up by other researchers, for example Ivor Lovaas who worked with severely disturbed autistic and mentally handicapped children. Lovaas *et al.* (1973) showed that not only was it possible to reduce life-threatening forms of self-injury, but that such disturbed behaviour patterns could be supplanted by adaptive behaviour which allowed the individual a greater degree of independence within his environment. Other researchers, such as Todd Risley (1974), showed that it was also possible to analyse systematically the controlling function of the patient's environment, in order to develop care settings which would allow more adaptive patterns of behaviour to flourish. These experiments pointed the way towards using scientific methods in the design of genuinely therapeutic milieux.

An Alternative Perspective

The outcome of these various psychological and social-systems studies was a strong contention that improvements in the quality of care might result from promoting a greater understanding of the principles of learning in nurse training and an appreciation of the nurse's role in the construction of 'learning environments'. As the behaviour therapy movement began to assert itself in the late 1960s and early 1970s, more recognition was paid to the role of the nurse as an agent of change. Psychologists such as Dave Peck (1973) argued that the role of 'behaviour change agent' was a natural one for all nurses but that it should be developed to a greater level of sophistication. Peck was suggesting a change in the whole climate of care. He wanted to see the stereotyped role of the nurse as a subservient, passive, infinitely patient provider of 'tender loving care' exchanged for a more active, constructive role; a role that would involve the facilitation of therapeutic change through the deployment of knowledge and skills about human functioning, drawn from the ever-growing reservoir of the behavioural sciences.

The Honeymoon

From our brief historical review it should be clear that *change* was about the only constant feature of that quarter century between the 1950s and the mid 1970s. Nurses had become aware of their therapeutic potential soon after the end of the Second World War. They spent the best part of two decades trying to bring it to fruition: often like a poor magician trying to produce a dove from a flurry of silk scarves. Some would say that the trick has yet to be performed, that nurses have not yet established in any precise or unique way what their therapeutic role is (Altschul, 1977). More importantly, it could be argued that although we have evidence that some nurses make their patients worse, we have little competing evidence that nurses can have a positive effect upon their patients' states. We do not believe that it is our remit to discuss such items here. We would acknowledge simply that although we accept readily that psychiatric nursing has come of age, others might take the view that it is still in its infancy. We take a more positive line for the following reasons:

(1) From the few examples already quoted it would appear that nurses have the *power* to influence patients. We share the concern of some of our eminent colleagues that this power is not always exerted in a positive direction. However, it also seems apparent that nurses need some kind of guidance if they are to avoid either becoming ineffective, or acting as a negative influence on their patients' lives. From our viewpoint, providing such guidance is a simple matter. The only problem is to budge those monolithic blocks of 'tradition' which obstruct our path.

(2) A number of studies have demonstrated clearly and scientifically the process by which nurses can translate their basic 'caring' orientation into a clearly defined therapeutic role. As we have observed, various researchers have been 'showing' us how to prepare nurses for such a role — indeed a variety of different therapeutic roles — since 1959. The only question which has not been fully answered is: 'When is the profession going to give such illustrations serious attention?'

We take a positive view for the simple reason that, despite all the debate and controversy over 'what is or is not nursing' and 'what is special about nurses', at the end of the day we have a vast army of people who meet with patients for allegedly professional purposes: let us concentrate our efforts on ensuring that such professional engagements are to the benefit of the client.

The Training of Nurses as Behaviour Therapists

The concept of the nurse as behaviour therapist is largely a British one. The first, and clearly the most famous, training programme was established at the Maudsley Hospital in London by the well respected professor of psychiatry and psychopathology, Isaac Marks, who originally trained with Eysenck in the 1960s. Marks's training programme set out to test the hypothesis that psychiatric nurses could be trained to function as key therapists. He was not interested in training adjunct or support therapists, as Ayllon and Michael had earlier described. His programme tried to prepare nurses to work autonomously, taking patients through all the stages of selection, assessment, treatment planning and implementation, and on through to discharge. A wealth of research data has been published to support the claim that these nurses could fulfil this therapeutic role *as well* if not better than psychiatrists and psychologists with whom they were compared (Marks, Hallam, Connolly and Philpott, 1977). The success of these nurses seemed to provide the seal of approval that the concept of the nurse as therapist needed. However, despite its success, this model of training still met with its detractors.

Marks, as we noted earlier, takes a rather conservative view of the efficacy of behaviour therapy. His training programme reflected this view, tackling mainly phobic and obsessional disorders unfortunately referred to as 'adult neurotics', a term not exactly on a par with the idea of holistic, person-centred psychotherapeutic care. Many nurses were unimpressed by the clear demonstration of the nurse therapist's effectiveness. Some appeared even to refuse to study the details of the training programme, continuing to depict these nurses as 'psychologists' assistants' (Wilson-Barnett, 1976); and others asserted that such 'neurotic problems' were only the tip of the psychiatric iceberg.

In the wake of the Maudsley experiment began another London-based training project, this time focused upon the mentally handicapped. Hilda Lewis House, a facility for severely mentally handicapped children and adolescents, and part of the Bethlem Royal Hospital, was used as the base for this programme. Mental-handicap nurses were taught to assess patients, to plan and carry out treatment or training programmes and also to pass on such skills to other staff or to parents and relatives. Clearly, this programme was concerned with training a different kind of 'nurse therapist'. This training project also received considerable recognition as a worthwhile addition to the skills and philosophy of mental-handicap nursing. A second training programme was established later in Devon, using the same syllabus of training; both programmes are still running at the present time. Surprising though it may seem, despite the absence of any alternative model of treatment and training for the mentally handicapped, no other training programmes based upon a behavioural model of nursing have flourished in England and Wales. Again it may be that despite the clear demonstration of the validity and potential of such a caring orientation, many nurses are unwilling to abandon their traditional roles.

Resistance and Resentment

The behavioural model which formed the basis for these training programmes of the early 1970s was a fairly eclectic one. Although many of the experimental projects with mentally handicapped or long-term psychiatric patients emphasised the use of an operant model of learning, many of the training techniques — especially those involving experience in groups, imitation learning and vicarious reinforcement — were drawn from the more complex social learning model of Bandura. The training programme devised by Marks depicted a behaviour therapy which was broadly based: indeed he was at pains to call it 'behavioural psychotherapy', indicating conceptual and practical links with other kinds of psychotherapeutic systems. The value of these training experiments was soon recognised, leading to the establishment of similar programmes in other English centres. In the wake of some of the important rehabilitation work done with long-stay psychiatric patients, which is discussed in another chapter, a course specialising in 'behavioural rehabilitation' was set up in Manchester in the late 1970s. It could be argued, therefore, that the model of behavioural nursing had been amply demonstrated, and was therefore deserving of the acknowledgement of the profession. However, as we noted earlier, many eminent nurses rejected not only the concept of the 'nurse as therapist' but also rejected the philosophy of behaviourism. One clear illustration of this gut-level rejection came from a respected writer on various aspects of psychiatric nursing, who commented that 'one area of psychiatry which concerns me and at times alarms me . . . (is) the growing use of Skinnerian or behavioural treatments . . . all in all there is a nasty smell of torture lurking behind the respectable cover of scholarship and learning' (Macmillan, 1979). This writer perhaps spoke for many nurses who wanted to stem the tide of an advancing science of human behaviour; believing that the old ways were the best ways. We would be at pains to point out that we are in no way satisfied with everything which is done in the name of 'behavioural treatment'. Indeed the example quoted by this writer was a clear illustration of the *abuse* of behavioural psychotherapy. Clearly it is important that restrictive or inhumane practices should be weeded out wherever they may be found. However, the argument that we have cited verged on the level of 'disinformation' favoured by the exponents of cold-war politics: an example of an 'abuse' of Skinnerian learning practices was used to sow the seeds of doubt in the minds of nurses. This doubt was capitalised upon by an emotional appeal for the adoption of a more 'humane' model of psychotherapy. We would hope that the case studies presented later will serve as illustrations of therapies which are humane in their orientation and application. If we were the rational beings which we believe we are, and if we lived in a world in which the demonstration of effectiveness (if not also of cost-effectiveness) was a truly important consideration, then the behavioural model of nursing would by now have ignited a chain of beacons that would have illuminated even the darkest corners of conservative nursing thought throughout the land. However, we are not quite that rational, nor are we particularly impressed by demonstrations of expertise or efficiency. We press this point in recognition of the obvious: that the behavioural model of nursing, which promised so much in the 1960s and demonstrated so much in the 1970s, is struggling to achieve anything like its true potential in the 1980s. This is not to say that it has not had its successes. It is merely a recognition of the fact that the reformation hoped for by Dave Peck and others has materialised only to a very limited degree.

Recently, there has been a wave of interest in 'humanistic' or 'holistic' psychiatric nursing (Beck, Rawlins and Williams, 1983). Such models often include the statutory 'passing reference' to the use of behavioural techniques. However, most emphasis is placed upon traditional interpersonal' forms of psychotherapy which, in research terms, are largely unsupported. At this stage in the development of psychiatric nursing it is important that nurses do not return to the 'mumbo-jumbo' world whence we came. A humane science of human behaviour — acknowledging the 'art' of its implementation — is possible. The case illustrations provided later in this book may serve to demonstrate this point.

And Now for Something Completely Different

We have acknowledged the seminal role of the two training programmes based in London in the early 1970s. These are both examples of true progress in nurse training and practice. However, both courses — and the later course on rehabilitation in Manchester — tended to emphasise a model of therapy pertinent to only one type of patient population. As a result there developed the practice of behavioural psychotherapy with 'adult neurotics' and the implementation of behaviour-modification programmes *either* with the mentally handicapped *or* with long-term psychiatric patients. By implication, if not by design, these programmes served to perpetuate the myth which had been developing over the previous decade: that behaviour therapy is appropriate to *only* an extremely limited range of disorders. We believed that it was necessary to look closely at such issues when we prepared the syllabus for our training programme in 1974. In one respect we wanted to avoid compromising ourselves in an ethical sense: by, for example, offering 'sophisticated therapy' to some patients and 'reductionist' therapy to the more disturbed and the more disadvantaged. We also wanted to investigate the possibilities of a more radical behavioural model: one that tried to look at *all* patients in the first instance as *people* with problems of social adaptation or psychological instability. Our goal was to help nurses to help such people become *more* proficient as 'social beings' and less distressed by their reactions to the world around them. *In no sense were we saying that we would help nurses to treat mental illness or mental handicap.* This course aimed to present a 'core training' in the assessment of patients with all manner of 'problems of living', and in the design and implementation of appropriate forms of remedial therapy. This training programme was shorter than the English courses, at only 6 months. This was seen as an incentive to Health Boards to second more nurses to the training programme, resulting in a more widespread appreciation of the behavioural model.

It is not our brief here to discuss our training programme. The philosophy of the programme and the technology of behaviour change that we teach have already been described in some detail (Barker, 1982). The most important feature of the course — how nurses applied the training in their interactions with patients — will be illustrated later in this book. Two features are, however, important. First of all our training attempted to train a wide range of nurses, with different levels of expertise and potential, to integrate the model of behaviour therapy into routine clinical nursing practice (McPherson, Barker, Hunter and Fraser, 1978). Secondly, we attempted to develop the relationship between nurses and psychologists which Ayllon and Michael had suggested more than 15 years earlier. In these two respects the training was unusual. It emphasised the dissemination of a radical, catholic model of behavioural psychotherapy, a model that did not discriminate in favour of or against any particular patient sub-group, and, more importantly, a model that was based entirely upon the collaboration of nurses and psychologists. As this book marks the tenth anniversary of this training programme, we are pleased to report that our goals have not changed markedly in either respect. Our efforts to shape a truly alternative model of nursing care, through an interdisciplinary partnership, seem to have stood the test of time.

Afterthoughts

In this chapter we have tried to give the reader an appreciation of the origins of contemporary behaviour therapy, and the route by which it has been adopted by the nursing profession. From our brief guide it should be apparent that what began as the academic study of behaviour in animals has been transformed, gradually, into an applied science of human psychotherapy. The way the model has broadened its focus is also of interest. The 'cold-war' days of the 1950s and 1960s when rigid boundaries were drawn between behaviour therapy and other forms of psychotherapy appear to be drawing to a close. We would still wish to retain our objectivity. It is important that any form of therapy establishes its validity through research findings. However, it is apparent that behaviour therapy can merge its boundaries with some other psychotherapies (cf. cognitive behaviour therapy) without losing any of its integrity or its credibility. It is important also to acknowledge that behaviour therapy has changed dramatically over the years because of its scientific tradition. Study after study has revealed weaknesses in either the theoretical model or in the technology of change. As a result, revisions have been made, leading to new models and to more sophisticated techniques.

The integration of behaviour therapy and nursing practice has become known as 'behaviour therapy nursing'. As our case studies will illustrate later, this is a widely ranging practice, dealing with a large variety of problems, in a varied patient population. However, we would contend that the 'scientific method' inherent in the model of behaviour therapy provides a valuable basis for planning and evaluating many other kinds of care and treatment. In this sense the behavioural model represents a reflection of the scientific method found in nursing-process reports. Here also there is an emphasis upon the planning of individualised care, and the rigorous evaluation of outcome. The behavioural model can add something further to this process, in the form of behavioural assessment and a wide range of behaviour-change techniques: methods of helping people which have already been evaluated and found to be of significant worth.

It has always been our belief, and it remains our main contention, that nurses cannot afford to ignore that store of knowledge and that broad technology which is commonly called behaviour therapy. Rather, we should say that they cannot ignore it without risking the delivery of a second-rate service to many patients. The 'behavioural' model of care and treatment has much to offer some patients, and something to offer virtually every patient. It even has something to offer nurses: the opportunity to evaluate critically the 'care' which they offer their patients and the opportunity to develop a therapeutic role which can be demonstrated rather than simply described on paper.

References

The publications marked by an asterisk (*) may prove difficult to locate in their original versions and, for that reason, the interested reader is referred to the summaries of these studies which appear in Alan Kazdin's excellent textbook entitled *History of Behaviour Modification: Experimental Foundations of Contemporary Research*, which was first published in 1978 by University Park Press, Baltimore, USA.

Altschul, A.T. (1977) 'Use of the Nursing Process in Psychiatric Nursing', *Nursing Times*, *73*, 1412–13

Ayllon, T. and Michael, J. (1959) 'The Psychiatric Nurse as a Behavioural Engineer', *Journal of the Experimental Analysis of Behaviour*, *2*, 323–34

Bandura, A. (1969) *Principles of Behaviour Modification*, Holt, Rinehart and Winston, New York

Barker, P.J. (1982) *Behaviour Therapy Nursing*, Croom Helm, London

Beck, A.T. (1976) *Cognitive Therapy and the Emotional Disorders*, International University Press, New York

Beck, C.M., Rawlins, R.P. and Williams, S.R. (1983) *Mental Health Nursing: An Holistic Life-cycle Approach*, C.V. Mosby, St. Louis

Borkowski, J. and Cavanaugh, J. (1969) 'Maintenance and Generalisation of Skills and Strategies by the Retarded', in N. Ellis (ed.), *Handbook of Mental Deficiency: Psychological Theory and Research* (2nd edn), N.J. Erlbaum, Hillsdale

Ellis, A. (1962) *Reason and Emotion in Psychotherapy*, Lyle Stuart, New York

Eysenck, H.J. (1952) 'The Effects of Psychotherapy: An Evaluation', *Journal of Consulting Psychology*, 16, 319–24

Eysenck, H.J. (1960) (ed.) *Behaviour Therapy and the Neuroses: Readings in Modern Methods of Treatment Derived from Learning Theory*, Pergamon, New York

*Fuller, P.R. (1949) 'Operant Conditioning of a Vegetative Human Organism', *American Journal of Psychology*, 62, 587–90

Gelfand, D.M., Gelfand, S. and Dobson, N.R. (1967) 'Unprogrammed Reinforcement of Patients' Behaviour in a Mental Hospital', *Behaviour Research and Therapy*, 5, 201–7

Hauser, M.J. (1978) 'Nurses and Behaviour Modification', *Journal of Psychiatric Nursing*, August, 17–18

Jones, M. (1952) *Social Psychiatry: A Study of the Therapeutic Community*, London, Tavistock

*Jones, M.C. (1924) 'The Elimination of Children's Fears', *Journal of Experimental Psychology*, 7, 382–90

Kazdin, A.E. and Wilson, G.T. (1978) *Evaluation of Behaviour Therapy: Issues, Evidence and Research Strategies*, Ballinger, Cambridge, Massachusetts

Klaber, M.M. and Butterfield, E.C. (1969) 'Stereotypic Rocking: a Measure of Institutional and Ward Effectiveness', *American Journal of Mental Deficiency*, 73, 13–20

*Liddell, H.S. (1938) 'The Experimental Neurosis and the Problem of Mental Disorder', *American Journal of Psychiatry*, 94, 1035–42

Lindsley, O.R. and Skinner, B.F. (1954) 'A Method for the Experimental Analysis of the Behaviour of Psychotic Patients', *American Psychologist*, 9, 419–20

Lovaas, O.L., Kobel, R., Simmons, J.Q., Stevens-Long, J. (1973) 'Some Generalisation and Follow-up Measures on Autistic Children in Behavioural Therapy', *Journal of Applied Behaviour Analysis*, 6, 131–66

Macmillan, P. (1979) 'Let the Punishment Fit the Crime?', *Nursing Times*, 75, 1657–8

McPherson, F.M., Barker, P., Hunter, M. and Fraser, D. (1978) 'A Course in Behaviour Modification', *Nursing Times*, 74, 1207–9

Mahoney, M. (1974) *Cognition and Behaviour Modification*, Ballinger, Cambridge, Massachusetts

Marks, I.M. (1979) 'Cure and Care of Neurosis', *Psychological Medicine*, 9, 629–60

Marks, I.M., Hallam, R.S., Connolly, J. and Philpott, R. (1977) *Nursing in Behavioural Psychotherapy*, Royal College of Nursing, London

*Masserman, J.H. (1943) *Behaviour and Neurosis: An Experimental Psychoanalytic Approach to Psychobiologic Principles*, University of Chicago Press, Chicago

Meichenbaum, D. (1977) *Cognitive-Behaviour Modification*, Plenum, New York

Mowrer, O.H. (1947) 'On the Dual Nature of Learning — a Reinterpretation of "Conditioning" and "Problem Solving"', *Harvard Educational Review*, 17, 102–48

*Pavlov, I.P. (1927) *Conditioned Reflexes: An Investigation of the Physiological*

Activity of the Cerebral Cortex, Oxford University Press, London

Peck, D.F. (1973) 'An Agent of Behaviour Change', *Nursing Times*, *69*, 139

Risley, T.R. (1974) 'Technology for the Comprehensive Care of Dependent People', International Practicum, B. Mod., University of Wales, Cardiff

Rosenthal, T.L. (1982) 'Social learning theory', in G.T. Wilson and C.M. Franks (eds.), *Contemporary Behaviour Therapy*, Guilford Press, New York

Skinner, B.F. (1938) *The Behaviour of Organisms: An Experimental Analysis*, Appleton-Century-Crofts, New York

*Thorndike, E.L. (1911) *Animal Intelligence: Experimental Studies*, Macmillan, New York

*Watson, J.B. and Rayner, R. (1920) 'Conditioned Emotional Reactions', *Journal of Experimental Psychology*, *3* 1–14

Wilson-Barnett, J. (1976) 'Reflections on Progress', *Nursing Times*, *72*, 24

Wolpe, J. (1958) *Psychotherapy by Reciprocal Inhibition*, Stanford University Press, Palo Alto

REHABILITATION IN PSYCHIATRIC AND
MENTAL HANDICAP HOSPITALS

Philip J. Barker and Douglas Fraser

The Psychiatric Hospital

The Nature of the Problem

A number of research workers have, over the past 25 years, drawn a
distinction between the deterioration in self-help behaviours and
social skills which is often observed to accompany a mental disorder
and the underlying disorder itself. Thus Gruenberg (1967) set out to
examine the elements of disturbed behaviour encountered in severe
mental disorders, which, he proposed, develop more or less
independently of the underlying disorders, are apparently preventable
and are the main way in which mental disorders place a burden upon
the community. In producing evidence for these proposals he argued
that the fact that similar patterns of disordered functioning are
associated with entirely different mental disorders leads one to
suspect that the disordered behaviour of psychiatric patients may
arise by mechanisms which are more or less independent of the
particular mental disorders in question: 'approaching the progressive
deterioration of pyschiatric patients from this point of view involves
us in an effort to distinguish the patterns of social behaviour from the
progress of a disease' (p. 1481).

Gruenberg formulated the concept of the 'social breakdown
syndrome' in order to describe these disabilities which are associated
with the psychoses but which are not necessarily a diagnostic
component of any specific psychosis. He describes the social
breakdown syndrome as a continuum in terms of which the severely
disordered manifest gross negligence of self-care skills and disruptive
behaviour, and the milder forms manifest only a slight diminution of
recreational activities without significant interruption of work
attendance and work performance. He points out that the social
breakdown syndrome is encountered both in patients who require
hospitalisation and in those who have been hospitalised for some
time, and argues that the syndrome may begin out of hospital and may
often be the main reason for hospitalisation being sought due to the

burden which it places upon relatives and upon the wider community. Thus the social breakdown syndrome differs from the concept of 'institutional neurosis' (Barton, 1959) in that its origins are sought outside of as well as inside institutions.

Gruenberg is rather vague in describing preventative measures which might be taken in the community setting, but in outlining measures which ought to be taken to prevent further deterioration following hospitalisation, he makes several prescriptions with which many present-day workers in the field of behaviour therapy would concur:

> ... when hospitalisation is required it will be least damaging if it is designed to maximise the patient's responsibility for himself ... the patient should be given every assistance in maintaining a self-respecting, self-governing role ... his home, work, recreational and community ties should not only be carefully protected but nurtured. (Gruenberg, 1967, p. 1485.)

The interested reader might wish to compare this advice with that given by Rob Durham in Chapter 5 of this book.

Wing (1967), in discussing schizophrenia, is less decisive than Gruenberg in drawing a clear distinction between the disorder itself and the accompanying deterioration in self-care behaviours and social skills. Indeed, he includes, in his category of 'negative symptoms of the primary handicaps' such deficits as poverty of speech and social withdrawal, and his category of 'secondary handicaps' is mainly concerned with the attitudes of others to the hospitalised patient and the patient's own attitudes towards hospitalisation. With reference to the latter, Wing observed that, with increasing length of stay in hospital, patients became progressively more indifferent to the prospects of discharge.

In later work, Wing and Brown (1970) do, however, concede that the social environment can have profound effects upon the negative symptoms of the primary handicaps:

> On the one hand, an under-stimulating social environment tends to increase symptoms such as social withdrawal, passivity, inertia and lack of initiative. This process is obviously seen best in the old-fashioned type of mental hospital, but it can quite easily occur in the community as well. On the other hand, there is the tendency to break down, with an effusion of florid symptoms, under conditions

of social over-stimulation. This second process is most frequently seen outside hospital, but it can certainly also be seen within it. (Wing and Brown, 1970, p. 21.)

Thus the emergence of the 'clinical poverty syndrome' (cf. Gruenberg's social breakdown syndrome), which comprises flatness of affect, poverty of speech and social withdrawal, is attributed by these authors to the poverty of the social environment which is most apparent within institutions. Such environmental poverty is equated with a lack of occupational opportunities, unfavourable staff attitudes, paucity of personal possessions and lack of outside contact. Wing and Brown conclude that the longer a patient has been in hospital the more likely he is to experience socially impoverished conditions and the more likely he is to be socially withdrawn and to show poverty of speech and flattening of affect (negative symptoms of the primary handicaps). Furthermore, with increasing length of stay the more likely a patient is to be indifferent about leaving hospital (the secondary handicap of 'institutionalism'). Such findings are paralleled, to a large extent, by the results of studies in institutions for the mentally handicapped which will be examined later in this chapter.

The Size of the Problem

Wing and Morris (1981) estimated that at the end of 1976 there were 83 939 in-patients in *English* psychiatric hospitals (1.81 per 1000 general population). Of these, 43 per cent were men and 57 per cent women. Nearly half of the total (49 per cent) were aged 65 years or more. Only 32 per cent had been in hospital for less than a year, and 46 per cent had been resident for more than five years; the remaining 22 per cent had relatively recently become 'long-stay'. Furthermore they pointed out that, in spite of therapeutic optimism, some people are still developing chronic disabilitities, and a 'new' long-stay group has been accumulating in hospital. The national figure — 40 people per 100 000 population resident in psychiatric hospitals for between one and five years, half of them under 65 years of age — gives a rough approximation of its size. Finally they give some indication of the total number of people who require some form of psychiatric rehabilitation which, in turn, raises the question of the adequacy of the current level of service provision for this client group:

It is difficult to estimate the size of the total group in receipt or in need of a psychiatric rehabilitation service since the information required is only available in local case registers which may not be representative of the national picture. However, an estimate based on the Camberwell Register gives a figure of 420 people per 100000 (210000 nationally) who, at the end of 1976, had been in touch with psychiatric services for more than a year, including a spell in some kind of residential or day accommodation. We do not have to specify an exact number of people with the kinds of disability under consideration in this book in order to be aware of the immensity of the problem and the scarcity of community resources devoted to it. (Wing and Morris, 1981, p. 8.)

While on the subject of the scarcity of community resources, we felt that we could not overlook David Hawks' incisive analysis of the prevailing ideology which has dictated that community care is a preferred alternative to hospitalisation for this client group:

The view that prolonged stay in hospital is to be avoided at all costs is not easily justified when it is considered that the environment into which many schizophrenics would be discharged is itself more institutionalized than the hospital. Brown *et al.* (1966) found that 21 of the first-admission schizophrenics studied by them who were either severely disturbed or unemployed during the last six months of the follow-up period spent 30 per cent of their daytime hours doing nothing. Institutionalism is not a prerogative of hospitals and at the present stage of development of after-care facilities in the community continued stay in hospital may be a preferred alternative to premature discharge. (Hawks, 1975, p. 279.)

On the policy of early discharge Hawks has this to say:

A study by Wing, Monck, Brown and Carstairs (1964) is of particular pertinence in that it indicates the extent to which a policy of early discharge can be pushed to the point of sending out patients suffering quite severe disturbances, and because it acknowledges the moral problem inherent in this policy. Of the 113 schizophrenic patients followed up, 51 per cent showed moderate symptoms when examined at the time of discharge and a further 17 per cent showed severe symptoms. At least 34 per cent were still actively deluded at the time of discharge. Despite the degree of disturbance they manifested, most of the patients wished to leave hospital, and while one-third of the relatives questioned expressed reservations none objected to the patients' discharge. Despite the fact that most of the patients were in contact with their general practitioners or with an out-patient clinic and that 38 per cent attended an Employment Exchange, 56 per cent deteriorated in clinical condition and 43 per cent were re-admitted. Half of those prescribed drugs did not take them as instructed, and half of those found work through the Exchange gave it up within a month or two.

The fact that relatives do not complain cannot be interpreted as justification for such a policy, rather is it to be taken as evidence of the obligation they feel and the low expectation they have of the services available. (Hawks, 1975, p. 281.)

As with the rest of his writing, Hawks's concluding comments require no further elaboration from our pens. Since we could not do justice to his work by summarising it and commenting upon it, we have taken the liberty of quoting extensively from it:

To return patients to the bosom of the community has a certain moral imperativeness which recommends its uncritical acceptance, as does the rejection of all forms of institutional care. There is at least some danger that these ends will be achieved not because of any clear evidence of the visibility of the alternative, but rather as a result of merely shifting the burden of care. It might be argued, that psychiatrists having assumed responsibility for the treatment and rehabilitation of the mentally ill have now discovered their impotence to effect a cure in at least a percentage of these patients. In recommending community care they are seeking to divest themselves of responsibility for these patients and instead are arguing that their adequate rehabilitation can only be effected in the community. Psychiatry's acceptance of a bio-social model of mental illness allows it on the one hand to proclaim society's responsibility for the development of mental illness and on the other hand to claim immunity when its "successful" treatments are vitiated by social considerations. If such an admittedly jaundiced view is adopted the recognition of the therapeutic role of the community is merely the most recent manifestation of a therapeutic nihilism never far submerged in psychiatry, where the management of chronic disorder embarrasses the medical conscience. (Hawks, 1975, p. 283.)

Rich food for thought and, in parts, rather painful for some to swallow. Let us now turn to an examination of the conventional in-patient management of this client group and of the development of behavioural approaches to rehabilitation.

Treatment

From the foregoing sections it may by now be apparent that we are in full agreement with the contention of Kazdin and Wilson (1978) which was referred to in Chapter 2 of this book that, with regard to the psychoses, the focus of attention of the behaviour therapist should be upon behaviours that may have contributed to the diagnosis rather than on the psychotic illness itself. This therefore involves us in an attempt to intervene in the following problem areas:

(1) deteriorated self-care behaviours;
(2) social withdrawal and lack of participation in leisure activities;
(3) impoverished job performance;
(4) delusional speech and ritualistic behaviour.

However, prior to reviewing the literature pertaining to these problem areas, it is worth bearing in mind that, in examining the conventional nursing management of patients in hospital, several studies have shown that patients' maladaptive behaviour is frequently reinforced by nursing staff and that adaptive behaviour may be ignored (Buehler, Patterson and Furniss, 1966; Gelfand, Gelfand and Dobson, 1967; Altschul, 1974; Paton and Stirling, 1974; Fraser and Cormack, 1975). For example, Gelfand and his colleagues noted that the more severely psychotic the patient was, the more likely it was that his prosocial behaviour would be ignored and his bizarre behaviour attended to and thereby reinforced. In the folklore of medicine there is an exhortation that the application of treatment procedures should, at the very least, do the patient no harm. Some of the conventional forms of management of psychiatric and mentally handicapped patients have not met even this minimum requirement, as the introductory sections of this chapter have demonstrated. With regard to the problem areas listed above, we shall now examine the contribution of behaviour therapy to the rehabilitation of psychiatric patients, and we will hopefully demonstrate that, rather than doing such patients no harm, its introduction has led to significant advances in this field. (For comparisons of behaviour therapy with other forms of rehabilitation practice, see Paul and Lentz, 1977; Stoffelmayr, Faulkner and Mitchell, 1979.)

(1) Deteriorated Self-care Behaviours. One of the earliest studies to address itself to this problem was that of Mertens and Fuller (1963), who chose to tackle the problem of shaving in a group of long-term psychotic patients in the hope that success in this area would enable them to develop treatment programmes for a range of self-care deficits, e.g. eating, dressing and personal grooming difficulties. Social reinforcement was used in addition to fruit, gum, snuff, cigarettes, candy and money, and after several weeks the following improvements were noted:

> the reluctance to come when called to shave was generally decreased;
> the patients developed increased attention to task in the course of the study;
> increased shaving skill was evidenced by a decrease in bizarre shaving responses such as shaving the head or eyebrows.

It was not until the introduction of the token economy in the mid-1960s that the wide range of self-care deficits characteristically shown by long-term patients was subjected to intensive and extensive programmes of behaviour therapy. Bandura (1969) has suggested that there are three main stages in the establishment of a token economy:

(a) Behaviours necessary for effective day-to-day functioning are specified, e.g. attention to personal hygiene, performance of simple domestic tasks and appropriate social responses.
(b) A unit of exchange is established, usually a plastic disc or token. The presentation of the token to the patient is made dependent upon his performance of the selected behaviours. Token presentation should be immediately contingent upon the occurrence of the desired behaviour and should be accompanied by praise and explanatory information.
(c) Tokens are made exchangeable for a variety of goods (sweets, cigarettes, etc.) and privileges (a long lie-in in bed, an afternoon off work, etc.)

An analysis of the token economy as a treatment modality will be presented in a later section of this chapter. In the meantime let us turn our attention to the results achieved in the area of self-care deficits by the application of token economy systems.

Two of the earliest studies in this area are reported by Schaefer and Martin (1966) and Atthowe and Krasner (1968). Schaefer and Martin reported substantial improvements in personal hygiene as a result of the application of token and social reinforcement, and in addition a significantly lowered readmission rate. Using a similar procedure, Atthowe and Krasner found that patient morale was increased, apathy was reduced (apathy was defined as the amount of time spent doing nothing) and self-care behaviours improved markedly. They also reported a higher discharge rate than had previously been the case.

However, some early doubt over whether or not the token economy was entirely responsible for such changes was raised by the work of Suchotliff, Greaves, Stecker and Berke (1970), who worked on improving personal grooming in chronically disturbed female patients. They found that an information-feedback procedure was sufficient to improve a range of personal grooming behaviours, and that the later introduction of a token economy led to no further changes. Nevertheless, the token economy system continued to be applied enthusiastically for some years with apparent success to such diverse aspects of self-care deficits as dressing and bed-making (Winkler, 1970); hair combing and face washing (Glickman, Plutchik and Lendau, 1973), and bathing, shaving and appropriate self-feeding (Fraser, McLeod, Begg, Hawthorne and Davis, 1976). However, in the last study, the question of the contribution of the token system *per se* to the therapeutic changes that were demonstrated was again raised:

... the work of Baker *et al.* (1974) suggests that behavioural change is not so much due to the specific token procedures as to factors which are introduced concomitantly with the establishment of a token economy. These may include an increase in the overall level of activity, an increase in the frequency of nurse-patient interactions and so on. It is obviously of crucial importance for the future development of behaviour modification programmes to discern which factor or combination of factors is responsible for behavioural change. (Fraser *et al.* 1976, p. 62.)

Studies pertaining to this crucial issue will be reviewed in the later section on the token economy. You may, however, be somewhat sceptical about the investment of so much time and effort in the reinstatement of basic self-care skills. If so, perhaps you will find some reassurance in the results of a recent study by Presly, Grubb and Semple (1982). They introduce their study by asserting that:

> In planning a rehabilitation unit for long-stay psychiatric patients, it seems essential to know what weight to place on a variety of factors which are generally considered of importance in this group, e.g. mental state, social behaviour, self care skills and capacity for work. There is, however, a dearth of information on the specific kinds of behaviour and on the levels of specific skills necessary for survival in the community on discharge from hospital, or more particularly, discharge to different types of alternative accommodation. (Presly *et al.*, 1982, p. 83.)

They therefore followed up, over a three- to four-year period, 51 long-stay psychiatric patients who had been admitted to a new rehabilitation unit. They found that the main difference between patients who succeeded in moving through the rehabiliation system and securing their discharge and those who failed at some point along the line lay in the area of self-care skills relevant to independent living. Presly *et al.* therefore concluded that a major focus of concern in the rehabilitation of long-stay patients should be the training of appropriate self-care skills, and that, at the very minimum, provision should be made for patients to cook their own meals and to launder their own clothes.

(2) Social Withdrawal and Lack of Participation in Leisure Activities. There have been a number of imaginative approaches to the problems of social withdrawal and lack of participation in leisure activities which are characteristically displayed by long-term psychiatric patients. If we may regard social withdrawal as a continuum, then at one end we have the patient who has a history of several years of complete mutism, and at the other we have the non-spontaneous speaker or the patient who only talks when he is spoken to and, even then, it is in a grudging manner as if he really needed to conserve the breath which he expels with each limited utterance. In the course of this review we shall examine treatment techniques applied at each end of this continuum as well as at the various points in-between.

Three mute female psychotic patients were treated by Sherman (1965) who used a combination of food reinforcement, shaping (reinforcing successive approximations to the desired behaviour) and imitative procedures, which involve the therapist in prompting the patient to copy the sounds that he is making. He succeeded in raising the word frequency of two of the patients from zero to over 1000 responses, and in the third patient he raised the percentage of questions answered from zero to 90 per cent. Nevertheless, success was not easily achieved in that each of the patients required over 90 sessions of intensive treatment!

Kale, Kaye, Whelan and Hopkins (1968) set out to achieve the more limited goal of establishing 'social greeting' patterns on a long-stay ward using a variety of operant procedures. After 100 brief sessions of treatment they had established this form of social interaction on the ward, and furthermore a follow-up study carried out three months after the end of treatment showed that the behaviour had been maintained.

The aim of a study by Milby (1970) was to increase the social behaviour of two long-term schizophrenics by praising responses such as talking to, working with or playing with another patient or a member of staff. In one patient the frequency of such responses was more than doubled, and in the other there was a 66 per cent increase in these response categories.

A controlled study of the use of operant conditioning in reinstating the speech of mute schizophrenics was published by Baker (1971). Eighteen patients were divided into two groups, and 25 individual sessions of treatment, each lasting 45 minutes, were given. The members of the experimental group were reinforced for responding verbally to questions whereas the members of the control group were reinforced for remaining silent. Since the results of the study clearly indicated that the patients who were reinforced for speaking improved more than those who were reinforced for silence, the effectiveness of the operant conditioning procedures was demonstrated and the members of the control group later underwent the speech reinstatement procedures.

Liberman (1972) reported a study of four female chronic psychotic patients who were described as withdrawn and verbally inactive. A variety of procedures was used to increase the amount of social conversation between these patients: token reinforcement, verbal reinforcement and remote prompting via a 'bug in the ear device' worn by the patients which enabled the therapist to communicate with them from the observation room. Reinforcement was successful in promoting a four- to five-fold increase in these patients' conversation rates — a finding that has important implications for those who are involved in attempting to increase the degree of participation in free-time leisure activities in long-term wards since many of these activities demand a fair degree of verbal interaction on the part of the participants and since conversation is, in itself, a leisure activity.

In a study of two near-mute chronic schizophrenic patients which was published in 1974, Thompson, Fraser and McDougall set out to investigate the possible superiority of instructional training procedures over the time-consuming technique of shaping by successive approximations. The treatment procedure, which also involved food reinforcement and modelling, was highly effective in reinstating speech in these patients in a relatively short time (ten 25-minute sessions), and the authors concluded that:

> ... where an adequate verbal repertoire can be assumed (i.e. verbal comprehension rather than verbal expression) a procedure involving instructions supplemented by imitative prompts with speech contingent reinforcement can be adopted in speech retraining programmes in preference to a procedure using response shaping by reinforcement of successive approximations. (Thompson *et al.*, 1974, pp. 87–8.)

It is worthy of note that the newly acquired verbal behaviour of the two patients in this study was maintained for a full year without any further treatment, after which time a successful attempt was made to develop conversational speech from the single-word responses which had earlier been reinstated.

The encouraging results of this study led to two further studies aimed directly at increasing speech output and, indirectly, at increasing the likelihood of participation in leisure activities. In the first of these studies (McPherson Cockram, Grimes, Fraser and Presly, 1979), 445 chronic schizophrenics living in hospitals serviced by the authors' Area Department were surveyed and it was found that 79 of them *never* spoke spontaneously to fellow patients, to staff or to visitors. Although they sometimes responded to questions, their answers were characteristically monosyllabic or incoherent in nature. A behavioural programme was therefore designed to be used by ward staff to teach patients to employ coherent sentences (elaborated when appropriate) in reply to factual questions about themselves and their surroundings. Twenty-one patients were selected for participation in this study and comparisons with a group of patients who were simply encouraged to speak but who did not participate in the behavioural programme indicated that a systematic approach to this problem is an absolute necessity if spontaneous speaking is to be re-established. The degree of the success of the study can be gauged from the authors' concluding remarks:

> Twenty-five brief sessions were sufficient to improve the patients to a level similar to that of patients with normal speech. The programme described would thus appear to be a useful addition to a rehabilitation programme aimed at improving communication and social skills in long-stay schizophrenic patients. (McPherson *et al.*, 1979, p. 231.)

The second study was that of a chronic schizophrenic patient who had spent 49 years in hospital and who had a history of 48 years of complete mutism. The study was reported by Fraser, Anderson and Grime (1981) and the treatment programme was carried out by a nurse working under the guidance of the senior author. In summary, it proved possible to take this patient, who had not spoken a single word for 48 years, and, by applying a variety of operant conditioning procedures, bring him to a level at which, after 40 hours of treatment, he was using sentences in response to questions. The patient was then included in a treatment programme similar to that which was reported immediately above, and his performance was rated as *above average* for the group of non-spontaneous speakers who were then participating in the programme!

We were once challenged as to the cost-effectiveness of many of the programmes of treatment which we have established for this patient group since few such patients can be expected to return to full economic productivity. We answered that the re-establishment of communication with these patients is a basic building block in the process of rehabilitation and resocialisation. What we are dealing with here is the re-enrichment of an impoverished quality of life and since our goals need not include the patients' eventual discharge from hospital, measures of cost-effectiveness seem sadly inappropriate.

(3) Impoverished Job Performance. In a series of experiments which they reported in 1965, Ayllon and Azrin attempted to improve the work performance of long-term patients by the introduction of a token economy system. A variety of jobs requiring varying degrees of experience and different levels of application were allocated to a group of long-stay patients of mixed diagnosis, e.g. serving meals; secretarial work; domestic work; dish-washing; assisting in the token

economy shop; assisting others in their self-care routines; acting as the cinema projectionist; giving guided tours of the token economy and acting as a hospital messenger.

From their findings Ayllon and Azrin concluded that the results of the six experiments demonstrated that the reinforcement procedure was effective in maintaining the desired performance levels. In each experiment the patients' performance levels fell to near zero when response-contingent tokens were withdrawn. On the other hand, the reintroduction of this reinforcement procedure restored performance almost immediately and maintained it at a high level for as long as the reinforcement procedure was in effect. In addition, the reinforcement procedure effectively maintained job performance both on and off the experimental ward (several of the jobs listed above were located in other parts of the hospital). The results of this study therefore offer considerable encouragement to those of us who are concerned to improve the work performance of the characteristically apathetic and withdrawn long-term patient.

This seminal study by Ayllon and Azrin was followed up by Sletten, Hughes, Lamont and Ognjanov (1968) who investigated the effect of the following variables upon the off-ward work performance of psychiatric patients:

(a) An operant conditioning approach in which preferred activities were permitted only when patients had earned enough tokens to be able to pay for them. During the time of application of this contingency, tokens were paid out either twice a day or three times a week.

(b) A conventional monetary reward system in which no attempt was made to regulate preferred behaviours and patients were simply paid for their work on an hourly basis.

(c) 'Off periods', when neither of the above contingencies was applied and patients were simply invited to carry out their work assignments.

Their findings suggest that the token system and the monetary reward approach are equally useful methods of improving work performance and that both were significantly better than simply inviting patients to participate in work activities. The frequency of token reinforcement (twice a day vs. three times a week) did not appear to have any differential effect upon work performance. It would therefore appear that the therapist who is concerned with tackling impoverished job performance has a straightforward choice between operating a token economy system and paying in cash. For further guidance on this subject please refer to the later section on the 'token economy'.

The effectiveness of monetary incentives was, however, further investigated by Walker (1979) in the setting of a community-based rehabilitation workshop. The aim of the study was to compare the effects of piece-rate payment, social reinforcement, piece-rate payment plus social reinforcement, upon the work performance of psychiatric patients. The work consisted of folding and glueing cardboard cartons, a task which is fairly typical of the work offered in many industrial therapy and occupational therapy departments.

The piece-rate group, the social reinforcement group, the piece-rate plus social reinforcement group, and the pay increase plus social reinforcement group were all found to be superior to the control and feedback group (who were paid simply for attendance at work) in terms of increased work performance and output. Walker therefore concludes that the findings of this study confirm that much can be done to improve the work performance of even severely ill chronic schizophrenics in an industrial situation by the systematic use of incentives. It should be remembered that, in many OT and IT units around the country, patients are paid simply for attendance at work; Walker's results suggest that impoverished job performance can only be tackled adequately if payment is made contingent upon work output.

(4) Delusional Speech and Ritualistic Behaviour. To review behavioural interventions in these problem areas might seem, at first sight, to be going well beyond our original brief of 'focusing upon behaviours that may have contributed to the diagnosis rather than on psychosis as such'. Nevertheless we would maintain that problems such as these, which are often thought to be the very essence of the psychotic process itself, may be maintained at an unnaturally high level by environmental consequences (e.g. staff attention). They should therefore be modifiable through the alteration of the contingencies which are observed to maintain them. This view of the problems of delusional speech and ritualistic behaviour brings them well within our brief.

Ayllon and Haughton (1964) selected three female psychiatric patients whom they described as showing 'very stereotyped symptomatic verbalisations'. In an attempt to demonstrate that such problems as delusional speech and persistent complaining were responsive to environmental consequences, they subjected these behaviours both to reinforcement and to extinction procedures:

> Reinforcement consisted of listening to or taking interest in the patient's verbalisations. In some instances this attention involved the offer of a cigarette or a piece of candy to the patient. Sometimes the nurse simply paid attention to the patient by lighting a cigarette herself and joining the patient. In general, the patient-nurse interaction followed a casual, social form, the primary object of which was to demonstrate interest in the patient.
>
> Extinction consisted of withholding social attention and the other tangible reinforcers already described. The nurses became, with some practice, quite skilful in appearing distracted or bored. Generally, the nurse was instructed to 'look away' and 'act busy'. This was easily accomplished by teaching the nurses to shift their attention to some other event taking place on the ward. (Ayllon and Haughton, 1964, p. 89.)

The case which is of most relevance to our review is that of Kathy:

> Kathy was a 47 year old female patient diagnosed as chronic schizophrenic. She had been in the hospital for 16 years. The patient's verbal behaviour centered around so-called 'delusions'. The content of her verbal behaviour was characterized by frequent references to 'Queen Elizabeth', 'King George', and the 'Royal Family'. A sample of her talk is as follows: 'I'm the Queen. Why don't you give things to the Queen? The Queen wants to smoke. . . . How's King George, have you seen him?' These self-references were traced through hospital records and had been reported over the preceding 14 years. The staff stated that references to herself as 'the Queen' had been virtually her only topic of conversation for the eight years immediately prior to this investigation. The patient had undergone a bilateral prefrontal lobotomy without apparent change in her verbal behaviour. As she was on a maintenance dosage of barbiturates when this investigation was initiated, this medication was maintained throughout. (Ayllon and Haughton, 1964, p. 90.)

During the first 75 days of the study 'psychotic verbal responses' were reinforced and non-psychotic speech was subjected to the extinction contingency in order to examine the controlling function of these environmental consequences. A rapid increase in psychotic speech was noted, along with an equally rapid decline in non-psychotic or normal speech. The procedure was then reversed for a 90-day period and non-psychotic speech was reinforced with cigarettes and attention from the nursing staff whereas psychotic speech was subjected to the extinction contingency. Upon withdrawal of reinforcement for psychotic speech, a rapid decrease in its frequency was observed with a corresponding increase in normal speech. The authors conclude this study as follows:

> Despite the patient's severe psychosis the verbal modification obtained represents a very encouraging step towards a more parsimonious view of the development of peculiar verbal behaviour in schizophrenic patients. These data suggest that unusual verbal repertoires can be shaped by the social environment. Therefore, the notion of aberrant verbal behaviour as indicative of inner processes that are malfunctioning may be unnecessary. At least to the extent that the community appears to exercise considerable control over this behaviour, we may understand the frequency of different classes of verbal behaviour as being dependent upon reinforcement contingencies found in the social environment. (Ayllon and Haughton, 1964, p. 92.)

This important demonstration of environmental control over what previously had been regarded as uncontrollable symptomatic behaviour was replicated in a number of studies for example, Wincze, Leitenberg and Agras (1972) examined the effects of token reinforcement and feedback upon the delusional speech of chronic paranoid schizophrenics. Six male and four female paranoid schizophrenic patients participated in the study. The results indicated that feedback (or correcting the inaccuracies in delusional speech) was effective about half the time in reducing the percentage of delusional talk, but that in at least three cases it produced adverse reactions (a not uncommon finding in studies employing this procedure). However, token reinforcement of non-delusional speech showed more consistency and reduced the percentage of delusional verbal behaviour in seven of the nine patients who underwent this procedure. The effects of both the feedback and the token reinforcement contingencies were quite specific to the environment in which they were applied and showed little generalisation to other settings within the hospital. This is again a common finding since, outside a patient's immediate ward environment, a variety of factors which may serve to maintain undesirable behaviour may be operating. For information on how to generalise treatment effects to other settings, the interested reader is referred to a paper by Walker and Buckley (1972).

A study that examined the effectiveness of two forms of behavioural intervention in reducing delusional speech, ritualistic behaviour and a range of other problem behaviours characteristic of long-term psychiatric patients was reported by Fraser, Black and Cockram (1981). The subjects of the study were nine male schizophrenic patients ranging in age from 30 to 58 years (mean age = 42.7 years), each with over 2 years' continuous stay in hospital (mean length of stay = 16.1 years, range 3 years 10 months to 27 years 2 months). They had been selected for transfer to a behaviour modification unit because, on the basis of a variety of behavioural measures, they had been found to be among the most deteriorated and institutionalised patients in the long-stay wards of a psychiatric hospital. As far as possible, medication was held constant for the duration of their stay in the unit.

Fraser and his colleagues attempted to assess the extent to which:

(a) verbal and written descriptions of desirable and undesirable behaviours (i.e. instructions) presented both as antecedents and as consequences of behaviour would prove effective in reducing the incidence of a wide range of inappropriate behaviour shown in three different settings:
   (i) at the patient's place of work;
   (ii) in the day-room of the ward during free recreation time;
   (iii) in the ward dining room during mealtimes;
(b) the application of a response-cost procedure, when paired with this instructions contingency, would prove effective in further reducing the incidence of inappropriate behaviour in these settings.

Response cost involved the withdrawal of tokens (previously earned for appropriate behaviour) contingent upon the performance of inappropriate behaviour (it is a system akin to the imposition of fines by the courts). The inappropriate behaviours that were the main focus of this study fell into three broad categories:

(1) behaviours displayed by most of the patients in all three settings, e.g. unprompted laughing, silent speech-like mouth movements, posturing, mannerisms, delusional speech, incoherent speech;
(2) behaviours displayed by most of the patients in specific settings, e.g. smearing spilled food on to their clothes, picking up food from the floor during mealtimes;
(3) behaviours displayed by individual patients, e.g. chewing cigarette butts, body rocking, persistently demanding cigarettes.

There was a baseline period of observation of the frequency of these problem behaviours which lasted for six weeks, and then the instructions contingency was put into operation for a period of 22 weeks; for a final period of six weeks, a response-cost procedure was superimposed on the instructions contingency.

Response cost was found to have little impact in further reducing the incidence of inappropriate behaviour over this final six-week period and, as the authors point out, it is:

> . . . a punishment procedure which sometimes leads to a temporary exacerbation of the problem behaviour which it is designed to control (Burchard and Barrera, 1972; Kazdin, 1975). In addition, as Kazdin (1972) points out, its application leads to passive avoidance learning in which the patient merely learns what not to do. In contrast, instructional training may be said to teach active avoidance learning, i.e. the patient learns to discriminate between alternatives and thus to display more appropriate behaviour. (Fraser, Black and Cockram, 1981, p. 265.)

On the other hand they clearly demonstrated that an approach involving the systematic application of an intensive programme of instructional training achieved considerable control over the frequency of a wide range of inappropriate behaviours shown by long-term schizophrenic patients. Their concluding comments, in which they refer to early experimental work on the nature of psychological deficits in schizophrenia, are worthy of reiteration:

> Buss and Lang (1965) and Storms and Broen (1969) argue that schizophrenics are likely to benefit from clear and detailed explanations, from extra information about the expectations of others and from informative feedback regarding the appropriateness of their behaviour. This assertion receives strong support from the results of the present study. (p. 265)

On the topic of experimental work on the nature of schizophrenic deficits, Hemsley (1977, 1978) has sought to examine the manner in which such deficits may limit the effectiveness of behavioural treatment programmes. He suggests that a minority of schizophrenics may show increased behavioural abnormality when confronted with treatment programmes which require of them more complex decision-making than they have previously been accustomed to. He views this type of patient as being in a state of 'information overload' and regards social withdrawal as a form of adaptation since social situations are the most likely source of response uncertainty and information overload. Wing (1975) had earlier proposed that social withdrawal and flatness of affect served a protective function in that they are, he suggested, a means of coping with severe thought disorder. He argued that if such patients are required to interact in the course of a treatment programme, they are likely to show an increase in florid symptomatology in the form of delusions, disordered speech or inappropriate behaviour. These assertions are sufficiently thought-provoking to temper the therapeutic zeal of even the most enthusiastic behaviour therapist. However, you should bear in mind that this effusion of florid symptomatology occurs in a minority of schizophrenic patients, that it is temporary in nature, and that even when a highly demanding programme of treatment is maintained (rather than being withdrawn when these undesirable changes are noted), many of these symptomatic behaviours are seen to remit as the patient adapts to a heightened level of stimulation.

The Token Economy

Since many of the studies reviewed above have involved the application of token economy procedures we now propose to examine critically the token economy as a therapeutic system.

As early as 1964, Ayllon and Azrin raised doubts about the conventional interpretation of the mode of action of reinforcement procedures. They concluded that food reinforcement for appropriate mealtime behaviour was initially ineffective because it ignored the major role played by the existing verbal repertoire of the patients concerned. They went on to propose that instructions alone might have been sufficient to produce a change in performance in the absence of food reinforcement. However, a further experiment led them to conclude that instructions can initiate behaviour but that reinforcement is needed to motivate and to maintain such behaviour. These findings led them to assert that a failure to utilise the existing verbal repertoire of humans (as had been the case in many of the studies prior to 1964) places great constraints on any attempt at changing behaviour by the application of reinforcement procedures. However obvious these findings may seem today, they marked a major step forward in our understanding of the process of reinforcement. They also led directly to the research on token economies which is discussed below.

Fraser (1978) argued that even if it is agreed that token economies achieve superior results when compared with traditional treatment methods, we are still left with the problem of how such results are achieved. As Gripp and Magaro (1974) point out in their review of token economy programmes: 'It is evident that self-care deficits can be overcome in a token economy and this may apply to relatively complex behaviour chains as well as discrete behaviours. However, it is not clear what aspect of the token economy context is responsible for improvements' (p. 209). The partialling out of the effective ingredients of a token economy would thus appear to be an issue of high priority if one is to attempt to establish the necessary and sufficient conditions for behavioural change.

One study that attempted some control over the variables which had thus far remained uncontrolled in the token economy was that of Heap, Bobbitt, Moore and Hord (1970). Self-care skills and grooming behaviour were the focus of treatment in this study.

Four sequential conditions, each of 14 days' duration, were applied:

(1) a baseline period of observation only;
(2) checking of behaviours informally and without comment;
(3) checking but with verbal reinforcement contingent on successful completion of target behaviours;
(4) checking plus verbal reinforcement plus token delivery upon successful completion of target behaviours.

The percentage of patients showing appropriate self-care behaviours was approximately 2 per cent during baseline. There were no significant changes during the second condition but there was approximately a 20 per cent increase during the third condition and approximately a 50 per cent increase during the fourth condition. Similar improvements were noted in grooming behaviour under the same four conditions. The results of this study appear strikingly in favour of the token/verbal reinforcement combination over verbal reinforcement alone. However, the cumulative effects of the treatment programme are not controlled for in this sequential design, that is, one does not know whether continuing verbal reinforcement alone for a sufficiently long period would have resulted in an equally large increase as was evidenced with the token/verbal reinforcement combination.

Baker, Hall and Hutchinson (1974) began their study of the token economy with some appreciation of possible uncontrolled variables:

> The particular ward may receive more attention from professional staff, with consequent improvements in staff morale and attitudes towards the patients. The nurses increase their efforts and provide a better standard of care for patients. They may now expect positive results. New activities and ward routines may be set up. In amongst all this, the hitherto neglected patient receives far more stimulation and attention than usual. (Baker *et al.*, 1974, p. 368.)

These authors selected seven patients, on the basis of several criteria, for removal from their original long-stay wards to a specialised token economy unit. They were observed in this setting for a period of six weeks. Following this, an activity programme was introduced in which patients were exposed to far more stimulation than usual; an occupational therapy programme was begun; trips to the cinema and to town were organised; social evenings were arranged. After three weeks, tokens were introduced non-contingently for a seven-week period. Contingent tokens were then introduced, being earned for the satisfactory performance of various ward tasks which gradually increased in number and variety. Contingent tokens were in effect for fourteen weeks, following which baseline conditions were reintroduced.

From their results Baker *et al.* (1974) concluded that there was little evidence that a specific token contingency was the main factor in changing the patients' target behaviours. The greatest change for most patients occurred during the early stages of the experiment. Although Baker *et al.* (1974) concluded that token reinforcement did not emerge as the critical therapeutic agent, they made no attempt to isolate the factors that were of greatest importance. Nevertheless, two possible critical variables that emerge from an examination of their programme are:

(a) an increase in the frequency of nurse-patient interactions, and
(b) a corresponding increase in the availability of social reinforcement.

Either variable or a combination of the two could be crucial in explaining the results of this study.

The most significant contribution to our understanding of the variables operating within token economy systems has been made by Dr Joseph Fernandez, a consultant psychiatrist who is based in Dublin (see Fernandez, Fischer and Ryan 1973a and b; Fernandez, 1978).

It is inevitably presumptious to attempt to summarise the findings from a substantial body of research such as that carried out by Fernandez over the past 16 years. Bearing this in mind, the major findings from his earlier studies (Fernandez, 1974) would appear to suggest that:

(a) changes in some target behaviours can be brought about by using instructions alone:
(b) the majority of target behaviours show most changes when instructions are combined with prompting and verbal reinforcement delivered by nursing staff;
(c) the one area which remained relatively unaffected by the application of these contingencies was social behaviour. Social behaviour, i.e. social interaction, and participation in recreational activities, changed substantially only when the contingent token condition was introduced.

Thus the results bear out some of the conclusions from earlier work by Ayllon and Azrin (1964) and the more recent study by Kazdin (1973), i.e. instructions alone are usually insufficient to effect long-term behaviour change and therefore require to be supplemented by verbal or tangible reinforcement or a combination of both.

However, more recent studies have led to a re-examination of these conclusions (see Fernandez, 1983; Fraser, 1983), and the role of token reinforcement in promoting the therapeutic changes which are often observed to follow the introduction of a token economy system is again in doubt.

... the token economy is seen to achieve its effect solely through the elaborate social information system which is embodied in its application and the conditioning theory of its mode of operation must, as a result, surrender to Occam's razor since there has been no reliable evidence to date that contingent token presentation is a critical therapeutic variable.

Briefly, the therapeutic process may be viewed as follows: in a social context the patient is systematically provided with information concerning his actions and their likely outcome for himself and for others. Behaviour change thus comes about through an informed appraisal of social consequences rather than via a hypothetical conditioning process or through an attempt to regain pleasures and privileges which are the patient's by right. In structuring a programme of rehabilitation along the lines suggested by these recent findings one would be inviting the patient to engage in a situation which involves a fair approximation to normal social exchange. One would also be providing reinforcers which are freely available in the outside community; approval, praise, encouragement and support, with no need of recourse to a highly contrived situation which requires an elaborate transititional period from tokens to these naturally occurring reinforcers if effective rehabilitation is ever to be achieved. It might still be contested that the token economy system as it has been implemented in psychiatric hospitals has justified techniques of deprivation and a situation of marked power imbalance by virtue of the results which have been achieved. However, I would wish to argue that we cannot continue to defend coercive systems by reference to their results since we have clearly demonstrated that programmes which involve no deprivation of basic rights and privileges achieve comparable results to those achieved in token economies. In treatment of any kind the procedures that cause least distress to the patient should always take priority. (Fraser, 1983, pp. 259, 260.)

Care of the Mentally Handicapped

Many of our observations regarding the care and treatment of the chronic psychiatric patient are relevant to our view of the care of the mentally handicapped. Although the origins of the problems affecting the two populations may be wholly different in character, the strategies of treatment and management which have been shown to be useful for the two groups have much in common. In this section we wish to consider the position of the mentally handicapped person in hospital, and the kind of problems that he presents which have proven amenable to behavioural intervention.

The Handicapped Population

The hospital for the mentally handicapped exists to accommodate people with varying degrees of intellectual and physical impairment, who cannot survive independently in the community, or who cannot be provided with satisfactory care in any alternative situation. Reasons for hospitalisation can be many and various, ranging from investigation of medical problems associated with mental handicap to social problems which might involve some form of 'stress relationship' between the individual and his family or local community.

It is a common misconception that the mental handicap hospital exists solely to provide medical and nursing care for handicapped people. This assertion was investigated by Leck, Gordon and McKeown (1967) in hospitals in and around the Birmingham area. They found that, of a total of 1 652 patients, only seven required on-going medical-nursing care and only one-half of the remainder required even basic nursing care; medical care of this latter group was exclusively concerned with the prescription of anticonvulsant or tranquilising drugs. The remaining patients required no formal nursing whatsoever. In her book, *Put Away*, Pauline Morris (1969) reiterated the view that, in general, traditional forms of nursing care were unnecessary for most patients. Surveying over 3 000 patients in hospital she found that although 68 per cent of staff saw their role in terms of the provision of nursing care *per se*, 38 per cent ranked the provision of social and habit training highly and 30 per cent were concerned to create a homelike atmosphere. Morris pointed out that the low staffing levels in the areas surveyed often meant that individualised treatment or the provision of social training as an aid to development was a virtual impossibility. More recently Oswin (1978) has suggested that although much attention has been focused upon the plight of the mentally handicapped, for many children in hospital little or no improvements have been made in the decade since the Morris study was instituted.

The Environment

Many of the problems involved in the provision of satisfactory care revolve around the ideologies as well as the physical environment of the institution. Although most hospitals have progressed a long way from the image of the restrictive institution typical of the last century, many continue to function as total institutions in that they represent the complete living experience of many residents. In order to evaluate the care service offered by the hospital, it is important to establish the extent to which it is institutionally oriented or patient centred. In a key study of this aspect of residential care, Raynes and King (1974) examined the kinds of practices applied in the management of mentally handicapped children. From this they were able to develop a scale which would assess the 'quality of care' in a variety of care settings for the handicapped. They found that although there were major differences between the residential units studied, such differences were not explained by the size of the unit or by differences in staff-child ratios. Instead, the role activities of the person in charge of the unit appeared to be most significant. Raynes and King pointed to the important interaction between the training orientation of the staff (their 'ideology') and the pattern of child care. Staff who had been trained to operate child-oriented patterns of care showed high degrees of verbal contact with individual children whereas nursing-trained staff were more task — or institutionally — oriented, with correspondingly lower rates of verbal contact with the children.

A Pragmatic Model

Grunewald (1974) has stated that the behaviour, rather than the degree of intellectual impairment, is the real problem of the handicapped person. Grunewald believes that behaviour is shaped as a result of the constant process of interaction between the individual and his environment.

> In practice we must always view mental retardation in relation to the person's environment . . . we do not have any mentally retarded people, but we do have retarded environments or surroundings . . . one is sometimes tempted to ask which is the most retarded, the person living here (in the collective ward) or the environment itself. (Grunewald, 1974.)

Official statements concerning services for the mentally handicapped may not be quite so radical, or positive, in outlook. However, they do echo the suggestion that the environment must be used to help the handicapped person achieve the goal of leading as normal a life as possible. The question has been repeatedly posed: should this be in hospital or in the community? No clear answer is evident at the present time. Although the advantages of a community care policy are by now widely accepted, it is clear that people can be institutionalised in the community as easily as they can in hospital. In a study comparing hostel and hospital staff, Campbell (1971) reported that 'total care' activities, which involved staff doing things for the resident that he might otherwise have done for himself, were much in evidence in the hostels studied. This underlines the claim that achievement of potential may well depend more upon the attitudes, training and ideologies of the staff than upon the physical setting of the handicapped person.

Although the social processes of the institution have nothing to do with the origins of the disparate conditions subsumed under the title of mental handicap, these processes, as opposed to the original aetiological factors, would appear to have a significant influence upon the behavioural performance of the handicapped person. The development of the behavioural approach towards the care and training of the mentally handicapped is based upon this assertion. In many ways the care and treatment of the severely disabled person in hospital are much the same, irrespective of whether the person is called mentally ill or mentally handicapped. Although adjustments are necessary to suit individual requirements, a common thread unites the approaches to both populations. In both cases the philosophy and technology of behaviourism are invoked to help the 'disabled' person lead a less distressing, more adaptive, life within the limitations of his existing physical or psychological 'pathology'.

Behavioural Assessment of the Mentally Handicapped

In sharp contrast to traditional diagnosis, behavioural assessment of the mentally handicapped de-emphasises the role of psychometric procedures (such as intelligence testing). Instead, more attention is given to repeated direct observation of the person, usually in his natural environment. From such assessment it is possible to identify targets for care or treatment and to establish whether or not such problems are situation specific. Does the person's behaviour change with a change of environment? Unlike traditional diagnosis, no attempt is made to isolate any historical causes. Instead, efforts are made to establish the role of environmental factors which may be cueing or signalling (antecedents) or reinforcing or maintaining (consequences) the pattern of behaviour. This information is crucial to the design of any treatment or training programme which will involve, in some way, the manipulation of the handicapped person's social or physical environment. The major distinction, therefore, between traditional and behavioural forms of assessment is that the latter is undertaken with the specific aim of planning and evaluating training or treatment programmes.

Labels and Labelling

The behavioural model stresses the uniqueness of the individual. This is especially true in mental handicap. Although labels such as 'severely mentally handicapped' may ease communication, they say so little about a person that they are virtually useless. Such labels can also be dangerous, especially if one believes that all 'severely mentally handicapped' people will behave in the same way and will have the same needs. This patent falsehood reduces the chances of more accurate perception of the function and needs of the individual (Bellack and Hersen, 1977). The behavioural model tends to avoid such classifications. Instead, priority is given to developing a list of adaptive behaviours and a catalogue of deficiencies, shown by the individual. Such a scheme would not only describe the person more fully than traditional diagnostic methods but would also provide the basis for setting care and training objectives.

The Mentally Handicapped Populations

Mental handicap has always been viewed as a medical syndrome. The causes of handicap are assumed, or shown, to be the outcome of neurological developmental delay or are ascribed to the influence of genetic or traumatic factors. Recently it has been suggested that two classes of handicap exist (Zigler, 1967). The first group is composed of the mildly and moderately handicapped individuals with IQ scores of 50 and above. This group, it is argued, may not be essentially different from people of higher intelligence: they represent an extreme on a normal intelligence continuum. The second group is composed of more severely and profoundly handicapped people with IQs below 40. These people are assumed to be different in terms of the causation of their mental handicap. It has been argued that a behavioural model may be an appropriate care-and-training framework for the first group, with the more severely handicapped people requiring a medical model of care.

In this chapter we shall review the use of behavioural approaches with both of these classes of mentally handicapped people. Although some of the newer developments, such as social skills training and the involvement of cognitive processes, obviously relate to the more mildly handicapped group, the value of a behavioural approach to more disabled people cannot be underestimated. Two of the case studies presented later in this book are concerned with people who have major primary handicaps (which would place them in the second of Zigler's groups) in addition to secondary handicaps acquired through long-term institutionalism. Although hardly a panacea, behavioural approaches may achieve unprecedented levels of success, where a range of medical, educational and custodial measures have failed.

Restructuring the Environment

Gardner (1971) has pointed out that a mentally handicapped person's failure to learn may be 'caused' by an insensitive environment. Where a handicapped person fails to learn, it could be argued that this is as much a result of ineffective teaching or training, as it is a function of learning disability. Bijou (1966) was one of the first to argue that the deficiencies of the environment might account for the deficiencies of the handicapped person. He argued that inadequate reinforcement could account for a failure to learn adaptive behaviour. On the other hand, unstimulating environments, a history of aversive experiences and reinforcement of inappropriate behaviour could account for the high incidence of maladaptive behaviour which often characterises this patient group. Where reinforcement is seen as 'inadequate', this could be either because the reinforcers used are not actually rewarding or because they are delivered 'non-contingently', with too much delay following the performance of the target behaviour. In other situations, reinforcement may be too little, too infrequent or too inconsistent. As we noted earlier, many handicap hospitals are organised specifically to manage or care for patterns of behaviour which are assumed to be part of the syndrome of mental handicap. It is not surprising, therefore, that the emphasis on managing such behaviour patterns tends to take priority over the development of more normal repertoires of behaviour. In this way the self-fulfilling prophecy of mental handicap is created.

The Major Targets

Although the behavioural model is unlikely to lead to a cure for mental handicap, there is ample theoretical and practical evidence to support its role in mental-handicap care (Birnbrauer, 1976). It is fair to say that the medical model has not led to any such cure either. As Albee (1969) noted, the mentally handicapped are more in need of teachers than doctors.

Practical Considerations

As we noted above, staff interaction with mentally handicapped people is often 'negative': responding to disruptive or dependent behaviour (Grant and Moores, 1977). To break down this pattern, experimental settings have studied the effect of small groups in which a staff member is responsible for only a few patients, providing materials, instruction and reinforcment in the form of individualised attention (Kelly, Holland and Webster, 1982). An alternative approach involves allocating two members of staff to work with a small group. One person acts as the 'room manager', keeping people busy, providing materials, and prompting, reinforcing or ignoring behaviour. The second person concentrates on an individual patient, training him apart from the group in a new skill (Porterfield, Blunden and Blewitt, 1980). In a recent study comparing these two approaches it was found that 'room management' and 'small groups' had much the same effect upon the promotion of on-task behaviour and staff-trainee interaction. However, room management promoted much more in the way of individual training: approximately four times as much as occurred in the small-groups situation (Crisp and Sturmey, 1984).

Self-care Skills

An extensive body of research has been applied to the area of the training of self-care skills: eating, dressing, washing and the use of the toilet, etc. Much of this research emphasises the 'habit-training' aspect of such skills training: acquiring behaviour in response to systematic prompting. However, a number of researchers have developed training systems that go far beyond basic habit formation.

Toilet Training. The traditional toilet-training approach involved training the handicapped person to eliminate upon being placed on the toilet (Ellis, 1963). This has largely been supplanted by efforts to promote the more complex skill of independent toilet use (Azrin and Foxx, 1971). Independent toileting involves a range of skills: identifying the need to use the toilet; finding a toilet; undressing; eliminating; using toilet tissue; dressing; flushing the toilet; and washing hands afterwards. This is a far cry from 'potty training'. The method developed by Azrin and Foxx is characterised by its use of an alarm to signal incontinence (the pants-alarm). These alarms help to pinpoint more accurately the times of the day at which incontinence takes place, during the initial baseline assessment stage. Variants of these alarms can be used in the toilet bowl itself to signal when appropriate elimination occurs. Indeed the main feature of their approach is its systematic structure. The handicapped person is usually given increased fluids during training, to increase his 'need' to use the toilet. The 'trainer' is on hand constantly during the early stages of training, prompting the patient to perform the various toilet-related behaviours and reinforcing either appropriate toilet usage or 'being dry', i.e. continent. The training package also carries some 'negative' features. When an incontinent incident occurs, the patient is required to perform an aversive or unpleasant routine, e.g. mopping up the wet floor, washing out wet clothing, showering and changing into fresh clothing. This is designed to weaken the chances of the reoccurrence of incontinence. It should be noted, however, that the programme is heavily weighted towards positive reinforcement. The increased-fluids regime is designed to increase the likelihood that the patient will use the toilet appropriately and will gain positive reinforcement, thereby strengthening this behaviour. Once the complex of toilet-related behaviours is established under 'controlled' training conditions, the patient is gradually shifted to less intensive forms of supervision. This allows him the opportunity to generalise his new skill to the everyday ward situation. Foxx and Azrin have extended the principles of this approach to cover nocturnal as well as diurnal enuresis. This is undoubtedly the training system of choice for most enuretic handicapped people (Foxx and Azrin, 1973).

Eating Skills. A variety of problems are evident in training handicapped people to eat, especially in a manner which conforms to accepted social standards. In common with other skills training exercises, a careful behaviour analysis is necessary to provide a framework which will make learning easier for the handicapped person. The task of eating is analysed, breaking the action of eating with cutlery into its various component parts. This task analysis is used as the basis for teaching. Most training programmes focus upon the provision of physical and verbal prompts to help the patient perform the various 'steps', e.g. of scooping food, lifting it to his mouth, eating, and returning the spoon to the plate to repeat the process. Gradually these prompts are faded, leaving the patient to perform more and more of the steps independently until the complete sequence is established.

However, mentally handicapped people who have spent much of

their lives in residential care may have learned, inadvertently, a range of inappropriate eating behaviours, which may require some retraining. Eating with fingers, stealing food, taking too long to eat, or gorging food are common problems. Programmes designed to reduce the incidence of such disruptive or antisocial mealtime behaviours again often use a package of techniques which are too complex to be described in detail here. Of particular relevance are the programmes that help to establish eating within acceptable time limits (Sanok and Ascione, 1978) and the elimination of disruptive behaviour at the meal table (De Kock, Mansell, Felce and Jenkins, 1984).

The Constructional Approach. Much of the attention of 'behaviour modification' programmes of the late 1960s and early 1970s with the mentally handicapped was focused upon extinguishing maladaptive patterns of behaviour. Goldiamond (1974) was one of the first to suggest that many of these problem behaviours might be resolved by extending the adaptive repertoire of the handicapped person. This 'constructional' approach concentrated its attention upon establishing and maintaining new or extended skills which naturally eliminated the handicapped person's need to engage in unacceptable behaviour. Apart from representing a more acceptable alternative for the handicapped person, this approach resolved many of the ethical dilemmas associated with the use of behaviour modification techniques designed to reduce or eliminate disruptive behaviour.

Lack of space prevents us from cataloguing the numerous studies which have been concerned with training the mentally handicapped person in self-care skills or with the modification of problem behaviour. As we noted earlier, the methods of behaviour change involved are similar to the techniques that are used with psychiatric patients, which were described earlier in this chapter. Readers who are interested in extending their knowledge of this area should, however, consult Whaley and Malott, 1971; Panyan, 1972; Kiernan, 1974; Perkins, Taylor and Capie, 1976; and Yule and Carr, 1981.

Social Skills

Many aspects of self-care skills could be seen as social skills. The manner in which we are required to eat, to dress and to comb our hair is socially determined. Many of the rituals involved in laying the table for dinner or using a public convenience are also socially determined. Here we wish to discuss more complex interpersonal skills. Strategies for training handicapped people in other social skills, such as using public transport, money handling, and self-care, are covered adequately by texts to which we have referred immediately above. In this section we wish to consider briefly the work that has been done fairly recently in training handicapped people in the art of communication and interaction with others.

It is clear that interest in the training of mentally handicapped people in interpersonal skills is of fairly recent origin (Bornstein, 1981). Despite many similarities between social skills training for the handicapped and for other populations, it is clear, with the former, that more attention has been paid to the behavioural aspects of skills training and less to the cognitive and perceptual aspects of interpersonal relationships. Although mentally handicapped people are acknowledged to experience difficulties in social problem-solving and in social-cue interpretation, little in the way of training has been offered so far in these areas. Instead emphasis has been placed firmly upon teaching the handicapped person to interact more effectively with (usually) other handicapped people.

Many mentally handicapped people show poor eye contact, excessive hand-to-face gesturing and poor conversational abilities. Bornstein and his colleagues (Bornstein, Bach, McFall, Friman and Lyons, 1980) increased the number of words spoken and improved the non-verbal behaviours (gestures, posture, eye contact, etc.) of a small group of moderately handicapped adults in a sheltered workshop. Earlier, Matson and Stephens (1978) had completed a similar exercise with four adults in an institution who also showed gross facial mannerisms and inappropriate affect. These patients were also classified as 'psychotic' for these reasons. In both cases a package of methods was used: instructions, modelling, social reinforcement, and role playing coupled with the provision of feedback following the role plays. At a more basic level, Whitman, Burish and Collins (1972) reported success in increasing the levels of social interaction in two hospitalised children. In a similar exercise, Twardosz and Baer (1973) increased the frequency of asking questions in two severely mentally handicapped, hospitalised adolescents. In both of these studies tangible reinforcement was used in conjunction with social reinforcement. However, it would appear that once we try to move beyond the stage of increasing simple social responses, the treatment package becomes more complex and the likelihood that change will be maintained after treatment diminishes. Holley (1980) worked with a group of seven severely and moderately mentally handicapped people in a hospital setting. Changes in non-verbal and verbal behaviour were reported following a course of intensive social-skills training, using modelling, role play, videotape feedback, social reinforcement and coaching. When a follow-up was done at eight weeks, some reduction in the gains made was reported.

As we have noted briefly above, two kinds of social-skills training have been emerging over the past decade. In the first, simple social interaction skills, often involving only one target behaviour (such as asking or answering questions), is taught either to individuals or to very small groups of severely handicapped patients. The second type incorporates many of the principles of social-skills training as applied to the treatment of psychiatric patients. A broad range of non-verbal and verbal skills is taught using a wide variety of techniques. This latter approach is generally available only to moderately or mildly handicapped people. It is not yet clear exactly how valuable such interventions are likely to be for the handicapped person. It is clear that unless the handicapped person can learn to extend his skills to situations outside the one in which he is trained, then he will make little progress. More importantly, some attention should be paid to training the patient to be able to respond to the subtle social cues that precede and accompany social behaviour. If social skills training with the mentally handicapped continues largely to ignore these issues, then it is debatable as to whether or not any advances have been made in this area in recent years.

Disturbed Behaviour

The term 'disturbed behaviour' is often thought to be synonymous with antisocial behaviour, which, in turn, refers to aggression as well as to a range of unacceptable behaviours that cause offence (such as masturbation in public) or disrupt on-going activity in the ward (e.g. shouting or screaming). Typically these problems have been tackled in one of two ways: either by adopting the constructional approach referred to earlier, in which case the person is trained to exhibit some mutually exclusive activity, or by decreasing the incidence of the offensive behaviour through more direct intervention. With regard to the latter, a range of methods has been employed. For example, reinforcement may be withdrawn for a limited period of time (time out from reinforcement) or withdrawn altogether (response cost). Both these techniques represent alternatives to the use of more distinctly punitive approaches that enjoyed some popularity in the past.

Other methods include that of Foxx and Azrin (1972) who

developed a method of overcorrection called 'restitution' which was designed specifically for people who 'upset' other people's environments. Instead of punishing the offender, the staff member merely required him to correct the disturbance he had caused, by for example replacing toys, books, pieces of furniture, etc and by restoring the living space to its original form prior to the disturbance. Traditionally the patient was required to repeat this restitutive act a number of times, thereby fulfilling the requirements of the overcorrection technique. This often involved him in spending up to 20 minutes 'restoring the environment'. A related technique was developed for people who were aggressive. This involved requiring the patient to go and lie down on his bed for approximately 20 minutes. This 'required relaxation' is assisted, at first, by staff prompting the patient to lie down and relax, and by holding his arms and legs down on the bed if necessary. Foxx and Azrin have extended the use of these overcorrection techniques to cover a wide range of antisocial and self-injurious behaviours: the ingestion of rubbish and faeces (Foxx and Martin, 1975) rumination and vomiting (Foxx, Snyder and Schroeder, 1979) and self-injury (Azrin, Gottlieb, Hughart, Wesolowski and Rahn, 1975).

Self-injurious behaviour refers to a broad array of behaviours that result in some kind of physical damage to the individual. Often such behaviours are repetitive and chronic and they tend to occur most often in more severely handicapped individuals. Head banging, face slapping, eye gouging, self-biting and the ingestion of rubbish are typical forms of self-injurious behaviour. Little is known about the causes of the problem. In some cases the behaviour may be related to acute pain, as in otitis media, or to some form of metabolic disorder (e.g. Lesch-Nyan syndrome) in which self-injury may be triggered by biochemical factors.

In many others the behaviour may be shaped inadvertently by staff or parents. Many of the treatments already mentioned have been used to good effect in 'managing' this problem. However, of special note here is the use of the Differential Reinforcement of Other Behaviour technique. In this case, reinforcement (e.g. attention) is withdrawn when the patient engages in self-mutilative behaviour; and a more adaptive response is immediately promoted and subsequently reinforced. This results in the shaping and establishment of a 'competing response': a behaviour pattern which is mutually exclusive to the original self-injury (see Wesolowski and Zawlocki, 1982). For readers interested in this area we would refer you to the

AABT Task Force Report (1982) where the various methods appropriate to the management of this problem are reviewed.

A Recent Innovation. The technique of facial screening has become increasingly popular in recent years for the management of both self-injurious behaviour and a number of antisocial acts occurring in the more severely mentally handicapped resident. It has been used with inappropriate sexual behaviour (Barrman and Murray, 1981), trichotillomania (Barrman and Vitali, 1982), screaming (Singh, Winton and Dawson, 1982) and self-injury (Lutzker, 1978). Although there are some slight variations in the report of its use, generally it involves tying a large terry-towelling bib around the neck of the patient. Each time he shows the maladaptive behaviour, the bib is lifted up and over his head and held firmly there, taking care not to restrict his breathing, until the behaviour has ceased for one minute. Although this recent innovation has been shown to be highly effective in reducing maladaptive behaviour patterns, it does rely upon one-to-one contact, and may be viewed as an unacceptable technique for anyone other than the severely mentally handicapped. However, it is clear that this technique carries no risk of harm to the patient, who often is being treated because of the harmful or disturbing aspects of his behaviour.

In this very brief review we have tried to illustrate three key areas in which the mentally handicapped person in hospital may receive training or treatment within a behavioural model. This is hardly the limit to the potential of the behavioural approach with handicapped people. We have emphasised only those key problems such as self-care and social skills deficits and antisocial or self-injurious behaviour which are commonly associated with institutional life. In addition, the mentally handicapped can experience all of the problems which the psychiatric patient and the normal person experience: especially anxiety and depression. These affective disturbances are beginning to be recognised and tackled within a behavioural model (see Matson, 1982). The behavioural approach also holds considerable promise in the area of teaching problem-solving skills (Guralnick, 1976) and as an adjunct to routine academic training (Whitman and Johnston, 1983). It is also encouraging that considerable strides have been made in the training of care staff (Hogg, Foxen and McBrien, 1981) and parents (Berry and Wood, 1981).

The Role of the Nurse

The role of the nurse in both the psychiatric hospital and the mental handicap hospital is very similar. Despite major differences between the two populations, a common thread emerges which emphasises the extension of the patient's adaptive behaviour repertoire and attempts to reduce levels of socially or personally disadvantageous behaviour. The nurse who is trained in behavioural methods may be involved in the delivery of behaviour therapy on a variety of levels. In the following section we would like to consider the different kinds of treatment setting that can be found, and the varieties of clinical role engaged in by the nurse behaviour therapist.

The Translation of Routine Care

We have already paid some attention to the importance of the environment in the delivery of care and its potential role in institutionalising the long-stay patient. Many of the studies which we have reviewed in this chapter have involved sophisticated manipulation of the patient's everyday routine. In some situations, such as the more complex token economy systems reported, virtually every aspect of the patient's day is co-ordinated into the training programme. Everyday living skills, social interaction, and occupational and educational activities may all be encompassed by the token-economy umbrella. In such situations the patient's 'routine' has been restructured in such a way as to offer both a living and a learning environment. Although token economies have often been misrepresented as simple mechanistic ways of motivating patients, many of the studies to which we have referred involve highly elaborate and complicated organisational systems designed to allow learning to take place, often on a variety of levels at once.

However, the token economy is not the only format which lends itself to integration within routine care. Especially within the mental handicap setting, the concept of 'curriculum planning' has been popular, whereby a range of self-care, social, recreational and educational activites are co-ordinated to provide levels of training and stimulation for a group of residents. It is clear that, with careful planning, this concept, which is borrowed from the educational sector, can easily convert the institutional routine into a dynamic learning environment.

The role of the nurse in such a situation can vary depending upon her status and the demands of the situation. At one extreme she may be the grass-roots clinician, involved heavily in the delivery of the training or treatment programmes, perhaps performing a dual function as both a ward charge nurse and 'the therapist'. At the other extreme a distinction may be drawn clearly between these two roles. In many settings the nurse behaviour therapist is largely a consultant figure, offering advice and training to colleagues who may well be less sophisticated in their understanding of the behavioural model or in the application of its technology. In the 'routine care' setting, the behaviourally trained nurse may help to plan the assessment of the patients and to design training or treatment programmes, and will then act as a co-ordinator and monitor of service delivery. This 'free range' role, in which the nurse may act as an adviser and consultant to several wards in a hospital, or to various teams of nurses, involves her in devoting considerable time to analysing assessment and treatment records; in monitoring progress, by graphing and charting information; in preparing material necessary for treatment programmes; and in training staff in the basic methods essential to the running of treatment programmes. Although many, if not all, of these roles may be performed by the on-ward clinician, clearly there are advantages in offering some nurses the opportunity to specialise in such a wide-ranging role. For example, if there are only one or two behaviourally trained nurses in a hospital, it might be argued that the adoption of 'consultant' role would have a greater overall impact than that of the ward-based clinician.

Where nurses have taken up this 'consultant' role, their activities have extended far beyond the realm of the delivery of clinical treatment or training programmes. As we have already noted, the role demands involvement in the management of staff, staff training, and some involvement in the ward organisation. We would add to this list involvement in forward planning of the hospital service in more general terms: collaborating with other members of the multidisciplinary team in establishing policy for the development of services, especially where a behavioural approach is indicated.

The Intensive Treatment Unit

Many of the problems presented by the long-term hospital resident cannot be overcome by even sophisticated manipulation of his 'routine' environment. Especially if such patients show highly disturbed patterns of behaviour of a chronic nature, it may be necessary to set up special facilities to meet these very special needs. Many hospitals for the mentally ill or handicapped have 'behavioural units', which specialise in the delivery of some form of intensive behavioural treatment. In some cases these units will offer a 'high-pressure' type of rehabilitation in which patients are trained to extend their skills within a short time-span to help expedite their discharge from hospital. In other cases the unit will house highly disturbed residents who, on their past record, are unlikely ever to live any kind of independent existence. In such a setting the aims are likely to be geared more towards reducing levels of distressing or dangerous behaviour than to the resettlement of residents.

There are a number of advantages associated with such intensive treatment settings:

(1) Where such a unit exists, it may be easier to identify and consolidate a specific caring orientation towards the residents. It will be agreed, generally, that the unit exists to offer behavioural forms of training and treatment, and in practice this function will be fulfilled. In a 'routine care' setting, where a mixture of different care models may exist, this inconsistency may obstruct the delivery of systematic training or therapy.

(2) Patients are usually selected carefully for inclusion in such a unit. This means that the whole business of assessment is more methodical, leading to the use of individual care plans for each patient and careful systematic monitoring of progress. In the routine care setting, assessment is likely to be more 'low key' and perhaps even haphazard in operation.

(3) Hopefully, an intensive treatment unit would tend to select staff as well as patients, since not all nurses have either the aptitude or the training to work in such a situation. Psychiatric and mental handicap nursing can be arduous activities. However, spending all day working intensively with (perhaps) highly disturbed patients can be soul-destroying. Clearly there is a great need to select staff who are equipped both technically and emotionally to deal with such pressures. In the routine care situation, the opportunity to hand-pick staff is less evident. Often an effort is made to convert staff to the value of the behavioural model, or attempts are made to introduce them to the methods of therapy through *ad hoc* training exercises. The weaknesses, not to say dangers, of half-hearted approaches such as these are obvious.

(4) Where an intensive treatment unit is established, with it own aims and objectives and a clearly articulated operational policy, it is much easier to evaluate the contribution which the behavioural

model makes to the welfare of the patients. It is, dare we say it, easier to be more 'scientific' about the whole business of training and treatment. In the routine care setting, with all its inconsistencies and with its seemingly unavoidable multiplicity of treatment and management methods, such a critical evaluation is often impossible.

(5) Finally, the existence of such a treatment facility offers an opportunity for all groups of staff to see the behavioural model in action. Just as some kinds of medical treatment can only take place under controlled (e.g. aseptic) conditions, so behavioural treatment and training for some residents is only feasible where consistency and commitment are the order of the day. It is clear that where such facilities have been established, the behavioural approach gains a fairer hearing and generally is evaluated more positively than is the case when it is implemented in a piecemeal or haphazard fashion.

The role of staff in an intensive treatment unit is crucial. Every nurse working in such a setting should have some training in behavioural methods, both in the philosophy and in the technology of behaviour change. However, it is imperative that the 'nurse leader' on the unit should possess an in-depth appreciation of the various technical, theoretical and ethical issues involved in the delivery of care. It should also be apparent that this kind of 'nurse behaviour therapist' also needs a significant quota of personnel management skills, in order to be able to respond to the needs of her nursing team who are engaged in the demanding role of routine clinicians.

Summary

In this chapter we have attempted to present some of the major issues concerning the application of the behavioural model in hospitals for the long-term psychiatric patient and the mentally handicapped. We have tried to indicate some of the important strategies of behaviour change that are relevant to these two populations, and the kinds of problems that typically would represent the treatment goals. Three major targets have been isolated in the succeeding discussion. First of all, we have described the various areas of skills training. The case reports by Peggy Griffiths and Lydia Stephenson, in Chapters 6 and 8 of this book, amply illustrate the role which careful analysis plays in assisting disabled and institutionalised people to extend their existing levels of adaptive behaviour. Secondly, we have emphasised the role of behavioural methods in motivating patients to develop new skills or to relinquish existing patterns of maladaptive behaviour. The case report by Chris Portues in Chapter 10 suggests how careful programming can take on a highly personalised flavour and thereby provide a motivational system designed to make a number of changes to the everyday behaviour of a long-term patient.

Finally, we have drawn attention to the areas of 'disturbed behaviour' which are commonly associated with the chronic psychiatric patient or the mentally handicapped person. We have shown how even quite intractable forms of behaviour disorder can respond to careful, consistent behavioural programming. In particular we have noted the value of a 'constructional approach', which leads the therapist in an interesting search for behavioural assets and prevents him from pouncing prematurely on the patient's behavioural excesses.

References

AABT Task Force Report (1982) 'The Treatment of Self-injurious Behaviour', *Behaviour Therapy*, *13*, (4), 529–54

Albee, G. (1969) 'Needed — a Revolution in Caring for the Retarded', *Trans-Action*, *8*, 37–42

Altschul, A.T. (1974) 'Relationships between Patients and Nurses in Psychiatric Wards', *International Journal of Nursing Studies*, *8*, 179–87

Atthowe, J.M. and Krasner. L. (1968) 'Preliminary Report on the Application of Contingent Reinforcement Procedures (Token Economy) on a "Chronic"' Psychiatric Ward', *Journal of Abnormal Psychology*, *73*, 37–43

Ayllon, T. and Azrin, N. (1964) 'Reinforcement and Instructions with Mental Patients', *Journal of the Experimental Analysis of Behaviour*, *7*, 327–31

Ayllon, T. and Azrin, N. (1965) 'The Measurement and Reinforcement of Behaviour of Psychotics', *Journal of the Experimental Analysis of Behaviour*, *8*, 357–83

Ayllon, T. and Haughton, E. (1964), 'Modification of Symptomatic Verbal Behaviour of Mental Patients', *Behaviour Research and Therapy*, *2*, 87–97

Azrin, N.H. and Foxx, R.M. (1971), 'A Rapid Method of Toilet Training the Institutionalised Retarded', *Journal of Applied Behaviour Analysis*, *1*, 89–99

Azrin, N.H., Gottlieb, L., Hughart, L., Wesolowski, M.D. and Rahn, T. (1975) 'Eliminating Self-injurious Behaviour by Educative Procedures', *Behaviour Research and Therapy*, *13*, 101–11

Baker, R. (1971) 'The Use of Operant Conditiong to Reinstate Speech in Mute Schizophrenics', *Behaviour Research and Therapy*, *9*, 329–36

Baker, R., Hall, J.N. and Hutchinson, K. (1974) 'A Token Economy Project with Chronic Schizophrenic Patients', *British Journal of Psychiatry*, *124*, 367–84

Bandura, A. (1969) *Principles of Behaviour Modification*, Holt-Rinehart-Winston, New York

Barrman, B.C. and Murray, W.J. (1981), 'Suppression of Inappropriate Sexual

Behaviour by Facial Screening', *Behaviour Therapy*, *12*, 730–5

Barrman, B.C. and Vitali, D.L. (1982) 'Facial Screening to Eliminate Trichotillomania in Developmentally Disabled Persons', *Behaviour Therapy*, *13* (5), 735–42

Barton, R. (1959) *Institutional Neurosis*, John Wright & Sons, Bristol

Bellack, A. and Hersen, M. (1977) *Behaviour Modification: An Introductory Textbook*, Williams and Wilkins, Baltimore

Berry, I. and Wood, J. (1981) 'The Evaluation of Parent Intervention with Young Handicapped Children', *Behavioural Psychotherapy*, *9* (4), 358–68

Bijou, S.W. (1966) 'A Functional Analysis of Retarded Development', in N. Ellis (ed.), *International Review of Research in Mental Retardation*, vol. 1, Academic Press, New York

Birnbrauer, J. (1976) 'Mental Retardation', in H. Leitenberg (ed.), *Handbook of Behaviour Modification and Behaviour Therapy*, Prentice Hall, Englewood Cliffs, NJ

Bornstein, P. (1981) 'Research Issues in Training Interpersonal Skills for the Mentally Retarded', *Education and Training of the Mentally Retarded*, *16* (1), 70–4

Bornstein, P., Bach, P., McFall, M., Friman, P. and Lyons, P. (1980) 'Application of a Social Skills Training Programme in the Modification of Interpersonal Deficits among Retarded Adults', *Journal of Applied Behaviour Analysis*, *13*, (1), 171–6

Brown, G.W., Bone, M., Dallison, B. and Wing, J.K. (1966) *Schizophrenia and Social Care*, Maudsley Monograph, No. 17, Oxford University Press, Oxford

Buehler, R.E., Patterson, G.R. and Furniss, J.M. (1966) 'The Reinforcement of Behaviour in Institutional Settings', *Behaviour Research and Therapy*, *4*, 157–67

Burchard, J.D. and Barrera, F. (1972) 'An Analysis of Timeout and Response Cost in a Programmed Environment', *Journal of Applied Behaviour Analysis*, *5*, 271–82

Buss, A.H. and Lang, P.J. (1965) 'Psychological Deficit in Schizophrenia: 1, Affect, Reinforcement and Concept Attainment', *Journal of Abnormal Psychology*, *70*, 2–24

Campbell, A.C. (1971) 'Aspects of Personal Independence of Mentally Abnormal and Mentally Subnormal Adults in Hospital and in Local Authority Hostels', *International Journal of Social Psychiatry*, *17* (4), 124–8

Crisp, A.G. and Sturmey, P. (1984) 'Organising Staff to Promote Purposeful Activity in a Setting for Mentally Handicapped Adults', *Behavioural Psychotherapy*, *12*, 381–99

De Kock, U., Mansell, J., Felce, D. and Jenkins, J. (1984) 'Establishing Appropriate Mealtime Behaviour of a Severely Disruptive Mentally Handicapped Woman', *Behavioural Psychotherapy*, *12* (2), 163–74

Ellis, N.R. (1963) 'Toilet Training the Severely Defective Patient: an S.R. Reinforcement Analysis', *American Journal of Mental Deficiency*, *68*, 98–103

Fernandez, J. (1974) 'Variables which Contribute towards the Behavioural Improvement Shown by Subjects in Token Programmes', Paper presented at the *4th Annual Conference of the European Association for Behaviour Therapy, London*

Fernandez, J. (1978) 'Token Economies and other Token Programmes in the United States', *Behavioural Psychotherapy*, *6*, 56–69

Fernandez, J. (1983) 'The Token Economy and Beyond', *Irish Journal of Psychotherapy*, *2*, 21–41

Fernandez, J., Fischer, I. and Ryan, E. (1973a) 'The Token Economy: a Living-Learning Environment', *British Journal of Psychiatry*, *122*, 453–5

Fernandez, J., Fischer, I. and Ryan, E. (1973b) 'Behaviour Modification Using Token Reinforcement', *Irish Journal of Psychology*, *2*, 34–56

Foxx, R.M. and Azrin, N.H. (1972) 'Restitution: a Method of Eliminating Aggressive

Disruptive Behaviour of Retarded and Brain-damaged Patients', *Behaviour Research and Therapy*, *13*, 153–62

Foxx, R.M. and Azrin, N.H. (1973) 'Toilet Training the Retarded', Research Press, Champaign, Illinois

Foxx, R.M. and Martin, E.D. (1975) 'Treatment of Scavenging Behaviour by Overcorrection', *Behaviour Research and Therapy*, *13*, 153–62

Foxx, R.M., Synder, M. and Schroeder, F. (1979) 'A Food Satiation and Oral Hygiene Punishment Programme to Suppress Chronic Rumination by Retarded Persons', *Journal of Autism and Development Disorders*, *9*, 399–412

Fraser, D. (1978) 'Critical Variables in Token Economy Systems: a Review of the Literature and a Description of Current Research', *Behavioural Psychotherapy*, *6*, 46–55

Fraser, D. (1983) 'From Token Economy to Social Information System: The Emergence of Critical Variables', in E. Karas, (ed.), *Current Issues in Clinical Psychology*, Plenum, New York

Fraser, D. and Cormack, D. (1975) 'The Nurse's Role in Psychiatric Institutions', *Nursing Times*, *71*, 125–32

Fraser, D., McLeod, W.L., Begg, J.C., Hawthorne, J.H. and Davis, P. (1976) 'Against the Odds: the Results of a Token Economy Programme with Long-Term Psychiatric Patients', *International Journal of Nursing Studies*, *13*, 55–63

Fraser, D., Anderson, J. and Grime, J. (1981) 'An Analysis of the Progressive Development of Vocal Responses in a Mute Schizophrenic Patient', *Behavioural Psychotherapy*, *9*, 2–12

Fraser, D., Black, D. and Cockram, L. (1981) 'An Examination of the Effectiveness of Instructional Training and Response Cost Procedures in Controlling the Inappropriate Behaviour of Male Schizophrenic Patients', *Behavioural Psychotherapy*, *9*, 256–67

Gardner, W. (1971) *Behaviour Modification in Mental Retardation*, Aldine-Atherton, Chicago

Gelfand, D.M., Gelfand, S. and Dobson, W.R. (1967) 'Unprogrammed Reinforcement of Patients' Behaviour in a Mental Hospital', *Behaviour Research and Therapy*, *5*, 201–7

Glickman, H. Plutchik, R. and Landau, H. (1973) 'Social and Biological Reinforcement in an Open Psychiatric Ward', *Journal of Behaviour Therapy and Experimental Psychiatry*, *4*, 121–4

Goldiamond, I. (1974) 'Towards a Constructional Approach to Social Problems', *Behaviourism*, *2*, 1–84

Grant, G.W.B. and Moores, B. (1977) 'Resident Characteristics and Staff Behaviour in Two Hospitals for Mentally Retarded Adults', *American Journal of Mental Deficiency*, *82*, 259–65

Gripp, R.F. and Magaro, P.A. (1974) 'The Token Economy Programme in the Psychiatric Hospital: A Review and Analysis', *Behaviour Research and Therapy*, *12*, 205–28

Gruenberg, E.M. (1967) 'The Social Breakdown Syndrome — Some Origins', *American Journal of Psychiatry*, *123*, 1481–9

Grunewald, K. (1974) 'The Guiding Environment: the Dynamics of Residential Living', in D.M. Boswell and J.M. Wingrove (eds), *The Handicapped Person in the Community*, Tavistock, London

Guralnick, M. (1976) 'Solving Complex Discrimination Problems: Techniques for the Development of Problem-solving Strategies', *American Journal of Mental Deficiency*, *81*, 18–25

Hawks, D. (1975) 'Community Care: an Analysis of Assumptions', *British Journal of Psychiatry*, *127*, 276–85

Heap, R.J., Bobbitt, W.E., Moore, C.H. and Hord, J.E. (1970) 'Behaviour Milieu

Therapy with Chronic Neuropsychiatric Patients', *Journal of Abnormal Psychology*, *76*, 349–54

Hemsley, D.R. (1977) 'What Have Cognitive Deficits to Do with Schizophrenic Symptoms?' *British Journal of Psychiatry*, *130*, 167–73

Hemsley, D.R. (1978) 'Limitations of Operant Procedures in the Modification of Schizophrenic Functioning: the Possible Relevance of Studies of Cognitive Disturbance', *Behavioural Analysis and Modification*, *2*, 165–73

Hogg, J., Foxen, T. and McBrien, J. (1981) 'Issues in the Training and Evaluation of Behaviour Modification Skills for Staff Working with Profoundly Retarded Multiply Handicapped Children', *Behavioural Psychotherapy*, *9*, (4), 345–57

Holley, J. (1980) 'A Social Skills Group with Mentally Retarded Subjects', *British Journal of Social and Clinical Psychology*, *19* (3), 279–86

Kale, R.J., Kaye, J.H., Whelan, P.A. and Hopkins, B.L. (1968) 'The Effects of Reinforcement on the Modification, Maintenance and Generalisation of Social Responses of Mental Patients', *Journal of Applied Behaviour Analysis*, *1*, 307–14

Kazdin, A.E. (1972) 'Response, Cost: the Removal of Conditioned Reinforcers for Therapeutic Change', *Behaviour Therapy*, *3*, 533–46

Kazdin, A.E. (1973) 'Role of Instructions and Reinforcement in Behaviour Changes in Token Reinforcement Programmes', *Journal of Educational Psychology*, *64*, 63–71

Kazdin, A.E. (1975) *Behaviour Modification in Applied Settings*, Dorsey Press, Illinois

Kazdin, A.E. and Wilson, G,T, (1978) *Evaluation of Behaviour Therapy: Issues, Evidence and Research Strategies*, Ballinger Publishing Co., Cambridge, Mass.

Kelly, B., Holland, J. and Webster, J. (1982) 'The Douglas Ward Activity Project', *Mental Handicap*, *10*, 16–17

Kiernan, C.C. (1974) 'Behaviour Modification', in A. Clarke and A.D.B. Clarke (eds), *Mental Deficiency: the Changing Outlook*, Methuen, London

Leck, I., Gordon, W.L. and McKeown, T. (1967) 'Medical and Social Needs of Patients in Hospitals for the Mentally Subnormal', *British Journal of Social and Preventative Medicine*, *21*, 115–21

Liberman, R. (1972) 'Reinforcement of Social Interaction in a Group of Chronic Mental Patients', in R.D. Rubin, H. Fensterheim, J.D. Henderson and L.P. Ullmann (eds), *Advances in Behaviour Therapy*, Academic Press, New York

Lutzker, J.R. (1978) 'Reducing Self-injurious Behaviour by Facial Screening', *American Journal of Mental Deficiency*, *82*, 510–13

McPherson, F.M., Cockram, L.L., Grimes, J., Fraser, D. and Presly, A.S. (1979) 'The Restoration of One Aspect of Communication in Chronic Schizophrenic Patients', *Health Bulletin*, *37*, September, 227–31

Matson, J.L. (1982) 'The Treatment of Behavioural Characteristics of Depression in the Mentally Retarded', *Behaviour Therapy*, *13* (2), 209–18

Matson, J.L. and Stephens, R.M. (1978) 'Increasing Appropriate Behaviour of Explosive Chronic Psychiatric Patients with a Social Skills Training Package', *Behaviour Modification*, *2*, 61

Mertens, G.C. and Fuller, W.B. (1963) 'Conditioning of Molar Behaviour in Regressed Psychotics: 1. An Objective Measure of Personal Habit Training with Regressed Psychotics', *Journal of Clinical Psychology*, *19*, 333–7

Milby, J.B. (1970) 'Modification of Extreme Social Isolation by Contingent Social Reinforcement', *Journal of Applied Behaviour Analysis*, *3*, 149–52

Morris, P. (1969) *Put Away*, Routledge, Kegan & Paul, London

Oswin, M. (1978) *Children Living in Long-stay Hospitals*, Spastics International

Medical Publication, London

Panyan, M.C. (1972) *New Ways to Teach New Skills*, H and H Enterprises, Kansas

Paton, X. and Stirling, E. (1974) 'Frequency and Type of Dyadic Nurse-Patient Verbal Interaction in a Mental Subnormality Hospital', *Intrnational Journal of Nursing Studies*, *11*, 135–45

Paul, G.L. and Lentz, R.J. (1977) 'Psychological Treatment of Chronic Mental Patients: Milieu versus Social Learning Programmes', Harvard University Press, Cambridge, Mass.

Perkins, E.A., Taylor, P.D. and Capie, A.C.D. (1976) *Helping the Retarded*, Institute of Mental Subnormality, Kidderminster

Porterfield, J., Blunden, R. and Blewitt, E. (1980) 'Improving Environments for Profoundly Handicapped Adults', *Behaviour Modification*, *4*, 225–41

Presly, A.S., Grubb, A.B. and Semple, D. (1982) 'Predictions of Successful Rehabilitation in Long Stay Patients', *Acta Psychiatrica Scandinavica*, *66*, 83–8

Raynes, N.V. and King, R.P. (1974) 'Residential Care for the Mentally Retarded', in D.M. Boswell and J.M. Wingrove (eds), *The Handicapped Person in the Communicy*, London, Tavistock

Sanok, R. and Ascione, F.R. (1978) 'The Effects of Reduced Time Limits on Prolonged Eating Behaviour of a Severely Disruptive Mentally Handicapped Woman', *Behavioural Psychotherapy*, *12*, 163–74

Schaefer, H.H. and Martin, P.L. (1966) 'Behaviour Therapy for "Apathy" of Hospitalized Schizophrenics', *Psychological Reports*, *19*, 1147–58

Sherman, J.A. (1965) 'Use of Reinforcement and Imitation to Reinstate Verbal Behaviour in Mute Psychotics', *Journal of Abnormal Psychology*, *70*, 155–64

Singh, N.N., Winton, A.S. and Dawson, M.J. (1982) 'Suppression of Antisocial Behaviour by Facial Screening Using Multiple Baseline and Alternating Treatment Designs', *Behaviour Therapy*, *13* (4), 511–20

Sletten, I.W., Hughes, D.D., Lamont, J. and Ognjanov, V. (1968) 'Work Performance in Psychiatric Patients (tokens vs. money), *Diseases of the Nervous System*, *29*, 261–4

Stoffelmayr, B.E., Faulkner, G.E. and Mitchell, W.S. (1979) 'The Comparison of Token Economy and Social Therapy in the Treatment of Hard-core Schizophrenic Patients', *Behavioural Analysis and Modification*, *3*, 3–17

Storms, L.H. and Broen, W.E. (1969) 'A Theory of Schizophrenic Behavioural Disorganisation', *Archives of General Psychiatry*, *20*, 129–43

Suchotliff, L., Greaves, S., Stecker, H. and Berke, R. (1970) 'Critical Variables in the Token Economy', *Proceedings of the 78th Annual Convention of the American Psychological Association*

Thompson, N., Fraser, D. and McDougall, A. (1974) 'The Reinstatement of Speech in Near-Mute Chronic Schizophrenics by Instruction, Imitative Prompts and Reinforcement', *Journal of Behaviour Therapy and Experimental Psychiatry*, *5*, 83–9

Twardosz, S. and Baer, D.M. (1973) 'Training Two Severely Retarded Adolescents to Ask Questions', *Journal of Applied Behaviour Analysis*, *6*, 655–61

Walker, H.M. and Buckley, N.K. (1972) 'Programming Generalization and Maintenance of Treatment Effects across Time and across Settings', *Journal of Applied Behaviour Analysis*, *5*, 209–24

Walker, L.G. (1979) 'The Effect of Some Incentives on the Work Performance of Psychiatric Patients at Rehabilitation Workshop', *British Journal of Psychiatry*, *134*, 427–35

Wesolowski, M.D. and Zawlocki, R.J. (1982) 'The Differential Effects of Procedures to Eliminate an Injurious Self-stimulating Behaviour (Digito-ocular Sign) in Blind

Retarded Twins', *Behaviour Therapy*, *13* (3), 334–45

Whaley, D.L. and Malott, R.W. (1971) *Elementary Principles of Behaviour*, Appleton Century Crofts, New York

Whitman, T.L. and Johnston, M.B. (1983) 'Teaching Addition and Subtraction with Regrouping to Educable Mentally Retarded Children: a Group Self-instructional Training Program', *Behaviour Therapy*, *14* (1), 127–43

Whitman, T.L., Burish, T. and Collins, C. (1972) 'Development of Interpersonal Language Responses in Two Moderately Retarded Children', *Mental Retardation*, *10*, 40–5

Wincze, J.P., Leitenberg, H. and Agras, W.S. (1972) 'The Effects of Token Reinforcement and Feedback on the Delusional Verbal Behaviour of Chronic Paranoid Schizophrenics', *Journal of Applied Behaviour Analysis*, 5, 247–62

Wing, J.K. (1967) 'Social Treatment, Rehabilitation and Management', in A. Coppen and A. Walk (eds), *Recent Development in Schizophrenia*, Headley Bros., Ashley

Wing, J.K. (1975) 'Impairments in Schizophrenia: a Rational Basis for Social Treatment', in R.D. Wirt, G. Winokur and M. Roff (eds), *Life History Research in Psychopathology*, University of Minnesota Press, Minneapolis

Wing, J.K. and Brown, G.W. (1970) *Institutionalism and Schizophrenia*, Cambridge University Press, Cambridge

Wing, J.K. and Morris, B. (1981) (eds), *Handbook of Psychiatric Rehabilitation Practice*, Oxford University Press, Oxford

Wing, J.K., Monck, E., Brown, G.W. and Carstairs, C.M. (1964) 'Morbidity in the Community of Schizophrenic Patients Discharged from London Mental Hospitals in 1959', *British Journal of Psychiatry*, *110*, 10–21

Winkler, R.C. (1970) 'Management of Chronic Psychiatric Patients by a Token Reinforcement System', *Journal of Applied Behaviour Analysis*, *3*, 47–55

Yule, W. and Carr, J. (eds) (1980) *Behaviour Modification for the Mentally Handicapped*, Croom Helm, London

Zigler, E. (1967) 'Familial Mental Retardation: a Continuing Dilemma', *Science*, *155*, 292–8

4 THE NURSE THERAPIST IN A PRIMARY CARE SETTING

Philip J. Barker and Douglas Fraser

Introduction

Traditionally, psychiatric nursing has been built around the provision of a hospital service. However, over the past twenty years various developments have been taking place within the community. In some cases this involves the provision of a service to maintain patients in the community following a period in hospital; in many cases a very long period indeed. In others the community-based service is designed to identify problems, and to offer help, at an early stage — before hospitalisation becomes necessary. This is often referred to as 'primary care'. We acknowledge that the term 'primary care' can have a very specific meaning, which may differ to some degree from our use of the term. We employ this expression to make a distinction between those 'chronic' problems that often necessitate hospital-based treatment, and the range of problems that can sometimes be tackled through some kind of community-based provision.

Over the last two decades community psychiatric nurses have established themselves as the first large group of specialist psychiatric nurses. Within the last decade major developments have taken place to offer specialist training which is commensurate with this specialist role. However, it is clear that these nurses are specialists only in so far as the location of their workplace differs radically from the traditional base used by most other nurses. It is not yet clear in what way the work which such nurses do in the community differs from that which takes place in the hospital. Even within community psychiatric nursing there exists a diversity of roles and models of care. Some of these facets of community nursing are influenced by the demands of various patient populations. In other cases, the ideological orientation which the nurse inherits from her training establishment is the guiding factor in determining her role relationship with patients. As a result we can see the emergence of sub-specialities within community nursing, of nurses who 'specialise' in the care of the elderly — often referred to as ESMI teams: the 'elderly severely mentally ill'; or who work with the post-rehabilitation population — those who have recently been discharged from hospital and are living in hostels or group homes. We also have those nurses who deal only with mentally handicapped people; perhaps even specialising within this sub-population itself. It is not our intention here to review the role of the community psychiatric nurse; nor to comment upon the value of specialist versus generic roles. We draw the reader's attention to this branch of psychiatric nursing merely to provide the setting for a discussion of the role of nurses who practise behaviour therapy within a primary care set-up. Such nurses — who may be members of community nursing teams, or 'primary care teams' in health centres — are, in practice, if not by definition, community nurses. However, the nature of their work and the principles of care and treatment which guide them may differ markedly from those of other community nurses. In this chapter we want to take a look at the kind of work which such a nurse might undertake, and at the relationship which she currently has and may, in future, enjoy with other community nurses.

The Primary Therapist

As we have noted earlier in the book, the concept of the nurse therapist has a fairly short history. The most precise description offered of the community-based nurse therapist is given by Marks, Connolly, Hallam and Philpott (1975). This is also the earliest such description that is supported by any research findings. We should note immediately that it is incorrect to refer to the nurses in the original Maudsley experiment as 'community nurses'. Many of the patients were, at least temporarily, hospitalised. It may be more accurate to call these nurses 'direct therapists' or primary therapists. They were the key workers in the presentation of treatment: in some cases the only professionals involved on a close or lasting basis with the patient. Marks *et al*, (1975) referred to these nurses as specialising in the treatment of adult neuroses. As we have noted elsewhere, the distinction between 'neurotic' and 'psychotic' patients, or conditions, is not always a helpful one in attempting to discriminate between those who should and those who should not be offered behavioural treatment. In our discussion here we shall only refer to the specific kinds of problem and the kinds of people who may be enrolled in therapy in a community context. Whether it is helpful to refer to such patients as 'neurotics' is arguable to say the least.

The concept of the nurse therapist articulated by Marks and his colleagues is similar to our own, at least in so far as it extends to work in a 'primary care' setting. The concept has also found favour in parts of North America (Latimer, 1980; O'Donoghue and Borgerson, 1980) as well as in Australia (Horne, McTiernan and Strauss, 1981). The nurses who were involved in the studies cited above work almost exclusively on a casework basis: acting as the primary therapist and designing and delivering the treatment package. Their role is distinctly different from that of those nurses working in in-patient facilities, who tend to work in groups, sharing the process of therapy often among members of a multidisciplinary team. This independent status registers another similarity to the community psychiatric nurse.

There are a number of reasons why nurses have been encouraged to take up this role of primary therapist. Perhaps one of the more accurate, but none the less unprepossessing, arguments is that nurses who are well trained as behavioural psychotherapists are cheaper than other kinds of psychotherapists (cf. Ginsberg and Marks, 1977). We take the view that such nurses are appropriate for a number of other reasons. First, providing that they are carefully selected before training, they will possess the kind of personal skills that are fundamental to the practice of any psychotherapy; skills that are not necessarily the birthright of psychiatrists and psychologists (cf. Robertson, 1982). It is also clear that many psychiatrists and psychologists who practise behavioural psychotherapy are often not content with a purely clinical role — cherishing desires to undertake research or educational commitments as an adjunct to their therapeutic role. In the nurse therapist we may have the makings of a full-time 'practitioner', who may significantly extend the service provision to patients. Perhaps, also, the nurse therapist may — by virtue of her less exalted status — be able to establish relationships with some patients, who — by virtue of their class or cultural affiliations — may encounter relationship problems with psychiatrists and psychologists (cf. Meldrum, McGowan, Higgins and Schaller, 1969). Our last reason is the most obvious. Nurses are already working as 'primary agents' in the community: in health centres, as part of community nursing teams. These nurses are already a significant aspect of the treatment service offered to patients. As Peck has observed, by offering a training in behavioural methods, we merely serve to reinforce their status as agents of behavioural change (Peck, 1973).

In principle, any behaviour problem which has been shown to be amenable to treatment by behavioural methods can be tackled in a direct therapy format, in a community setting. However, practical considerations dictate that certain problems, occurring in certain individuals, are more likely to respond to therapy. In this first section here, we shall discuss the various classes of disorder which research suggests are suitable targets for behaviour therapy.

The Key Targets

A group of four disorders exists which, in the light of contemporary research, can be treated by behavioural methods *alone*. We would emphasise that although behavioural methods have been shown to be successful in reducing the effect of these disorders, this does not mean that these methods are always used (alone or in conjunction with other forms of treatment). However, at least in principle, behaviour therapy is the treatment of choice for these disorders.

Simple Phobias

Simple or specific phobias are those disorders that are characterised by fear *and* avoidance of specific situations: e.g. heights, certain animals, lifts. Typically, the patient does not show anxiety in any setting other than the phobic situation. However, in some cases the patient may avoid two or more situations. Some of these phobias are exaggerations of natural fears — such as fear of insects, snakes, or being trapped. In others, the fear may be of wholly innocuous stimuli — e.g. of birds or kittens. In such cases the fear may have generalised from another feared situation, in the manner described in Chapter 2; or may have been directly conditioned through some form of 'traumatic learning'.

Generalised Phobias

Although such phobias are thought to have two distinct forms: social phobias — where the patient is afraid of contact with people, and the so-called 'agoraphobic syndrome', where the patients report fear and avoidance of a wide range of situations, it is common for the latter to be accepted as including elements of social phobia, travel phobia, and high levels of anxiety experienced at any significant distance from a safe base, such as home. Although much common ground exists between one 'agoraphobic' and another, it is clear that the distress experienced by one patient may not be found in another when faced with similar situations. For instance, one patient may find standing in a bus queue 'intolerable', but may relax as soon as she gets on the bus; another may have to get off the bus earlier than planned in order to escape from intolerable levels of anxiety.

Obsessional Disorders

These patients also experience high anxiety and exhibit avoidance behaviour. However, the key feature here is the performance of some repetitive behaviour — such as repeated hand washing to avoid contamination, or repeated checking of doors and locks to avoid burglary (compulsive rituals); *or* some form of repetitive thinking — e.g. recalling or imagining some unpleasant scene (obsessional ruminations). Behavioural methods have been successful in reducing the severity of severely handicapping ritualistic behaviour. Although the success rate with ruminations is much less impressive, it is often more successful than physical methods of treatment such as psychosurgery.

Psychosexual Disorders

A range of sexual difficulties has been successfully treated by behavioural methods. Impotence and premature ejaculation in men, and vaginismus and anorgasmia in women, have been treated by a broad range of methods, which focus upon the education (or re-education) of the partners in sexual behaviour. At the same time they are assisted to reduce the levels of anxiety that inhibit the successful performance of sexual intercourse.

The Treatment of Anxiety

A common feature of each of the above disorders, is *anxiety*, which may also present as a problem in its own right. Two forms of *exposure* represent the commonest techniques in the treatment of anxiety. In both cases the patient is required to perform some 'approach' behaviour which inhibits the avoidance strategies he would normally employ. In *graded exposure* (or desensitisation) the patient is encouraged to face or approach his most feared situation in gradual stages: beginning at a level where anxiety is minimal and can be easily managed. Spider phobics might study pictures of spiders, or an agoraphobic might enter the corner shop and buy one item before leaving. As his anxiety diminishes at one stage, the patient progresses gradually to stages that evoke higher and higher levels of anxiety.

Alternatively, in *flooding*, the patient is encouraged to face his most threatening situation immediately — jumping in at the deep end. The spider phobic is required to handle a live spider and the agoraphobic to enter a supermarket when it is busy. In this form of treatment the patient is required to remain in the situation until his anxiety begins to abate. Both graded exposure and flooding may be conducted in imagination (imaginal desensitisation or flooding) or in real-life situations (*in vivo*). The graded exposure technique was first developed by Wolpe (1958) and has been successful with a range of anxiety-based problems. Leitenberg (1976) suggested that this graded approach was 'demonstrably more effective than both no treatment and every psychotherapy variant with which it has been compared'. Within the last decade, *in vivo* exposure in the course of which the therapist *models* the approach behaviour has become increasingly popular. Through modelling the patient not only has access to social support, but may also benefit from the encouragement to imitate the therapist's (or another patient's) actions. Flooding developed from a dynamic psychotherapy technique which required the patient to imagine highly disturbing fantasies (Stampfl and Levis, 1967). This approach aims to extinguish the patient's fear at the highest level, thereby accelerating the speed of progress when compared with the graded exposure method. However, it comes as no surprise to find that patients often reject the more rapid method in favour of the more relaxed approach. In recent years there has been a marked trend towards *in vivo* exposure with modelling for many anxiety/avoidance problems. Frame and Turner (1984), however, showed that patients could do this alone, thereby reducing the 'costs' of therapist time. Chambless, Foa, Graves and Goldstein (1982) have suggested that although *in vivo* exposure is very popular, especially with agoraphobics, flooding in imagination is just as effective, and is less time consuming for the therapist.

In recent years there has been a tendency towards the use of complex packages of treatment, involving a range of techniques. In many cases this trend has been criticised on the grounds that the therapy may be unnecessarily complicated. However, in many cases patients often need more than simple exposure if the gains made during therapy are to last after contact with the therapist has ceased. Sartory, Rachman and Grey (1982) have recently noted that many patients experiencing fear are, after treatment, able to reinstate their fears by simply recalling fear-evoking events. This suggests that patients may need to learn how to handle their 'mental pictures' of feared situations, as well as their behaviour under such conditions. Findings such as these have offered support for the development of cognitive adjuncts to exposure treatment (see also Mathews, Gelder and Johnston, 1982).

Adjunct Therapy

A number of other disorders can also be resolved, to varying degrees, by behavioural methods. However, in such cases the behaviour therapy usually acts as an adjunct to some other form of treatment: such as drug therapy, or membership of some self-help group. A broad range of disorders can be tackled under this 'adjunct therapy' umbrella. However, since a mixture of methods is involved, the evidence in support of the behavioural approach is obviously less than conclusive. Consequently, we shall confine ourselves to a brief description of the various problems, while referring to the methods that show promise.

Generalised Anxiety

Anxiety states — of free-floating anxiety — account for a substantial proportion of the acute psychiatric population. Such patients can be distinguished from those suffering from phobic states by the apparent absence of any obvious 'trigger' for their anxiety. Often such patients display strong cognitive features: *imagining* things going wrong or their failure to cope with impending events, or 'reporting back' to themselves in an exaggerated, catastrophic fashion. Such patients contribute to the escalation of their anxiety through their 'self-talk', the commonly observed result of which is the 'fear of fear'. Flooding (imaginal) has been shown to be highly successful in extinguishing such anxiety, where highly specific memories evoke the anxiety, such as traumatic memories (Forbank and Keene, 1982). Where the anxiety is more generalised, a combination of 'coping self-instruction' with an adjustment of the patient's thinking style appears to hold most promise (Woodward and Jones, 1980).

Social Anxiety

Although this has been mentioned as a variant of agoraphobia, it frequently presents as a separate problem. The patient tends to avoid interpersonal situations, in which he is required to interact with people, either individually or in groups. In many cases such patients are 'chronically shy' and may also lack the skills of interpersonal communication essential to a comfortable social role. Social skills training has been shown to be helpful in such cases (Trower, Bryant and Argyle, 1978) and assertion training may be of value (Alberti and Emmons, 1970). However, in many situations, graded exposure *in vivo*, and the self-instructional 'coping' methods mentioned earlier are invaluable (Halford and Foddy, 1982). In common with the trend towards 'packages' of techniques for other anxiety disorders, some writers have suggested that a combination of social skills training, exposure and cognitive restructuring may be necessary in most cases of interpersonal-skill difficulty (Stravynski, 1984).

Depression

Depression — either alone or in association with generalised anxiety — is one of the major problems in psychiatry. Such problems — for surely we are talking about a *range* of depressive disorders rather than a single condition — have responded erratically to physical methods of treatment and to traditional forms of psychotherapy. Within the last decade a substantial body of evidence has been accumulated to suggest that in selected cases various behavioural and cognitive change methods can be helpful in at least reducing the severity of such disorders. Beck and his colleagues (Beck, Rush, Shaw and Emery, 1980) have popularised a 'cognitive therapy' package which employs a range of behavioural and cognitive restructuring methods. However, some writers have suggested that behavioural methods *alone* can be effective (Wilson, Goldin and Charbonnea, 1983). In particular there are the reinforcement-based methods of Lewinsohn (1969) and their combination with self-reinforcement and behavioural assignments in the self-control approach of Kornbluth and Rehm (1983).

Eating Disorders

Patients who refuse to eat or who overeat have always been popular targets for behaviour therapists. However, their efforts rarely met with more than short-term success. In recent years a trend towards more complex packages of treatment has been evident in this field too. Dietary education, self-control strategies, membership of self-help groups and the role of exercise have all been evident. Perhaps the most important aspect of such problems is their potential life-threatening nature. This is true of severe obesity, and also of anorexia (where the patient, usually female, starves herself) and of bulimarexia (where the patient alternates between bingeing and vomiting followed by starvation). Obesity is often the result of a biological predisposition which is accelerated by inappropriate eating and activity patterns. Treatment often involves ingenious attempts to reverse the pattern, and to maintain change across time. It has been suggested that anorexia and bulimarexia may have more complex origins. The patient may begin dieting following rejection: this may be perceived or actual. Boskind-Lodahl and Sirlin (1977) report that nearly all of the patients in their study began to binge after being rejected by men. The binge made them feel out of control, guilty and even more ugly. This led to a renewed compulsion to lose weight, by fasting or purging or both. Once the pattern begins, dieting produces a psychological boost. However, the patient may also have to respond to biological pressure to eat — resulting in bingeing (Slade, 1982). Recently one particular package of techniques has shown considerable promise in maintaining appropriate eating patterns and weight gain. Holmgren (1984) reports the use of self-control, dietary training, body awareness and the provision of general social support and occupational therapy. This 'first stage' exercise leads to more long-term psychotherapy intended to maintain changes in eating behaviour and in the self concept.

Similar strategies appear to hold the most promise for weight reduction, with the inclusion of aerobic exercise to change the patient from a sedentary, food-fixated lifestyle to a more active diet-conscious one.

Alcohol Abuse

Alcohol abuse has also fascinated behaviour therapists, who devoted much energy to trying to treat the problem through aversive methods. Success was often achieved easily under treatment conditions but relapse was frequently evident as soon as the patient returned to the 'real world' with all the natural inducements to return to previous drinking patterns. This seemed to suggest that total abstinence was the only solution for the alcoholic. Recently, researchers in the United States and in this country have suggested that an alternative is possible, at least for some patients. 'Controlled drinking' involves a package of techniques, emphasising the drawing up of a contract between patient, therapist and often members of his family, and the systematic acquisition of self-control strategies which allow drinking in moderation, rather than complete abstinence. Although this approach presents a refreshing alternative to total abstinence, its clinical use is as yet fairly restricted (see Heather and Robertson, 1981, for a detailed review).

Habit Disorders

A number of different problems can be subsumed under the heading of habit disorders. Trichotillomania is a fairly exotic term used to describe a simple activity — pulling out one's own hair. Often this behaviour occurs against a background of anxiety or interpersonal discord. The problem is, however, responsive to a specific habit-reversal technique, which increases the patient's awareness of the process involved in hair pulling, thereby helping him or her to control its occurrence (Fleming, 1984). Insomnia is another problem which can be associated with other disorders, such an anxiety or depression. Where specific thoughts or anxiety problems are keeping the patient awake, then these must naturally be the focus of treatment. However, where no such obvious features are evident, the disorder may be regarded as a habit disorder which may be amenable to change by means of modifications to the sleeping routine (see Lacks, 1983, for a review of this area).

Marital Discord

Interpersonal problems within relationships can result from unasser-tiveness on the part of one partner, but in many cases involve a breakdown of the relationship on both sides. A number of behavioural contracting methods have proven useful in helping couples — not necessarily married ones — to re-establish balance or enjoyment in relationships which had become one-sided or stale. This approach is often combined with sex therapy or with the treatment of alcoholism, where it exists in only one partner. One of the more clearly defined packages is Azrin's 'reciprocity counselling' method (Azrin, Naster and Jones, 1975), which helps the couple to learn that there are practical alternatives to the self-defeating round of arguments and silences. More recently, Piercy (1983) has reported a 'penny game' which is intended to break the common cycle of 'you win, I lose'. This is used in conjunction with regulation skills and marital assertion training. This form of 'conjoint therapy' has also proven useful and popular where violence is a feature of the relationship (Taylor, 1984; see also Nomellini and Katz, 1983).

Current Trends

The disorders that were briefly described above have commonly been seen as representative of psychiatric disorder, or, at the very least, as indicative of some kind of psychological 'hang-up' in need of psychotherapeutic resolution. Interest in developing new or improved technologies of behaviour change for these problems is well illustrated in the contemporary behaviour-therapy journals. However, one of the most interesting developments of the last decade has been the attention paid to psychological problems which are secondary to other disorders of a more physical nature. High blood pressure has been shown to respond to relaxation training (Agras, Schneider and Taylor, 1984), and chronic pain has become a key area of interest from both a theoretical and practical perspective (Keefe, 1982). Again, packages of techniques have found most favour. Figueroa (1982) has found that self-relaxation and pain management conducted in groups is significantly better than either traditional psychotherapeutic support or self-monitoring methods. However, perhaps the use of various forms of biofeedback best illustrates the variety of 'new ground' which can be broken; in the control and stabilisation of diabetes mellitus (Guthrie, Moeller and Guthrie, 1983); dental anxiety (Denny, Rupert and Burrish, 1983); and carpal tunnel syndrome (Silverstein, 1983). Nevertheless, it should also be noted that the less technical methods of anxiety management have also proven to be useful in dealing with such physical disorders (Rose, 1983).

It is self-evident that patients who suffer from serious physical disorders or who anticipate surgical investigation will experience some degree of anxiety. It is encouraging to note that in some areas behavioural methods are being deployed to tackle these problems. However, it is also clear that many problems (such as diabetic instability) may stem from the behavioural mismanagement of his biological system by the patient himself, and may be responsive to systematic training in self-control techniques. Similarly, patients suffering from a range of cardiovascular disorders may be maintaining their problems by their lifestyles, or by the nature of their reactions to their disorders. Programmes of behavioural and cognitive change appear to hold promise for the management of the psychological problems that frequently accompany such disorders.

The Process of Therapy: Relationships

The relationship between the nurse and her patient in the primary care setting differs markedly from that of her colleagues in the hospital. In a few cases the nurse may have the support of another therapist, for example when running groups or conducting conjoint therapy with couples. However, in all other instances she will work alone with the patient. This direct therapist role marks a radical departure for nurses. Traditionally, nurses have always had the support of colleagues — nurses and others — in their routine management of the patient. The atmosphere and structure of the psychiatric hospital often lends further support which is absent in the case of the primary care nurse. This is especially so where she operates from a general-practice health centre, or visits the patient in his own home. The primary care nurse stands alone: a practitioner supported only by her skills and knowledge and the status afforded her by the patient himself. It should be apparent that such a role is not appropriate for every psychiatric nurse. In many cases the demands may prove too daunting for even the most capable of clinicians.

The relationship between patient and therapist cannot be distinguished from the process of therapy itself. Behaviour therapy has frequently been described by its critics as a mechanistic process. We cannot agree with this view. Although patients in a primary care setting may be motivated to overcome their difficulties, a major responsibility lies with the therapist to promote and to capitalise upon the patient's motivation for change. The therapist must also promote a positive relationship with the patient from the very outset. Patients are unlikely to submit to potentially distressing procedures, or to undertake assignments outside the clinic, if they do not hold the therapist in high regard. The need to cultivate this positive relationship begins at the first meeting, if not earlier; for instance, when appointment letters are sent to the patient.

The Stages of Therapy

The therapy programme can be broken down into a series of interlinked stages. Initially, an assessment is undertaken. Here the patient gets a chance to introduce the therapist to his problems; at the same time allowing her a chance to find out what kind of individual lies behind these problems. The assessment may take only a single session. In more complex cases this may run to three or four sessions. The information supplied in the course of assessment will help in the planning of the treatment programme which, in turn, will be evaluated from its introduction through to its conclusion. Close attention is therefore paid to the evaluation of the effects of therapy. The patient and therapist review the programme in detail, retaining and expanding those aspects which appear to be useful, and amending or omitting those tactics which have been ineffective. Towards the end of the treatment these evaluation sessions will be devoted to a discussion of ways in which the therapist can withdraw from the treatment programme while allowing the patient to take greater responsibility for the solution of his own problems. In what follows we shall consider some of the practical issues involved in the delivery of these stages of therapy.

The First Encounter

The patient is given free rein to discuss his problems: the therapist guides him through short, non-threatening questions and will occasionally, in the interests of accuracy, summarise what has been said. From this type of conversation an idea of the patient's presenting problems, and something of his life in general, should emerge. The therapist will pay particular attention to putting the patient at ease and to communicating an atmosphere of support, acceptance and confidence. By briefly summarising what the patient has said during the conversation, she can show her grasp and understanding of what he is saying. She can also demonstrate her willingness to appreciate the significance of his problems. In addition to establishing the nature of his major problems, this session will also be devoted to revealing the patient's expectations concerning treatment. What does he think that the therapist is going to do to help him? Does he envisage an active or a passive role for himself in his own treatment? The therapist is also trying to impose some kind of order on the list of problems supplied by the patient. Which is the most problematic? Which might be tackled first? This first encounter offers an opportunity to establish a collaborative relationship between patient and therapist. Traditionally the patient's role in medical care has been viewed as wholly passive in nature. The therapist takes the initiative and the patient simply accepts the treatment offered. Experience has shown that psychiatric patients who are allowed or encouraged to adopt a passive role in treatment often relapse once the active ingredients of the treatment programme are withdrawn. For this reason a trend has been established, within behaviour therapy, to encourage a more evenly balanced working relationship between patient and therapist. The patient is given a clear message from the outset that he will be expected to play a major part in helping himself overcome his problems of living. The therapist will supply the necessary information and guidance to help him realise these goals. Mahoney (1974) has described this relationship in terms of the personal-scientist model. He suggests that psychotherapy involves the patient finding out more about himself. Armed with such information he is then encouraged to experiment with his own functioning in order to change himself or to resolve his problems of living. In a sense the patient subjects his own attitudes and behaviour to experimental manipulation. He establishes a single case study and adopts the dual role of experimenter and experimental subject. Our experience shows that the establishment of this type of working relationship is appropriate for almost all primary care patients. Its main virtue may lie in the fact that, from the very outset, the patient is being prepared for life without the therapist.

Developing the Assessment

Once the therapist has established the problem areas, more detailed assessment can begin. In most cases a range of options is available, involving global methods (completion of questionnaires or rating scales); self reports (the patient makes notes and observations on facets of his own behaviour); and further interviewing in the course of which the therapist will take more detailed notes on the patient's problem behaviours. Usually from the end of the very first session the patient can begin collecting short diary-type notes on the occurrence and severity of his problems. Where do they occur, how often and to what extent do they disrupt his life? At first these diary notes may be fairly cursory in nature. As therapy progresses, and the patient becomes more confident, these notes may be expected to become more detailed and rigorous. The therapist is required to make judgements during the sessions: what is the patient's main problem? Why does he believe this to be the case? Often tape recordings of sessions can be replayed and used as a basis for arriving at more considered opinions on the nature and extent of the presenting problems. This approach allows a more detailed analysis of the progress of each session. It also frees the therapist from note-keeping during the session. However, this approach is not appropriate for every patient, nor indeed for every therapist. Rating scales or questionnaires may be used to measure specific problems (such as anxiety or depression), or they may assess thinking styles, or more general patterns of behaviour (such as assertiveness). By the end of the assessment phase the therapist will have established a rank ordering of the patient's problems and determined their relative severity and frequency, and will be beginning to think about ways in which they might be tackled.

Designing the Treatment Programme

Although the therapist may have a favoured tactic for resolving a particular problem, there is an advantage in offering the patient a choice of treatments. For instance, if he suffers from social anxiety, he might be offered a choice between treatment on an individual basis or in a group with other socially anxious patients. The phobic patient may be offered a choice between a graded exposure programme and flooding — where the rigours and benefits of each approach are honestly spelled out. Although the patient may be influenced by the therapist in making a choice between alternative forms of treatment, the final choice is his. Taking such a decision may be the first real demonstration of his collaborative role in therapy.

Although some aspects of the design of the treatment programme may be decided during these face-to-face sessions, this type of planning may take place in the comfort of the therapist's office. Time is needed to establish, perhaps in some detail, how the programme will operate. Equipment may have to be sought for use in treatment. A programme for a spider-phobic may require an assortment of black-and-white and colour photographs of spiders, as well as toy spiders, dead and live spiders and perhaps a video recording on the natural history of the arachnids. Kirby's study, which is presented in Chapter 9 of this book, illustrates a programme of treatment in which a range of such props was employed. In other cases technical equipment, such as biofeedback devices, may need to be employed. Home-instruction audio tapes, for example for relaxation or those that carry instructions for homework assignments, may need to be recorded. In addition, assessment forms for use by the patient or the therapist may need to be designed and printed. Although the therapist may have a supply of such materials, especially those that are used with some regularity, in many cases some degree of individualisation of materials used in treatment is both desirable and necessary. This means that some time must be allowed between sessions for the preparation of such materials.

The therapist usually corresponds with the referral agent, most commonly a general practitioner or psychiatrist, at the end of the assessment stage. She is by now able to summarise her findings and to outline the intended course of therapy. She may also ask for further information about concurrent medical or psychiatric treatment, or about treatment which the patient has received in the past. It is good practice for the therapist to keep the patient informed about the passage of such information. At the next session the patient will have the opportunity to discuss the details of his treatment plan. The emphasis of this discussion is placed on the practical details of the programme: what the patient will be expected to do; what the therapist may be expected to contribute and, finally, what the outcome of this undertaking is likely to be.

Treatment Sessions

These are usually broken down into three sections. First of all the patient is given a chance to 'report back' on his homework assignments. Then the therapist will brief him on the next stage of the therapy, which will occupy the bulk of the session. Finally they will talk about the patient's next homework assignment, discussing how he should arrange this to ensure his success. The patient is expected to carry out the prepared assignments, using the strategies he has discussed, and, if necessary, rehearsed, within the sessions. The therapist also needs to do some homework between sessions; reviewing the progress of the treatment plan, corresponding with other professionals, and making preparations for the next session.

Treatment is most often an individualised affair. The patient sees the therapist in private and receives help which is tailored to suit his individual needs. In some cases the patient's spouse may be included in a conjoint-therapy exercise. In the case of problems such as social anxiety, social-skills deficits, or alcohol abuse, the treatment might be presented in a group setting to allow exposure to others, to encourage the development of coping skills or to arrange mutual support from others experiencing similar deficiencies. Sessions may be held in the clinic at first, but may soon be extended to take place in cafes, pubs, shopping precincts, etc., where the 'real world' of the patient can be confronted.

Reducing Therapist Involvement

In the early stages, treatment sessions may be fairly lengthy and at frequent intervals. The patient may be seen several times a week at first, although once weekly is more usual. The patient who continues to work and live in the community may lack the support and encouragement which the hospitalised patient receives. For this reason therapy must be stolidly supportive otherwise some patients with severe problems may break down completely and require hospital care. Initial sessions rarely last for less than an hour. This is not a lengthy period considering that a review of homework, the conducting of formal therapy and planning for the next stage of treatment must all be squeezed into the 60 minutes. During the early stages the patient may be given the opportunity to contact the therapist between sessions by phone when he meets special problems or more commonly to seek advice and reassurance prior to tackling a demanding assignment. However, if dependency upon the therapist is to be avoided, this 'hot-line' facility must be used sparingly and only in selected cases.

When there are clear signs that progress is being made, sessions may be spaced at fortnightly and then at progressively longer intervals. Once the patient has received all the necessary coaching in coping skills or in problem analysis within sessions, the time saved may be translated into more discussion time related to homework. How has the patient coped with various events? How might he cope better? In this way the patient begins to take increasing responsibility for analysing and resolving actual and potential problems. As therapy enters its final stage, the importance of the therapist as a 'change agent' is minimised and the role of the patient as his own agent of change is emphasised. Certainly the therapist remains 'on hand' to contribute encouragement and a degree of technical assistance. However, the collaborative relationship has led to something of a role reversal: the patient may now be more active in discussing problems and their solution than is the therapist. The patient may even take the responsibility of summarising his own progress by making a chart or graph, thereby confirming his therapeutic gains. Finally, the formal sessions will be discontinued and the patient will be asked to report back for follow-up or booster sessions. During this phase he may be invited to keep in touch with the therapist by means of brief telephone calls or, as Ablett suggests in Chapter 7, by sending detailed tape-recorded messages. Such measures may ease the problem of severing links with the patient.

Settings

Therapy may take place in a variety of situations. Psychiatric out-patient clinics are a popular venue for the simple reason that this is often where community psychiatric services are based. Frequently the clinic is located in a district general hospital, but it may alternatively be part of a large psychiatric hospital. Where the clinic is based at a general hospital, this may hold considerable advantages for the patient who is distressed by the stigma of suffering from a psychiatric disorder. The other advantage of operating from such a base is that it allows the nurse therapist to share experiences and information with other members of the team. The patient's case notes can be readily consulted and the medical, social-work or psychology staff who may be involved with the patient can be consulted on an informal basis to discuss each member's involvement with the patient. Where the nurse works outside such a shared facility, communications are likely to be more difficult and more formal in nature.

Health centres have become a popular venue for behaviour therapists in recent years. In this setting treatment can appropriately be called primary care, since this is the patient's first port of call when he begins to experience difficulty. In some settings the general practitioner is perhaps more likely to short-circuit the psychiatric referral route by referring to a trained nurse therapist those patients who appear to have a problem that might be amenable to behaviour therapy.

The provision of treatment services from either of these two established facilities (the general hospital out-patient department and the health centre) has obvious advantages. However, where a patient is literally housebound by his difficulties, it may be appropriate, at least in the initial sessions, to visit him at home. Although this may be comfortable for the patient, it is not necessarily desirable. If a housebound patient succeeds in his efforts to attend a clinic session, then, even before the session has begun, he has achieved a success. Where the patient is visited at home, this success is denied him.

In general we would advocate selecting the situation which best suits the presenting problem. Often this will not be the situation selected by the patient. For instance, most agoraphobics would happily settle for a string of home visits, rather than having to attend clinics. Where sessions are conducted *in vivo*, they will usually be preceded by clinic-based preparatory sessions. However, the actual therapy may take place anywhere: it is what takes place within therapy that is important; where it takes place is a matter for negotiation.

Professional Relationships

The nurse therapist who is conducting behaviour therapy with a psychiatric patient may be the key therapist, the person who is doing most to help the patient overcome his problems. However, she is unlikely to be the only person professionally involved. A doctor will usually have referred the patient for treatment in the first instance. This may be the GP or a psychiatrist. The patient may be receiving supportive medical treatment, in the form of anxiolytic or anti-depressant medication, from this doctor. A social worker may also be involved, especially where there is a problem with other members of the patient's family, such as children, or where there is a history of criminal behaviour, such as drug abuse. In some cases community nurses may also be involved, especially if the patient has recently been discharged from hospital. There is clearly a need for close liaison between the different professionals who contribute towards the management of a particular case.

What form should such liaison take? As we have noted already, the nurse therapist may have an opportunity to discuss the progress of treatment on an informal basis with other professionals. Beyond this there is clearly a need for regular reporting of progress in letter form. Copies of such reports would be sent to all professionals involved in the management of the patient. These reports should be factual summaries of what is planned, or has been achieved in therapy. Every effort should be made to omit from such reports anything that is based upon speculation rather than upon detailed observation and analysis of the problem. The reports in this sense should be highly factual. In addition to these written reports, some record of the progress of therapy should be maintained in casenote form. These notes, which should be compiled on a session-by-session basis, will be helpful if someone else needs to step in to take over the case, or if the patient is re-referred at a later date.

Summary

It should be apparent that the work of the nurse therapist in a primary care setting differs markedly from that of her colleagues in the hospital setting. Although she may be a member of a community nursing team based in a psychiatric hospital, she may equally well be a member of a psychology service based in a district general hospital. Although the former would have some contact with a team of community nurses and the latter would have some contact with psychologists, both may tend to spend most of their working week alone, dealing with patients in a variety of treatment settings.

From our brief review of the literature it is clear that the behavioural model of treatment has a significant contribution to make to the resolution of a wide variety of problems. Although behaviour therapists have achieved a reputation for their treatment of phobic and obsessional disorders, there is still a reluctance to acknowledge their role in the treatment of other disorders. Indeed there exists a strong reliance upon the provision of nebulous forms of supportive psychotherapy or a reliance upon drug treatments which, as is arguably the case with the benzodiazepines, may create more serious problems than the ones they were designed to relieve.

We are anxious to point out in concluding this chapter that the role of the nurse therapist in community care is largely undeveloped. Although some commentators (cf. Marks, 1973) have reported on the successful deployment of nurse therapists, this exercise was conducted with a highly selected patient population. It has been our experience that nurse therapists, can, and indeed do, work with much more complex cases in which straightforward phobias or anxiety disorders are not clearly evident. This has led to the development of a multifaceted approach involving the use of cognitive as well as behavioural therapy. The three cases reported later in this book (by Ablett, Kirby and Harkin) illustrate this point. However, a number of issues have still to be resolved. Should such nurses be part of community nursing teams, or should they be members of nurse behaviour-therapy teams which exist separately from the community nursing service but work in close collaboration with their soulmates in clinical psychology? Clearly we have a preference for the latter option since this is the model of practice which we have pioneered.

The multifaceted role of the nurse therapist has already been suggested as the model for community psychiatric nursing. Carr, Butterworth and Hodges (1980) recommend a broad-based service offering consultative, educational, medical, clinical and psychotherapeutic roles similar to those of the nurse therapist. In many senses this merely highlights the similarities that we indicated earlier. In our view the simplest way to conceptualise the role of the nurse behaviour therapist in primary care is as a nurse specialist. The psychotherapeutic methods used by such a nurse are likely to distinguish her from other community nurses. Although many reports of community psychiatric nurses suggest that they can be involved in the use of behavioural methods, this in no way indicates that they are skilled behaviour therapists. It is our contention that the achievement of such a role requires extensive training, a great deal of commitment, and years of practice. It may be more acceptable to view the nurse behaviour therapist as a specialist within the community nursing establishment. It is, however, clear that some overlap will continue to exist between the two groups. However, such an overlap currently exists between social workers and community nurses (Hunter, 1980). Overlap between services combined with increasing specialisation within services is no bad thing if it leads to a development rather than a duplication of the services concerned.

References

Agras, W.S., Schneider, J.H. and Taylor, C.B. (1984) 'Relaxation Training in Essential Hypertension', *Behaviour Therapy*, *15* (2), 191–6

Alberti, R.E. and Emmons, M.L. (1970) *Your Perfect Right*, Impact Press, San Luis Obispo

Azrin, N.H., Naster, B.J. and Jones, R. (1975) 'Reciprocity Counselling: a rapid learning based procedure for marital counselling', in C.M. Franks and G.T. Wilson (eds), *Annual Review of Behaviour Therapy, Theory and Practice*, Brunner/ Mazel, New York

Beck, A.T., Rush, A.J., Shaw, B.F. and Emery, G. (1980) *Cognitive Therapy of Depression*, Wiley, New York

Boskind-Lodahl, M. and Sirlin, J. (1977) 'The Gorging Purging Syndrome', *Psychology Today*, March, 50–2, 82–5

Carr, P., Butterworth, C.A. and Hodges, B. (1980) *Community Psychiatric Nursing*, Churchill Livingstone, Edinburgh

Chambless, D., Foa, E.B., Graves, G.A. and Goldstein, A.J. (1982) 'Exposure and Communication Training in the Treatment of Agoraphobia', *Behaviour Research and Therapy*, *20* (3), 219–31

Denny, D.R., Rupert, P.A. and Burrish, T.G. (1983) 'Skin Conductance Biofeedback and Desensitisation for Reducing Dental Anxiety', *American Journal of Biofeedback*, *6* (2), 82–7

Figueroa, J.L. (1982) 'Group Treatment of Chronic Tension Headaches: a Comparative Treatment Study', *Behaviour Modification*, *6* (2), 229–39

Fleming, I. (1984) 'Habit Reversal for Trichotillomania: a Case Study', *Behavioural Psychotherapy*, *12*, (1), 173–80

Forbank, J.A. and Keene, T.M. (1982) 'Flooding for Combat Related Stress Disorders', *Behaviour Therapy*, *13* (4), 499–510

Frame, C.L. and Turner, S.M. (1984) 'Self-exposure Treatment of Agoraphobia', *Behaviour Modification*, *9* (1), 115–22

Ginsberg, G. and Marks, I.M. (1977) 'Costs and Benefits of Behavioural Psychotherapy: a Pilot Study of Neurotics Treated by Nurse Therapists', *Psychological Medicine*, *7*, 320–1

Guthrie, D., Moeller, T. and Guthrie, R. (1983) 'Biofeedback and its Application to the Stabilisation and Control of Diabetes Mellitus', *American Journal of*

Biofeedback, *6*, 88–95

Halford, K. and Foddy, M (1982) 'Cognitive and Social Skills Correlates of Social Anxiety', *British Journal of Clinical Psychology*, *21* (1), 17–28

Heather, N. and Robertson, I. (1981) *Controlled Drinking*, London, Methuen

Holmgren, S. (1984) 'Phase I Treatment for the Chronic and Previously Treated Anorexia Bulimia Nervosa Patient', *International Journal of Eating Disorders*, *3* (2), 17–36

Horne, D.J., McTiernan, G. de L. and Strauss, N.H.M. (1981) 'A Case of Severe Obsessive-Compulsive Behaviour Treated by Nurse Therapists in an In-patient Unit', *Behavioural Psychotherapy*, *9* (1), 46–54

Hunter, P. (1980) 'Social Work and Community Psychiatric Nursing — a Review', *International Journal of Nursing Studies*, *17*, 131–9

Keefe, F.J. (1982) 'Behavioural Assessment and Treatment of Chronic Pain: Current status and Future Directions', *Journal of Consulting and Clinical Psychology*, *50* (6), 896–911

Kornbluth, S.J. and Rehm, L.P. (1983) 'The Contribution of Self-reinforcement Training and Behavioural Assignments to the Efficacy of Self-control Therapy for Depression', *Cognitive Therapy and Research*, *7* (6), 499–528

Lacks, P. (1983) 'The Effectiveness of Three Behavioural Treatments for Different Degrees of Sleep Onset Insomnia', *Behaviour Therapy*, *14* (5), 593–605

Latimer, P. (1980) 'Training in Behaviour Therapy', *Canadian Journal of Psychiatry*, February, 26–7

Leitenberg, H. (1976) 'Behavioral Approaches to Treatment of Neuroses', in H. Leitenberg (ed.), *Handbook of Behaviour Modification and Behaviour Therapy*, Prentice Hall, Englewood Cliffs, NJ

Lewinsohn, P.M. (1969) 'Depression, a Clinical Research Approach', *Psychotherapy: Theory, Research and Practice*, *6*, 166–71

Mahoney, M.J. (1974) *Cognition and Behaviour Modification*, Ballinger, Cambridge, Mass.

Marks, I.M. (1973) 'The Psychiatric Nurse as Therapist — Developments and Problems', *Nursing Times*, 30 August, 137–8

Marks, I.M., Connolly, J., Hallam, R. and Philpott, R. (1975) 'Nurse Therapists in Behavioural Psychotherapy', *British Medical Journal*, *111*, 144–8

Mathews, A.M., Gelder, M.G. and Johnston, D.W. (1981) *Agoraphobia: Nature and Treatment*, Tavistock, London

Meldrum, M.J., McGowan, H. Higgins, J. and Schaller, D. (1969) 'Nurse Psychotherapists in a Private Practice', *American Journal of Nursing*, *69*, 2412–15

Nomellini, S. and Katz, R.C. (1983) 'Effect of Anger Control Training on Abusive Parents', *Cognitive Therapy and Research*, *7* (1), 57–68

O'Donoghue, F.P. and Borgerson, M.B.C. (1980) 'Training and Utilisation of Nurse Therapists in a Behaviour Therapy Clinic', *Canadian Journal of Psychiatry*, *25*, 212–14

Peck, D.F. (1973) 'An Agent of Behavioural Change', *Nursing Times*, 30 August, 139

Piercy, F.P. (1983) 'A Game for Interrupting Coercive Marital Interaction', *Journal of Marital and Family Therapy*, *9* (4), 435–6

Robertson, I. (1982) 'Behavioural Concepts and Treatments of Neuroses: Comments on Marks and Wilson', *Behavioural Psychotherapy*, *10* (2), 179–83

Rose, M.J. (1983) 'The Effect of Anxiety Management Training on Control of Diabetes Mellitus', *Journal of Behavioural Medicine*, *6* (4), 381–95

Sartory, G., Rachman, S. and Grey, S.J. (1982) 'Return of Fear: the Role of Rehearsal', *Behaviour Research and Therapy*, *20* (2), 123–33

Silverstein, L. (1983) 'Biofeedback Training (BFT) for Carpal Tunnel Syndrome', *American Journal of Biofeedback*, *6* (2), 111–17

Slade, P. (1982) 'Towards a Functional Analysis of Anorexia Nervosa and Bulimia Nervosa', *British Journal of Clinical Psychology*, *21* (3), 167–79

Stampfl, T. and Levis, D. (1967) 'Essentials of Implosive Therapy: a Learning-Based Psychodynamic Behavioural Therapy', *Journal of Abnormal Psychology*, *72*, 496–503

Stravynski, A. (1984) 'The Use of Broad Conversational Targets in Social Skills Training to Promote Generalisation of Gains to Real Life', *Behavioural Psychotherapy*, 12 (1), 61–7

Taylor, J.W. (1984) 'Structured Conjoint Therapy for Spouse Abuse Cases', *Social Casework*, *65* (1), 11–18

Trower, P., Bryant, B. and Argyle, M. (1978) *Social Skills and Mental Health*, Methuen, London

Wilson, G.T. (1982) 'Adult Disorders', in G.T. Wilson and C.M. Franks (eds), *Contemporary Behaviour Therapy*, Guilford Press, New York

Wilson, P.H., Goldin, J.C. and Charbonnea, M (1983) 'Comparative Efficacy of Behavioural and Cognitive Treatment of Depression', *Cognitive Therapy and Research*, 7 (2), 111–24

Wolpe, J. (1958) *Psychotherapy by Reciprocal Inhibition*, Stanford University Press, Stanford, CA

Woodward, R. and Jones, R.B. (1980) 'Cognitive Restructuring Treatment: A Controlled Trial with Anxious Patients', *Behaviour Research and Therapy*, *18*, 401–7

5 CREATING THERAPEUTIC ENVIRONMENTS

Robert C. Durham

Introduction

Most readers of this book will probably have mixed feelings on the subject of 'creating therapeutic environments'. On the one hand, an interest in behaviour therapy may well have stemmed in part from a belief that changes in the ward environment can be of considerable benefit to patient functioning. On the other hand, clinical experience in changing even small aspects of institutional environments may well have involved a good deal of frustration and disappointment. Though there is much that can usually be done to improve the 'therapeutic atmosphere' on many wards, there are also many obstacles that need to be overcome in making the necessary changes. Nurse therapists do not of course have any special sensitivities or claim to knowledge on these matters; most people who work on hospital wards for the mentally ill or handicapped are aware of the powerful influence for good or ill that the institutional environment exerts on the daily lives of both staff and patients. Indeed, the need to prevent the processes of institutionalisation and to maintain a reasonable quality of life have become part of at least the implicit goals of all the various professions who work in hospital settings. Many of Goffman's (1961) ideas about the dehumanising effects of 'total' institutions' — the lack of privacy, rigid daily routines, the social distance between staff and residents — have become a part of our professional consciousness.

There are, however, several reasons why nurse therapists in particular do need to develop a clear understanding of the various aspects of institutional life that both constrain and facilitate the implementation of desirable treatment programmes. Suppose, for example, that a nurse therapist is asked by a ward to design an individual treatment programme for a patient with poor social skills and occasional aggressive behaviour. Suppose, furthermore, that the ward has few permanent staff and provides a generally poor quality of life for its residents. Should she accede to this request and concentrate her efforts on one individual, or would it be more appropriate (and more ethical) to renegotiate the referral and focus her energies on a programme to improve the overall quality of life of all the patients? If she does decide to design an individual treatment programme, what is the likelihood that the ward staff will be willing or able to carry it out? If the programme fails, will this be interpreted as a failure of behaviour therapy or of her own clinical skills, or will it be attributed to other factors such as inherent problems in the organisation of the ward? In order to resolve these questions, which can undoubtedly pose quite acute personal and professional dilemmas for the nurse therapist, it is necessary to have a clear understanding of the nature of the environment in which treatment programmes operate.

In the first place, although the demands made upon the nurse therapist will be primarily to treat specific clinical problems, it is important that she places such demands within the broader perspective of the overall quality of care enjoyed by the patients on the ward. In regard to social skills deficits, for example, it may be that improvements in the degree of social stimulation provided by the ward as a whole may be a more appropriate response to the referral than would an individual programme of social skills training (cf. Durham, 1983). In some cases it may not be cost effective to devote scarce professional resources to one individual when a more broadly based intervention might lead to positive changes for a large number of patients. There may also be moral issues to consider. If the nurse therapist believes that making improvements in the general therapeutic environment should be a higher clinical priority than that of designing a treatment programme for the individual patient referred, then she certainly has some professional obligation to point this out and perhaps renegotiate the original referral. In all these cases it is necessary to assess the therapeutic environment objectively and to decide whether or not change is possible. One important aspect of this assessment is a clear idea about what this rather elusive notion of 'a reasonable quality of life' means in everyday clinical practice, and we begin this chapter with a discussion of this issue.

The second question raised by our imaginary example underlines the importance of another aspect of the assessment process referred to above, namely the ability and willingness of the ward staff to meet the demands that a treatment programme may make on their personal and organisational resources. There will inevitably be circumstances in which it is reasonable to conclude that, because of inadequate staffing levels, poor ward communications, or some other constraining factor, it is simply not possible to implement the treatment programme that is required for the problem referred. Indeed, in many institutional settings it is clear that everyday clinical practice lags some way behind the kinds of treatment regime that clinical research studies have shown to be efficacious. For example, although our knowledge of the kind of therapeutic interventions that decrease symptomatic behaviour and improve social functioning in long-stay patients is at a reasonably advanced stage (e.g. Hersen and Bellack, 1978; Rimm and Masters, 1979), it is also true to say that there have been many difficulties in realising the promise of these new approaches. Clinical research projects demonstrating effective treatment approaches all too frequently fail to become a routine part of clinical work once the momentum of research has passed (cf. Hall and Baker, 1973). There will be few behaviour therapists working in institutional settings who could not cite numerous examples of the difficulties of setting up and maintaining treatment programmes that were of demonstrable benefit to the patients concerned. The reason for this state of affairs, of course, is that treatment programmes do not take place in a vacuum; in fact their effectiveness is crucially dependent upon a whole variety of factors: communication across shifts, number of permanent staff, nursing management support, dependency needs of the patients, staff morale, to name but a few. Thus, in order to make sensible decisions about the feasibility of implementing ward-based treatment pro-grammes, it is important that the nurse therapist be familiar with the considerable literature that exists on the various factors that affect the nature of institutional care. The next two sections of the chapter are concerned with this area, first by way of discussing some of the general ways in which institutional processes affect treatment programmes, and secondly by describing some of the minimum conditions necessary for implementing and maintaining individual treatment plans.

The third question posed by our hypothetical referral concerns the way in which the failure of a treatment programme may be interpreted by the therapist and the ward staff. This touches on a much more personal matter, the self-esteem and indirectly the motivation of the nurse therapist herself. It is entirely natural of course to feel some pressure to demonstrate one's professional competence when responding to a referral. Much of our personal and professional self-esteem is based on a feeling of competence, and most people are sensitive as to how their work is evaluated and interpreted by other people. However, although such pressures and concerns are shared by all disciplines working in the psychiatric field, and are in part an inevitable consequence of the change from a custodial to a treatment-oriented approach, they are in some ways much more acute in behaviour therapy, especially as it is applied to the treatment of chronic problems in institutional settings. The very nature of this approach, with its emphasis on the systematic application of well-defined treatment techniques to carefully specified problems, tends to make the relative failure of a treatment programme readily apparent and more easily attibutable to a lack of competence on the part of the therapist. The openness of behaviour therapy, however creditable from a clinical and scientific point of view, invites critical scrutiny from others and hence creates pressures on the therapist. This would not be a problem if patients always responded positively to this approach, but in reality, of course, behavioural treatment, like all other methods of treatment, rarely proceeds exactly according to plan. Progress is usually slow, and punctuated by a variety of major and minor setbacks; treatment strategies may need to be revised, and even completely changed as therapy progresses. Moreover, the treatment plan itself may demand from the therapist and the ward staff an active involvement with the patient that has to be sustained over a long period of time. This can be inherently stressful and unrewarding if the patient concerned is passive, apathetic, verbally abusive, or disturbed and unpredictable in his or her behaviour. In fact, most therapeutic interactions with institutionalised patients are one-sided; they have to be sustained in spite of the attitudes and behaviour of the patients. It is therefore important to take account of the personal stresses that may be associated with individual treatment programmes, and in the final section of the chapter, two aspects of coping with stress are briefly discussed.

Basic Elements of a Therapeutic Environment

In recent years a growing consensus has emerged concerning the essential ingredients of an institutional environment that promotes for its residents a reasonable quality of life and that provides an appropriate level of care and individual treatment. This consensus has been shaped by a variety of influences. Perhaps the most obvious of these has been the very considerable changes that have taken place over the last 30 years in our conception of the nature of madness and psychiatric disorder. The advent of effective psychotropic medication, the increasing influence of social and community psychiatry, and the increasing sophistication of scientific explanations of psychiatric disability and mental handicap have all resulted in a very much more positive and optimistic attitude to treatment and rehabilitation. Innovative approaches to institutional care ranging from the therapeutic community movement initiated by Maxwell Jones (1952) to the token economy approach of Paul and Lentz (1979) have not just defined specific forms of social treatment for specific problems, but have also underlined the general importance of providing institutional patients with social stimulation, normative roles and expectations, feedback, and individual support (cf. Fraser, 1983, and Shepherd, 1984). Similarly, the principles of community psychiatry and the increasing use of day-care facilities, out-patient treatment, residential hostels, and group homes, have blurred the distinction between hospital and home and vigorously challenged the notion that the mentally ill and mentally handicapped are unable to appreciate or cope with life outside the institution (cf. Stein and Test, 1978). One consequence of this emphasis on rehabilitation and resettlement has been a much greater awareness of the skills that are needed to live in the community, and the subsequent development of training programmes to prepare patients for life outside the hospital (see, for example, Durham, 1982, and Goldstein, Sprafkin and Gershaw, 1976). The concept of 'normalisation' (cf. Wolfensberger, 1972) and the attempts to translate this into a set of guidelines for everyday clinical practice (see, for example, Wolfensberger and Glenn, 1975), are also a direct result of the policy to move the centre of care from the hospital to the community. These developments have inevitably led to changes in the traditional hospital environment so that it more closely approximates the character of everyday life, although the funding for the necessary professional resources in the community has been grossly inadequate (McPherson, 1983).

Another important influence on the nature of a therapeutic environment has stemmed not so much from positive developments in treatment and rehabilitation but from a growing awareness of the adverse effects of living in an institutional environment. We have already mentioned the work of Goffman (1961) whose vivid descriptions of the 'total institution' have done much to stimulate a reappraisal of practices that had very much been taken for granted. An attempt to operationalise Goffman's ideas so as to study the nature of institutional care in more formal, scientific terms was made by Tizard and his colleagues (see King, Raynes and Tizard, 1971) and has led to the notion that management practices can be described as being either 'institutionally oriented' or 'client-oriented'. They found clear evidence in a study of the type of care provided for severely mentally handicapped children that 'client-oriented' practices, which existed mainly to meet the needs of individual clients, were associated with more frequent and warmer interactions between staff and patients than were 'institutionally oriented' practices, which existed mainly to serve the needs of a smooth-running organisation. Furthermore, these differences could not be accounted for by the severity of the handicaps of the children, the size of the units, or the staffing ratios, although they were associated with the backgrounds of the staff and the type of training they had received. These results have recently been replicated by Shepherd and Richardson (1979) in a study of local-authority day centres for the adult mentally ill. Writing from a rather different perspective, Barton (1976) has described the typical institutional practices that can give rise to what he has termed 'institutional neurosis', by which he means a state of apathy, dependency and loss of initiative. There is certainly a growing awareness that there is a price to be paid for caring for people in institutional settings, although it is important to appreciate that it is not just hospital environments that are responsible for ill-effects. Recent research has revealed many subtle and unexpected ways in which our health can be affected by the environment in which we live (see, for example Insell and Moos, 1974; Canter and Canter, 1979).

A third influence on institutional practices has been the strident, though at times ambivalent, voice of the general public. Newspaper and television accounts of 'scandalous' conditions in hospitals for the mentally ill and mentally handicapped have appeared with depressing regularity over the last 20 years. The poor quality of care that has been revealed by these accounts, as well as by the reports of official investigations (e.g. SE Thames RHA, 1976) has usually resulted in some degree of public condemnation, and this has undoubtedly contributed to some changes in attitude towards institutional care. As the residents of these insitutions have gradually come to be viewed as people with problems, illnesses and handicaps, rather than as figures of fear and ridicule, there has been a growing willingness to evaluate their quality of life using similar moral standards to those employed in everyday life. One such standard, a variation of the 'golden rule', is to judge as unacceptable those conditions of care that one would not be prepared to accept if a close relative (or oneself) were a resident in the institution.

Though the above criterion overlooks many of the problems and complexities of caring for the mentally ill and handicapped, it does, none the less, constitute a useful starting point for thinking about the overall goals of care. It encourages the belief that institutional care should provide as 'normal' a quality of life as possible, and that deviations from this need to be justified. The following guidelines, which draw freely on all the various influences mentioned previously, have been written in this spirit. They constitute an attempt to describe the practices that contribute to a reasonable quality of life in institutional settings, and make no reference to those factors that constrain or limit the implementation of these practices. This has been done deliberately in the belief that it is usually more productive to have a clear idea of what *might be* and to ask the question 'Why not?' than to proceed primarily on the basis of seeking explanations for *What is*.

Recognition and Support of Each Person's Individuality

Birthdays are marked with a card and a small celebration. A note is taken of the birthdays of close relatives, and the patient is encouraged to send them birthday cards. Each patient is encouraged to buy his or her own clothes, cosmetics, shaving lotion, etc. Personal possessions such as photos of relatives, pot plants, mementoes, coffee mugs, and pictures, are encouraged and visible on the ward. When first admitted to the ward, a detailed assessment is made of each patient's special likes and dislikes, idiosyncratic habits, hobbies, usual sleep routines, food preferences, etc., and as far as possible he or she is encouraged to retain these habits on the ward. Each patient is addressed by the name by which he or she prefers to be called (first name or second name, Mr, Mrs or Miss).

Maximum Opportunity for Contact with the Outside World

Visitors and volunteers are welcomed and encouraged. Visiting times are flexible and there are no restrictions on numbers. Patients have easy access to telephones and postal services. Trolley telephones are used if necessary, and pens and writing paper are readily available. There is an adequate choice and supply of books, magazines, and daily newspapers. Transportation to the local community is readily available and patients are encouraged to use it. Staff are insured to transport patients in private or hospital cars. Group outings are kept to a small number of people whenever possible. Use of local community facilities is actively encouraged (e.g. library, swimming pool, cinemas, parks). Members of staff keep in regular contact with relatives (with patients' permission) in order to give them information and support, and to encourage visits.

Opportunities for Learning, Work and Recreation

Patients have a planned programme of weekday activities with individual routines whenever possible. There are adequate library services with a sufficient quantity and range of up-to-date books and cassettes, including 'talking' books and large-print books where appropriate. There are adequate recreational materials such as games and gardening facilities. Television is available in a room separate from the living room. Incentive payment schemes in relation to sheltered work are operated so that payment is related to productivity. Skills training in work, community living, reading, writing and so forth are provided when appropriate. Alcohol in small quantities is available if there are no medical contraindications.

Clear Ward Communications

New patients are provided with information on the organisation and function of the ward, and are given a general orientation to the daily routine and staff expectations. There is an up-to-date noticeboard of daily events and future activities. Signs on the ward are clear, courteous, and readable, with colours and large letters used where necessary. Where appropriate, patients are given a copy of their own timetable and are encouraged to keep their own diary of appointments. There are regular staff meetings to discuss general difficulties and possible solutions.

Maximum Degree of Choice and Responsibility

Each patient is encouraged to do his or her own laundry, bedmaking and basic household chores. There are opportunities to buy and cook the food of one's choice. Each patient is encouraged to buy his or her own clothes (including underclothes) and shoes, to have a hairstyle of his or her own choosing, and to decide whom to sit next to at mealtimes. Menus are used if possible. Patients carry their own cash and can open bank and savings accounts. They are involved as much as possible in planning their own treatment programme. Locked doors and physical restraints are kept to a minimum. Sanctions for antisocial behaviour are communicated clearly to all patients. As far as possible, each patient is responsible for taking his or her own medication.

Home-like Atmosphere and Daily Routine

Meals are served at 'normal' times and at small tables, with tablecloths and teapots, etc. used wherever possible. Rising and retiring routines are at 'normal' times, and account is taken of individual preferences. There is adequate privacy in bathing, toileting, and personal care. The ward is decorated with fresh paint, warm colours, carpets and pictures. There is adequate space for the number of patients on the ward. Thre is individual storage space and locks are provided. Excessive noise and smells are kept to a minimum (e.g. by oiling wheels and regular cleaning). The temperature, lighting, and ventilation are at comfortable levels. Patients are able to see out of the windows when seated.

Recognition of Needs for Friendship and Sexual Relationships

Opportunities for mixing with the opposite sex in public and private are provided. Individual needs for physical affection and sex are responded to in a sensitive and understanding manner. Sex education and contraceptive advice are given if needed.

Individual Help and Support

Each patient has the opportunity for individual contact with a member of staff on a regular, planned basis, in order to receive support, identify specific problems, monitor progress, and discuss personal treatment plans. Routine medical and dental care are available, including the provision of dentures, eye glasses, hearing aids, etc. as needed.

General Constraints on Patient-centred Care

In the previous section we described some basic characteristics of a therapeutic environment from a fairly idealistic standpoint, and emphasised the importance of two guiding principles that have emerged from the clinical and research literature: normalisation and the provision of patient-oriented as opposed to institutionally oriented care. In everyday clinical practice of course, there are always several factors which to varying degrees inhibit or prevent the implementation of the kind of quality of life and attention to individual patient needs that we described, and these are reviewed in this section. We are therefore turning our attention to the second stage of assessment, in which the essential task is to try to understand the ward environment from the point of view of the staff and the institutional context in which they work. This involves a careful investigation of the function and organisation of the ward, the nature of staff-patient interaction, and the physical and personal resources that are available. The object of this process is to arrive at some sensible conclusions about the kind of changes that would improve the quality of care and the likely obstacles to making such changes.

When assessing the reasons why a particular ward is unable to implement certain aspects of a patient-centred system of care, several points should be borne in mind. First, it is helpful to try to avoid making hasty judgements that are based on stereotyped notions of how all clinical settings should operate. There has been a tendency in psychiatry, as Orford (1982) and Kennard (1979) have pointed out, to judge clinical settings with reference to certain 'ideal types' that may be quite unrepresentative of the large range of clinical settings that exist, and which may lead to quite unrealistic conclusions about the virtues or shortcomings of a particular setting. Thus, the 'total institution' described by Goffman (1961) is sometimes taken to represent all that is undesirable about institutional care, and is contrasted unfavourably with 'therapeutic communties' such as that described by Maxwell Jones (1952), which are then held up as the ideal model on which institutional care should be based. The danger with such a 'black and white' approach is that it overlooks the many differences in the organisation of care that are necessitated by the needs of different patient populations, and it takes no account of how local circumstances may influence the resources available to meet these needs. The Henderson unit at Belmont Hospital, for example, as described by Maxwell Jones (1952) and Rapoport (1960), was specifically concerned with young adult psychiatric patients with problems of repeated antisocial behaviour, and it is clear that several key aspects of the approach that was developed were a reflection of the particular needs and capabilities of this population. It would be a mistake to suppose that a similar approach would be either desirable or possible with, say the chronic adult mentally ill or the psycho-geriatric population; certain principles of the 'therapeutic community' ethos might well be applicable but only in so far as they are interpreted as general guidelines. As Kennard has pointed out in his useful review of therapeutic communities in practice (Kennard, 1979), an attitude that 'democratisation', for example, is an essential feature of all therapeutic environments can lead to the inhibition of the necessary flexibility that is required to respond effectively to the variety of problems that arise in everyday clinical work. In such a case it would be better to be guided by the more general principle that patients should be actively encouraged to participate in the life of the community.

Secondly, our knowledge of the institutional and organisational variables that tend to promote a high quality of care are based very largely on correlational studies which are not able to identify with any certainty the causal relationships that exist among these variables. It is rarely possible to single out one particular factor from the many that are always involved, and suggest that it alone is primarily responsible for the problems that have been observed. Thus, most of the important research in this area, such as that of Rutter and his colleagues on schools (Rutter, Maughan, Mortimore, Ouston and Smith, 1979), Wing and Brown (1970) on mental hospitals, and King *et al.* (1971), on hostels and hospitals for the mentally handicapped, has involved making very broad comparisons among different institutions on a variety of measures of the quality of care provided, the facilities available, and the ways in which the staff are organised. From complex statistical analyses of these measures it is possible to develop hypotheses about the kinds of factor that seem to be associated with high levels of care, but the cause-and-effect relationships between the variables frequently remain unexplained. Subtle interactions between a host of obvious and not so obvious factors are likely to constitute the 'real' explanation of shortcomings in any particular setting, and it is wise to be cautious when applying the findings of this type of research. With these points in mind we can now proceed to a brief review of some of the key issues, beginning with those aspects of institutional care that are generally outside the control of ward staff, such as staffing levels and the design of the buildings, and then moving on to subjects such as staff attitudes and ward organisation, which are less clear cut but more amenable to change.

Location, Size and Facilities

The location of a clinical setting has an obvious effect on its relationships with the community. It does not take sophisticated research methods to know that patients who live in a large hospital situated some distance from the nearest town will have difficulty maintaining close links with family, friends, and the familiar surroundings of their local neighbourhood. Poor bus services and long distances to travel will tend to decrease the frequency of passes home, and inhibit family and friends from visiting, thus increasing the dependency of patients on hospital facilities for work and recreation and making more difficult the kind of community skills training programmes that the process of rehabilitation requires. Rehabilitation and resettlement require the collaboration of social work services, out-patient clinics, community services, and hospital-based services, and it is inevitable that the isolation of hospital from community will tend to retard the development of good working relationships between them. Of course, hospitals can still be isolated from the community even if situated in the middle of a town; high forbidding walls and a large unattractive building are a potent symbol of the community's desire to keep contact to a minimum, and a constant reminder to patients of the stigma of being mentally ill or handicapped. Size is clearly an important factor here, since large buildings with a large number of patients are likely to be much more obtrusive in any location.

The size of an institution is an important variable for a number of other reasons. There is a strong, though not inevitable, tendency for large institutions to adopt bureaucratic and centrally administered systems of management in which the people with the most power and influence are least involved in the day-to-day work with the patients or clients. This can then lead to a situation in which the staff with the most contact with patients, and hence the most influence for good or ill on the quality of care provided, perceive themselves to have the lowest status in the institution and only minimal involvement in the decision-making process. The feelings of powerlessness that stem from this perception can have an extremely corrosive effect on the motivation that is needed to maintain client-centred patterns of care, with the result that clinical practice becomes increasingly geared to the convenience and needs of the staff rather than the patients. This process, which is well illustrated in the research of Norma Raynes and her colleagues (Raynes, Pratt and Roses, 1979), can, however, be mitigated by management practices that de-emphasise centralised decision making and attempt to maintain regular supportive contact with the direct-care staff. Thus, even large institutions can maintain a high quality of care if they consist of autonomously managed units in which the staff are involved in formulating operational policy and have some influence on the day-to-day running of the unit. Raynes, Pratt and Roses (1974) argue that living units with more than 30 patients are not able to sustain a high quality of patient care, and in general it would seem that, above a certain size, patient-centred care is simply not possible. Small-sized living units are not of course any guarantee of a high quality of care, and it should not be supposed that there is any direct relationship between numbers of patients and quality of care, apart from a general tendency for a greater degree of involvement and activity among staff and patients in smaller units (Bella, 1976).

Inappropriate or poorly designed facilities can also place formidable obstacles in the way of nursing staff. With the best will in the world it is very difficult to provide patients with privacy if, for example, toilet and bathroom facilities are communal, the bedroom area consists of a large dormitory, and there is only one small living room. Separate living areas for the pursuit of different activities (e.g. watching television, playing records, listening to the radio, reading, writing, sitting quietly, and so on) are of considerable importance; the sight of a large number of patients all sitting in one room with the television permanently switched on is an inherently depressing one. Expensive structural alterations, however, are not always needed to alter the character of an environment. Much can often be achieved with inexpensive partitions, imaginative decorations, and small items of furniture.

Number and Permanence of Staff

As with the number of patients being cared for, it is clear that below a certain ratio of staff to patients it is difficult if not impossible for staff to provide patient-centred care. There is no clear consensus as to what this limiting ratio is, and obviously a great deal depends on other factors such as the dependency needs of the patients. In Britain the current Department of health and Social Security guidelines suggest a ratio of one member of staff to every three patients, although Sutton (1981) has argued that this is insufficient to carry out active rehabilitation programmes. Moreover, simple ratios can be very misleading since it is the ratio of permanent, trained staff to patients that is of most importance. Constantly changing members of staff can have a very powerful undermining effect on any attempts to organise patient-centred patterns of care (cf. Hall and Baker, 1972), as can a low ratio of trained to untrained nursing staff. Conversely, it is also clear that good staff-patient ratios are no guarantee of a good quality of care; it is the manner in which staff are managed and organised that is of most importance, as we shall discuss below.

Service Obligations

The function of a clinical unit within the mental handicap and psychiatric services is clearly an important influence on care since this affects such matters as admission and discharge policies, selection of staff, relationship with other clinical units, and, most importantly, the type of patients cared for. People suffering from severe senile dementia, from chronic schizophrenia, from adolescent behaviour problems or from varying degrees of mental and physical handicap will differ greatly in their ability to communicate rationally and in their capacity to make choices and understand treatment plans. Within these broad groupings the presence of people who are very disturbed, aggressive, or socially disruptive will powerfully influence the atmosphere on the ward and the amount of time that the staff are able to spend on routine care. In addition, wards with an obligation to admit acutely disturbed patients will find it more difficult to sustain patient-centred patterns of care than wards which provide non-urgent help to a selected group of patients. Kennard (1979) discusses this point at some length in connection with many 'therapeutic communities' which have often had a freedom to be selective about staff and patients that has not been enjoyed by less specialised clinical settings. It is simply easier to attend to individual needs and to maintain a cohesive therapeutic atmosphere if there is not a constant rotation through the unit of disturbed and unwilling residents.

Attitudes, Organisation and Management

So far in this section we have discussed some fairly clear-cut obstacles to implementing patient-centred patterns of care. Whether or not a ward is able to meet the challenge that these obstacles present, and create a therapeutic environment in spite of the difficulties, depends a great deal on other, less tangible factors such as staff attitudes, ward organisation, and styles of management. Although usually considered as separate issues, these factors are in practice very closely interwoven. A useful place to start in assessing the factors is with the function of the ward as perceived by the staff. Are the nursing staff able to describe the function of the ward in terms of its overall clinical objectives and therapeutic ideology, its relationship with other hospital and community services, and its admission and discharge policies? Are their views shared by the medical staff and members of other disciplines involved with the ward such as occupational therapists, social workers and clinical psychologists? If the staff are not clear about these matters, or if there is evidence of serious ambiguities or disagreements in the views expressed, this will undermine the unity of purpose that is necessary if the staff are to work together effectively. A sense of shared purpose does not mean that everyone on the ward should always agree with each other but it does mean that there should be a general consensus concerning overall policy and objectives.

A related set of questions can be asked about the nature of the ward routine. Is there a daily timetable of ward activities which provides for a variable routine of social, recreational, therapeutic, and work-like activities? Does this routine include regular opportunities for the staff to meet together to discuss patient progress, to formulate treatment plans, to review ward policy, and to provide mutual support? What provision is made for regular staff-patient meetings? Are there arrangements for regular in-service training sessions? The answers to these questions will indicate a good deal about the ward atmosphere, the attitudes of staff to each other and the nature of their working relationships. Thus, the absence of a clearly worked-out weekly timetable may well indicate that little thought has been given to the particular needs of the patients, and that both patients and staff spend little of their time actively engaged in constructive activities. This in turn may reflect the fact that ward rules and regulations are centrally determined and that there is little autonomous decision making.

Another important aspect of ward organisation concerns the allocation of staff duties and the ways in which these duties are monitored and reviewed. Are the staff given specific therapeutic tasks to carry out in relation to individual patients or groups of patients? Are some of these tasks based upon individual treatment plans that include a list of key problems and treatment goals? Do individual members of staff have special responsibilities for particular patients on the ward, or is patient care primarily organised in terms of set routines that apply to all patients without reference to individual care plans?

Finally, and perhaps most importantly, is the need to assess the nature of the relationships between staff and patients and among the staff themselves. How much time is spend in conversation with individual patients in a supportive counselling role? Are patients given prompts and feedback in a sensitive or an authoritarian manner? How much evidence is there of warmth, humour and support in staff-patient relationships? Very similar questions might also be asked about the relationships between the staff. Are staff able to communicate with each other openly and comfortably, or is there a rigid hierarchical line of authority between staff at different levels? Is personal initiative and individual responsibility encouraged by senior staff? To what extent do senior staff model the therapeutic skills that are needed to work effectively with the patients? Such questions are not easily answered with only brief acquaintance of a ward, and clearly there are no hard and fast rules about effective interpersonal relationships. However, it does seem reasonably clear from the clinical and research literature that high levels of patient-centred care will be associated with staff who are actively involved with their patients so as to communicate positive but realistic expectations, provide help and support when required, prompt and reinforce appropriate behaviour and give clear feedback when necessary. A low level of staff-patient interaction, and few obvious examples of these therapeutic processes, will invariably reflect some basic deficiencies in the quality of staff-patient relationships. The manner in which the clinical team is led can most easily be observed during the handover between shifts, or during case conferences or other kinds of group meetings. Of crucial importance here is the style of leadership adopted by the charge nurse and medical staff (as well as senior members of other disciplines), and in particular the degree to which the very necessary qualities of efficiency, firmness and objectivity are successfully combined with the equally necessary qualities of warmth, sensitivity, and openness. Although the former 'tough-minded' approach is necessary for effective clinical work with difficult problems, the 'tender-minded' approach is also needed to defuse the inherent stresses of the work, and to maintain the motivation and involvement of all members of the team. Leadership which lacks one or other of these contrasting approaches can be a major constraining influence on the provision of patient-centred care (cf. Watts and Bennett, 1983).

Ward Organisation and Individual Treatment Programmes

The major conclusion to be drawn from the previous section is that a large number of different factors interact so as to affect the degree to which patient care is centred on individual needs and problems. This general perspective is important for the nurse therapist for two reasons. First, it can point to the type of changes that need to be made in order to improve the quality of care, and, secondly, it can highlight the inherent difficulties that the staff have to overcome constantly in their day-to-day work. In the long term these contrasting insights into the nature of institutional settings are of great importance in working towards gradual change. In the short term, however, patients are referred from wards with less than ideal resources and facilities, and decisions have to be made about the feasibility of specific treatment programmes. It is the purpose of this section to describe five key aspects of ward organisation that influence the ability of the staff to implement and maintain individual treatment plans of the kind commonly used in behaviour therapy. Such plans generally involve several members of the ward staff in observing and recording one or more aspects of a patient's behaviour and in carrying out some therapeutic intervention on a regular basis. Moreover, these activities usually occur on a daily basis and often need to be changed or modified in the light of the patient's progress. They therefore require an organisational system that emphasises the importance of clear communications about very specific issues, regular discussion and review, accountability in regard to implementing particular tasks, training in therapeutic skills, and a general consensus regarding overall policy and professional roles. Although these requirements are obviously not unique to behavioural treatment programming and might well be thought of as being essential to all clinical settings, they can be surprisingly hard to achieve in everyday clinical practice. What follows is an attempt to operationalise these requirements in terms of five key aspects of ward functioning. Their importance in terms of the successful implementation of treatment programmes is reflected in the order in which they are discussed.

(1) Regular Meetings

Rationale. These are needed to discuss special clinical problems, appropriate goals, and treatment plans for individual patients, and to review progress on a reasonably regular basis. They are also important in providing an opportunity to discuss particular difficulties that may have arisen in implementing the treatment plan so that solutions can be worked out that are acceptable to all concerned.

Comment. If the regular patient review meeting on the ward, which is usually led by the consultant, includes nursing care plans as an explicit focus of at least part of the meeting, then it makes sense to use this forum to discuss treatment plans. However, if this is not the case, perhaps because the meeting mainly consists of a brief review of an individual patient's medication and mental state, some other regular meeting will need to be organised. Such a meeting can take a number of different forms; the important point is that it should be attended regularly by as many staff as possible who are involved with the patient. It may be very useful for someone to keep a record of the decisions that are made so that staff who are unable to attend can keep up to date with current developments.

(2) Care Co-ordinators/Primary Therapists

Rationale. This involves each patient on the ward being assigned to a permanent member of the nursing staff who takes responsibility for co-ordinating their nursing care, getting to know them as closely as possible, and advocating on their behalf when necessary. This helps to promote accountability for implementing treatment plans, and encourages among staff a sense of personal involvement, responsibility and purpose. It also helps to ensure that all patients on the ward receive some regular support and attention.

Comment. This type of system is an addition rather than an alternative to the usual manner of care in which the charge nurse has overall responsibility for nursing care on the ward, and all nurses can potentially be involved with any of the patients. Its main purpose is to get round the nearly impossible task on traditional wards of each nurse being expected to know in detail the personal needs and idiosyncrasies of all patients on the ward. In practice it is much easier and more productive for each nurse to become closely involved with a small group of patients while at the same time maintaining a general involvement with all of them. It may be helpful for one person from each shift to work together as care co-ordinators or for a trained nurse to be paired with a nursing assistant.

(3) Statement of Ward Function and Policy

Rationale. A written document describing the function of the ward, the admission policy, daily routine, ward organisation and general therapeutic approach helps to provide all staff with clear expectations in regard to their professional role on the ward. It also helps to promote a sense of common purpose and group identity, and facilitates the orientation of new and temporary staff.

Comment. This kind of document should ideally be written by a senior member of the nursing or medical staff following consultations with everyone who is professionally involved with the ward. However, if this is not possible, a similar type of document focusing more narrowly on operational policy in regard to nursing care will also be extremely valuable. Whatever the scope of the document, it is important to organise regular but infrequent meetings to review and if necessary revise policy in the light of changing circumstances.

(4) Systematic Record Keeping

Rationale. Some form of problem-oriented record keeping, to which all staff have access, is necessary if treatment programmes are to be implemented in a systematic and co-ordinated manner by staff working on different shifts. It also enables new or temporary members of staff to acquaint themselves rapidly with the salient characteristics of each patient and his or her treatment.

Comment. The nursing process, which embodies the concept of a problem-oriented approach to record-keeping and treatment planning, is still in the early stages of development, and there is a good deal of controversy about the ideal form it should take (cf. Kratz, 1979). From the point of view of behavioural treatment programmes the essential requirement is a brief account of the nature of the problem, the treatment plan being used, and the progress made from week to week. It may be easiest to keep such a record in a readily accessible format such as a loose-leaf ring binder to which flow sheets can be added as appropriate.

(5) In-service Training

Rationale. Some form of in-service training is necessary to provide staff with the opportunity to learn the clinical skills that are needed to implement treatment plans effectively, and to enable them to keep abreast of new approaches to treatment and rehabilitation. If conducted imaginatively, it can go a long way towards increasing staff morale and creating a climate of mutual respect and understanding among members of the team.

Comment. There are a variety of ways of organising such training (cf. Sims, 1981; Milne, 1982) ranging from informal sessions on the ward to a systematic training programme for all hospital staff. It is likely to be most effective if it is mainly concerned with practising specific skills for dealing with specific problems, and actively involves the participants in the learning process.

If the above aspects of ward organisation are missing in varying degrees, it will be necessary either to exclude the possibility of implementing a treatment programme that involves ward staff, or, alternatively, to attempt to build into the ward organisation some or all of those elements that are missing. Which course of action to adopt will of course depend on a number of other factors such as time available, severity of the referred problem, and the attitude of the ward staff to making the necessary changes. There is in addition a third alternative, which is to proceed with the treatment plan, perhaps in a modified form, but to implement it without involving the staff. This may be quite feasible for some problems such as specific anxieties or specific deficits in self-care or social skills, but is likely to be of little value for more pervasive difficulties. The important point is to be clear about which of the alternatives is most appropriate in the circumstances.

Personal Coping Strategies

In the introduction I referred briefly to some of the stresses that can result from being responsible for the design and implementation of treatment programmes, and from sustaining therapeutic relationships with disturbed and unresponsive patients. Implicit in the sections that have followed has been a third potential area of stress that is associated with initiating changes of an organisational kind. It is inevitable that nurse therapists who work in institutional settings will become involved in attempts to change the way the 'system' operates, and working at this wider level does perhaps require a greater adjustment in professional role than that required in designing treatment programmes or seeing individual patients. It means coming to terms with the limitations of one's individual power and learning to accept the fact that institutional change is a gradual process. It also demands a good deal in the way of tact and patience, and puts a premium on the art of diplomacy and negotiation with people who may hold views quite contrary to those expressed in this chapter. (Head-on collisions with the guardians of the *status quo* are rarely of much value!) Expressing this in the terminology of cognitive-behavioural therapy it means that the nurse therapist needs to learn a set of coping strategies that will enable her to function effectively in this particular role. In this final section of the chapter, two aspects of coping with stress are discussed that are relevant to the nurse therapist's involvement in organisational change, as well as to her work in designing and implementing treatment programmes.

Learning to Challenge 'Automatic Thoughts'

There is a growing literature in both general psychology and behaviour therapy on the value of training patients in coping skills for dealing with personal problems and stressful situations (cf. Goldfried, 1980), and on the ways in which people naturally cope with stress in their everyday lives (cf. Lazarus and Launier, 1978; Pearlin and Schooler, 1978). Curiously, this valuable body of knowledge has rarely been discussed in terms of alleviating the stresses and strains of those people responsible for creating therapeutic change, and yet it is of course as relevant to the therapist as it is to the patient. If cognitive-behavioural theory and therapy are effective with some of the problems experienced by the residents of institutions, it should also be effective with some of the (much less severe?) problems of the staff of these institutions. In short, there may be a great deal to be learned in certain circumstances from applying cognitive-behavioural therapy to oneself. There are a great variety of ways of coping with stress, but some of the insights of cognitive therapy (e.g. Beck, 1976) may be particularly relevant to coping with the stresses of working in institutional settings. For example, some of the frustration that can result from initiating organisational change may stem from 'seeing' the changes that one is trying to bring about as being 'obviously desirable' or 'basically just common sense'. After all, isn't much of this chapter fairly obvious? Of course nursing staff should communicate clearly to each other about individual care plans. Of course patients should be encouraged to keep in contact with the outside world. And so on. Thoughts such as these may seem entirely reasonable and appropriate responses to the gap that typically exists between actual practices and desirable practices; they may be accepted unquestioningly, perhaps at a level just below conscious awareness. In terms of cognitive therapy, however, they may be just the kinds of 'automatic thought' that give rise to a sense of frustration and tension that undermines morale and inhibits effective problem-solving. The reason for this is that such thoughts actually contain so-called 'thinking errors' in which the 'reality' of the situation is interpreted in a distorted manner; thus, instead of approaching the gap between actual and ideal practices with a reasonable and realistic set of expectations about what can and cannot be achieved in the circumstances, the therapist perceives the situation in terms of unrealistic and over-demanding expectations that make effective action very difficult. Thus, she ignores the large body of evidence which suggests that most staff in institutions find change to be an unwelcome and painful process. Indeed, from a historical point of view, it is clear that many aspects of current medical and nursing practice that now seem entirely appropriate, and are very much taken for granted, were at one time daring innovations that were only accepted after a prolonged period of struggle and controversy. Moreover, it is generally not reasonable to assume that other people will tend to hold broadly similar views to one's own, and in this particular context it is almost always unhelpful to feel strongly that other people *should* do so. Such an attitude is likely to result in conflict and a further entrenchment of opposing points of view, whereas a more objective and realistic perspective would be more likely to maintain motivation and morale in spite of setbacks and frustrations.

Maladaptive thinking processes may also play a role in the difficulties of sustaining an active involvement with long-stay patients, and they almost certainly contribute to the detached, cynical and negative attitude towards institutionalised patients that is characteristic of the 'staff burnout syndrome' (cf. Cherniss, 1980). Thus, for example, abusive behaviour may be taken personally when in fact it is due to the patient's experience of very distressing auditory hallucinations. An apathetic and socially unresponsive patient may trigger off feelings of anger, irritation, or anxiety that are a result of 'automatic thoughts' that the patient is lazy, ungrateful, selfish, or even deliberately obstructive. The failure of a patient to respond quickly to a treatment programme that required a good deal of effort to set up may engender unpleasant feelings of personal incompetence, or, conversely, may result in the therapist giving up prematurely on the basis that the patient is either 'incurable' or totally institutionalised. And yet on closer examination such thoughts may reflect a very 'black and white' and over-simplified picture of the real reasons why patients behave in the way that they do. They have more to do with our own needs to feel appreciated, competent, and in control of our relationships with other people, and our defensive reactions when these needs are not met. Instead of anticipating difficulties and seeking solutions that are based on an understanding of the individual patient concerned, we too easily tend to react on the basis of our preconceived ideas of how we think he or she *should* behave. Rather than learn how to cope with the anxieties and ambiguities of working with people who are psychologically disturbed or handicapped, we find it easier to avoid contact and to attribute the difficulties to the person's illness or undesirable personality traits.

The process of detecting and changing distorted and unhelpful ways of thinking is not of course an easy matter, as any cognitive therapist will readily testify. It involves a willingness to become aware of 'automatic thoughts' that may be associated with signs of stress, and an ability to challenge these thoughts with more reasonable and realistic ways of perceiving the same situation. The problem in doing this is that we tend to have an emotional investment in the correctness of our own individual view of the world that makes us cling to our assumptions and beliefs with considerable tenacity. Moreover, our cognitive processes have a built-in confirmatory bias (cf. Glass and Arnkoff, 1982). To overcome this inherent resistance to change, a special effort has to be made to step outside one's own picture of reality and to understand the world from different perspectives. The importance of understanding other people's points of view is strongly emphasised by Margaret Garland (1983) in her sensitive and insightful account of her experiences as a ward sister in a medium- to long-stay ward of a mental hospital. There is no simple way of gaining such understanding, but it can clearly come from a variety of different sources. Reading books, talking with colleagues, attending conferences, as well as working with patients, are all valuable in developing appropriate perspectives on working in institutional settings and hence in learning to use cognitive therapy procedures for coping with stress.

The Importance of Social Supports

Just as psychological research has emphasised the value of learning to use specific techniques in coping with stress, it has also pointed to the importance of a person's social supports in reducing the effects of stress (e.g. Henderson, 1977; Brown and Harris, 1978). Nurse therapists who 'go it alone' are likely to experience more stress than nurse therapists who develop relationships with colleagues in which they can share difficulties, discuss solutions, and receive emotional support. This can be particularly important in implementing organisational change, where the presence of a small group of reasonably like-minded people may be crucial to the success of the enterprise (cf. Fairweather, Sanders and Tornatsky, 1974; Georgiades and Phillimore, 1975). The cultivation of supportive relationships with colleagues, in both nursing and other disciplines, is likely to pay large dividends in the long run even if this involves a considerable amount of time and effort. Although this may appear to be just common sense, it is surprising how difficult this may be to achieve in practice. Differences in ideology, shortages of time, professional defensiveness, and other factors, may all conspire to increase social isolation among staff who all work in the same clinical setting (Cherniss, 1980). As with other coping strategies, it is necessary to make a special effort to build social supports into the organisation of everyday work.

Conclusion

The central thesis of this chapter is that the quality of the therapeutic environment as a whole is a crucial factor in determining the viability and effectiveness of behavioural treatment programmes. It is therefore important that nurse therapists (and indeed other therapists) understand the nature of the clinical setting in which they work, and much of the content of this chapter has been concerned with describing the various factors that need to be taken into account in this regard. In the first place we considered some factors that have influenced our current notions of what is meant by the 'quality of life', and we went on to describe in some detail the ways in which this rather general concept can be realised in everyday practice. The principles of normalisation and patient-centred care clearly provide useful reference points when working in this area. However, in considering what kind of life we should aim to provide for the long-term residents of our institutions, we are also concerned with moral issues. Nursing care which seeks to preserve human dignity in spite of very difficult circumstances is not just important from a clinical or psychological standpoint; it is also an expression of a deeper set of values about the kind of society that is worth striving for.

In the second place we considered the various ways in which the nature and organisation of institutional care can affect the quality of life of the residents and the ability of the staff to implement individual treatment programmes. Though some negative aspects of institutions are not amenable to change, it is equally clear that various aspects of staff organisation and ward management are changeable, and it is hoped that this chapter has given some positive guidance about such matters. In particular we have emphasised the importance of systems of organisation that encourage among ward staff good communications, mutual support, and a sense of personal involvement with, and responsibility for, individual patient care. Finally, we suggested that the implementation of behavioural treatment programmes may involve a fair degree of stress for the staff involved, and that particular attention needs to be paid to helping them develop effective coping strategies.

The creation of a therapeutic environment is not an activity which has a beginning or an end; it is rather a continuous process which requires attention to many different factors at the individual, organisational, and physical level. There is much research that needs to be done on the interrelationships of these factors and it is likely that current practice will seem as outdated to the clinicians of 25 years time as the practices of 25 years ago seem to us now. However, in the immediate future the real challenge lies not so much in developing new approaches to care and treatment but in putting into everyday clinical practice the knowledge that we already possess.

References

Barton, R. (1976) *Institutional Neurosis*, 3rd edn, John Wright & Sons, Bristol

Beck, A.T. (1976) *Cognitive Therapy and the Emotional Disorders*, International Universities Press, New York

Bella, D.A. (1976) 'Relationship of Institution Size to Quality of Care: A Review of the Literature', *American Journal of Mental Deficiency*, *81*, 117–24

Brown, G.W. and Harris, T. (1978) *Social Origins of Depression*, Tavistock, London

Canter, D. and Canter, S. (eds) (1979) *Designing for Therapeutic Environments: a Review of Research*, Wiley, New York

Cherniss, C. (1980) *Staff Burnout: Job Stress in the Human Services*, Sage Studies in Community Mental Health, Sage, London

Durham, R.C. (1983) 'Long-stay Psychiatric Inpatients', in S. Spence and G.W. Shepherd (eds), *Developments in Social Skills Training*, Academic Press, London

Durham, T.M. (1982) 'Community Living Skills Training in Psychiatric Rehabilitation', *British Journal of Occupational Therapy*, *45* (7), 233–5

Fairweather, G.W., Sanders, D.H. and Tornatsky, L.G. (1974) *Creating Change in Mental Health Organisation*, Pergamon Press, New York

Fraser, D. (1983) 'From Token Economy to Social Information System: The Emergence of Critical Variables', in E. Karas (ed.), *Current Issues in Clinical Psychology*, vol. 1, Plenum Press, New York

Garland, M. (1983) *'The Other Side of Psychiatric Care'*, Macmillan Press, London

Georgiades, N.J. and Phillimore, L. (1975) 'The Myth of the Hero Innovator and Alternative Strategies for Organisation Change', in C.C. Kiernan and F.D. Woodford (eds), *Behaviour Modification with the Severely Retarded*, Associated Scientific Publishers, Amsterdam

Glass, C. and Arnkoff, D. (1982) 'Think Cognitively: Selected Issues in Cognitive Assessment and Therapy', in P.C. Kendall (ed.), *Advances in Cognitive-Behavioural Research and Therapy*, vol. 1, Academic Press, New York

Goffman, E. (1961) *Asylums: Essays on the Social Situation of Mental Patients and Other Inmates*, Anchor Books/Doubleday, New York

Goldfried, M.R. (1980) 'Psychotherapy as Coping Skills Training', in M.J. Mahoney (ed.), *Psychotherapy Process*, Plenum Press, New York

Goldstein, A.P., Sprafkin, R.P. and Gershaw, N.J. (1976) *Skills Training for Community Living*, Pergamon Press, Oxford

Hall, J.N. and Baker, R.D. (1972) 'Practical Difficulties in the Implementation of Token Economy Programmes', paper presented at the *Second European Conference on Behaviour Modification, Wexford, Ireland*

Hall, J.N. and Baker, R.D. (1973) 'Token Economy Systems: Breakdown and Control', *Behaviour Research and Therapy, 11*, 253–63

Henderson, S. (1977) 'The Social Network, Support and Neurosis: the Function of Attachment in Adult Life', *British Journal of Psychiatry, 131*, 185–91

Hersen, M. and Bellack, A.S. (1976) 'Social Skills Training for Chronic Psychiatric Patients: Rationale, Research Findings, and Future Directions', *Comprehensive Psychiatry*, 559–80

Insell, P.M. and Moos, R.H. (1974) *Health and the Social Environment*, Lexington Books, Toronto

Jones, M. (1952) *Social Psychiatry: a Study of Therapeutic Communities*, Tavistock Press, London

Jones, M. (1976) *Maturation of the Therapeutic Community: an Organic Approach to Health and Mental Health*, Human Sciences Press, New York

Kennard, D. (1979) 'Limiting Factors: the Setting, the Staff, the Patients', in R.D. Hinshelwood and N.P. Manning (eds), *Therapeutic Communities: Reflections and Progress*, Routledge & Kegan Paul, London

King, R., Raynes, N. and Tizard, J. (1971) *Patterns of Residential Care*, Routledge and Kegan Paul, London

Kratz, C.R. (ed.) (1979) *The Nursing Process*, Bailliere Tindall, London

Lazarus, R.S. and Launier, R. (1978) 'Stress-related Transactions between Person and Environment', in L.A. Pervin and M. Lewis (eds), *Perspectives in Interactional Psychology*, Plenum Press, New York

McPherson, F. (1983) 'Long-term Care — An Introduction', in E. Karas (ed.), *Current Issues in Clinical Psychology*, vol. 1, Plenum Press, New York

Milne, D.A. (1982) 'A Comparison of Two Methods of Teaching Behaviour Modification to Mental Handicap Nurses', *Behavioural Psychotherapy, 10*, 54–64

Orford, J. (1982) 'Institutional Climates', in J. Hall (ed.), *Psychology for Nurses and Health Visitors*, British Psychological Society and Macmillan Press, London

Paul, G.L. and Lentz, R.J. (1977) *Psychosocial Treatment of Chronic Mental Patients: Milieu vs Social-learning Programs*, Harvard University Press, Harvard, Mass.

Pearlin, L.I. and Schooler, C. (1978) 'The Structure of Coping', *Journal of Health and Social Behaviour, 19*, 2–21

Rapoport, R.M. (1960) *Community as Doctor: New Perspectives on a Therapeutic Community*, Tavistock Press, London

Raynes, N.V., Pratt, M. and Roses, S. (1974) Final Report: Organisational Structure and Care in Institutions for the Retarded, US Department of Health Education and Welfare, Grant HD 04147 Mimeo., Cambridge, Mass.

Raynes, N.V., Pratt, M. and Roses, S. (1979) *Organisational Structure and the Care of the Mentally Retarded*, Croom Helm, London

Rimm, D.C. and Masters, J.C. (1979) *Behaviour Therapy: Techniques and Empirical Findings*, Academic Press, New York

Rutter, M., Maughan, B., Mortimore, P., Ouston, J. and Smith, A. (1979) *Fifteen-thousand Hours: Secondary Schools and Their Effects on Children*, Open Books, London

SE Thames RHA (1976) Report of Committee of Inquiry, St Augustine's Hospital, Chatham, Canterbury, South East Thames Regional Health Authority

Shepherd, G.W. (1984) *Institutional Care and Rehabilitation*, Longman, London

Shepherd, G.W. and Richardson, A. (1979) 'Organisation and Interaction in Psychiatric Day Centres', *Psychological Medicine, 9*, 573–9

Sims, A. (1981) 'The Staff and their Training', in J.K. Wing and B. Morris (eds), *Handbook of Psychiatric Rehabilitation Practice*, Oxford University Press, Oxford

Stein, L.I. and Test, M.A. (1978) 'An Alternative to Mental Hospital Treatment', in L.I. Stein and M.A. Test (eds), *Alternatives to Mental Hospital Treatment*, Plenum Press, New York

Sutton, G. (1981) 'The Organisation and Administration of Nursing Services for Long-stay Patients', in J.K. Wing and B. Morris (eds), *Handbook of Psychiatric Rehabilitation Practice*, Oxford University Press, Oxford

Watts, F.N. and Bennett, D.H. (1983) 'Management of the Staff Team', in F.N. Watts and D.H. Benett (eds), *Theory and Practice in Psychiatric Rehabilitation*, Wiley, Chichester

Wing, J.K. and Brown, G.W. (1970) *Institutionalism and Schizophrenia: a Comparative Study of Three Mental Hospitals, 1960–68*, Cambridge University Press, Cambridge

Wolfensberger, W. (1972) *The Principle of Normalisation in Human Services*, National Institute for Mental Retardation, Toronto

Wolfensberger, W. and Glenn, W. (1975) *Program Analysis of Service Systems (PASS 3)*, National Institute for Mental Retardation, Toronto

PART TWO: CASE STUDIES

INTRODUCTION

In the preface to this book we discussed briefly the content of each of the following case studies. We explained that these studies had been selected to demonstrate the range of problems which are, at present, thought to be amenable to behavioural intervention. This does not mean, of course, that only the problems described in this section are suitable targets for behaviour therapy. As we discussed in Chapter 2 the range of behaviour therapy is much wider than the six problem areas covered here. The six studies presented in this section serve only as examples of some of the targets of the behaviour therapist: problems which occur commonly in any nursing situation, and therefore which may be of considerable relevance to nurses interested in the behavioural model of care.

We should also like to emphasise that the methods of assessment and treatment which are used in the following cases are not by any means the only possible strategies at the disposal of the behaviour therapist. The techniques described portray the method by which one individual, the therapist, attempts to meet the needs of another individual, the patient. Since therapists can vary greatly in their theoretical orientation to therapy and in the way in which they conduct it, the *practice* of behaviour therapy can vary enormously from one practitioner to the next. The nature of therapy is, of course, also greatly influenced by the presentation of the patient. For these reasons we would invite the reader to focus attention upon the *process* of therapy in the following case studies; rather than upon the practice of the specific techniques described. As we have noted above, the methods of assessment and behaviour-change described in the studies are not the only possible strategies which might have been adopted. For this reason the reader should concentrate upon the relationship between the design of the therapy programme and the needs of the patient concerned. Although it may seem something of a paradox we believe that by attending to the process of therapy the reader will gain a deeper understanding of the practice of therapy, than by attending solely to the practical details of the techniques used in the management of the case.

We believe that the person who is equipped only with a set of assessment or behaviour change techniques may be able to offer only

145

a restricted form of therapy. The person who has an awareness of the process of therapy is less restricted, being able to adapt his/her approach and the techniques involved, to suit the demands of the situation. For this reason our training programme has always tried to emphasise that behaviour therapy is greater than the sum of its parts (i.e. its inherent techniques). In the cases which follow nurses illustrate how, through rigorous assessment, they tried to make sense of particular problems of living. Although the approaches vary from one case to another, each illustrates how the assessment 'bred' the selection of particular strategies for behaviour-change. The resultant programmes emphasise the selection of targets which were meaningful to the patients concerned. The pursuit of these goals of therapy are described in equally rigorous terms as the nurses try to evaluate the overall value of their therapeutic programmes.

Although the cases selected have, in the main, successful outcomes, this was not a key requirement for selection. We hoped to be able to show other nurses what are the true possibilities of the behavioural approach within psychiatric and mental handicap nursing. In some cases success may be measured in terms of discharge, the recommencement of 'normal living' or the gratitude of the patient. However in others, 'success' may be measured in terms of arrested deterioration. Our aim in this second section is modest: to *suggest* the possibilities for the nurse in the mental health field. The task of *demonstrating* the 'art of the possible' we leave to our colleagues through the medium of their case reports.

P.J.B./D.F.

6 THE TREATMENT OF BATHING AND EATING PROBLEMS IN A MENTALLY HANDICAPPED WOMAN

Peggy Griffiths

Introduction

Women's magazines tell us a certain bath product 'makes a woman feel good all over . . . and it shows!'; that a body spray, if we try it, will 'make the nicest things happen to us'.

With regard to food, the magazines give us countless recipes: 'meals to make you feel good'; 'Enjoy yourselves with x's casseroles', we are instructed; and television tells us that y's cereals 'have extra vitamins'.

To refrain from washing, to have 'BO', is a social offence in our culture: it is something our best friends are reluctant to tell us about. Slimming diets in their many forms are fashionable, and anorexia nervosa is on the increase, but we regard people who do not enjoy their food as a nuisance as dinner guests. However, when considering any maladaptive behaviour with someone who lives in an institution, one has to take into account what Goffman (1961) says about institutional life in which 'each phase of the member's daily activity is carried on in the immediate company of a large batch of others, all of whom are treated alike and required to do the same things together'.

When the subject of this study was referred for bathing and eating problems, she presented as someone living in a barren institution, who could not understand the exchange of tokens in a programme carried out 5 years previously; who was so distractable that psychological testing could not decide if she was mildly, severely or profoundly mentally handicapped; who, according to those who knew her well, had no particular interests in life. For these reasons it seemed of prime importance to the author that, before any programme could be considered, a suitable reinforcer would need to be found for her.

The *Oxford English Dictionary*, in its definition of the word 'reinforce' uses the phrase, 'to strengthen'. Hemsley and Carr (1980) say

Reinforcement is not peculiar to behaviour modification, but is widely used in everyday life. Few of us would go regularly to work if we were not paid. Teachers and parents expect to help children learn by encouragement, praise and prizes. Reinforcement may be defined as any event which when it follows a behaviour strengthens the probability or increases the frequency of that behaviour's occurrence.

Ayllon and Azrin (1968) in their chapter 'Discovering Reinforcers' stress that 'by observing what the individual does when the opportunity exists, those activities that are very probable at a given time will serve as reinforcers'. Thus cigarettes were used by these authors to reinforce various behaviours of patients who had a high probability of smoking; cartoon movies were used by Baer (1962) as a means of reinforcing children for indulging in activities other than thumb-sucking.

For any event (whether smiles, candy, gum, praise, money or attention) to be called a reinforcer, Van Etten, Arkell and Van Etten (1980) say the target behaviour must increase in rate, duration or intensity. There are few universal reinforcers. Events that are reinforcing for one person may not be reinforcing for another. For example, Isaacs, Thomas and Goldiamond (1960) used chewing gum as a reinforcer to reinstate verbal behaviour in a hospitalised mute psychotic patient. During the early stages of the experiment when no response could be obtained from the patient, a packet of chewing gum accidentally fell out of the therapist's pocket. This brought an immediate response from the patient in form of eye movement. Thus a reinforcer was accidentally discovered and was subsequently used successfully. As you will see later, such chance discoveries can play a prominent part in the development of a behaviour therapy programme.

The Subject

Betty, at 33, is a slim, 1.65 m-tall (5 ft 5 in) attractive brunette, showing off her good figure well with her 'ballerina-like' walk. Initially the first give-away that there is 'something different' about Betty is when she opens her mouth, revealing her 'Epanutin gums' (hypertrophy of the gums). With her bright, dark-brown eyes and expressive face, her speech (or rather lack of it) comes as a surprise. Though she may say the odd word quite clearly, mostly her speech is a language of her own, and her gesturing and mime are often easier to comprehend. Betty's attention is difficult to capture. She often appears to be caught up with something that occurred earlier and all her energy is involved in the urgency of telling you something you cannot possibly understand. She often seems to feel that she has said something funny as she can go into peals of laughter while 'talking'. However, once her attention is captured (capturing it being the difficult part), she is a keen pupil and eager to please, and she shows she has a good comprehension of complicated language and a sense of humour.

Betty's childhood was spent in what was then called Rhodesia. At the age of 12 she entered institutional life permanently, her mental handicap, severe epilepsy and temper tantrums constituting the reasons for her admission. Her father died when she was 29 and her mother currently visits infrequently.

Until age 22 she lived in a ward in which she was expected to do little for herself: she was bathed, dressed and escorted everywhere. At 22 she was promoted to a 'pre-rehabilitation' ward, in which people were expected to be capable of learning to dress and bathe, and to shop in the hospital cafeteria. This ward is somewhat typical of the upgraded old grey institutional type, with 24 beds in a dormitory all sporting continental covers and teddies on the beds. There are bus runs, coffee mornings, and hospital disco evenings, and there is one hour of swimming per week. Clothes are individualised, although what is worn for the day is decided by ward staff. Bathing is carried out on Tuesdays and Thursdays after lunch (for Betty and half of the ward complement). This is done collectively: i.e. all 12 women undress together, wait in line for one of the three baths prepared by the nurses; and then dry and dress together.

As a preliminary evaluation for a token economy scheme, Betty was referred when aged 26 to a psychologist for IQ testing and American Association for Mental Deficiency (AAMD) ratings. The psychologist reported: 'Intellectual assessments were carried out in order to give an indication of Betty's level of functioning on a standardised test instrument: the results suggest that her performance is within the severely to profoundly handicapped range.'

In terms of adaptive behaviour as measured on the AAMD scales, Betty is below average in all areas of functioning, including basic skills of independent living. On the maladaptive side, Betty scores above average on such items as violent and destructive behaviour, antisocial behaviour, rebellious behaviour and unacceptable vocal habits.

The group token economy scheme was designed to improve personal hygiene skills, table manners and bedmaking. After a few months the unanimous staff decision was that Betty should be withdrawn, 'as her increase in temper tantrums was seen as attributable to the fact that she could not understand the value of the tokens, nor the delayed exchange system, which was in operation at the time'.

In 1978, when Betty was nearly 30, the first Everyday Living Skills Inventory (ELSI: Barker, Docherty and Tosh, 1976, unpublished) was done by nursing staff. ELSI is an assessment of skills fundamental to everyday survival and independence, which is designed to discover the degree of dependency a patient may have on care staff. It is divided into such areas as general hygiene, simple language, dressing and mealtime behaviour. The level of ability is rated on a scale from 0 (refuses to perform the behaviour) to 5 (requires verbal prompting to initiate the behaviour). The manner of recording is visual, and the assessment evaluation record sheet makes it possible to assess any change that has taken place between one assessment and the next. Some relevant results of three ELSIs completed by ward staff on Betty are shown in Table 6.1.

Table 6.1: Results of ELSIs Completed on Betty

	ELSI		
	1	*2*	*3*
Instruction following	3	5	5
Attention to task	3	5	5
Bathing	0	0	0
Clothing appearance	4	5	5
Bed making	2	5	5
Table laying	0	0	0

* *1:* 10 August 1978; *2:* 22 May 1979; *3:* 17 June 1980.

ELSI Scores on Three Separate Occasions

Around the same time as the first ELSI was completed, the first small group programme for personal hygiene organised by nursing staff was started. It appears that Betty bathed satisfactorily for some members of staff, but not for others. This programme lasted for 6 months.

A second small group programme called 'Achievement Potential' then commenced. This involved daily washing, before breakfast, after dinner and after tea. From the ten available recording sheets studied,

Betty's reliability in carrying out the required behaviour was clearly in question.

Supplementary Information and Subjective Impressions

Betty has a certain sophistication of movement and social interaction. Her figure and the way she wears her clothes have a more 'normal' appearance, in the author's opinion, than one generally finds in a mentally handicapped population. She can carry on a 'conversation' across the dinner table, and if one is out of earshot, from her gestures and interest one would think that the 'conversation' was understood and meaningful to both parties. Her 'language' sometimes sounds strangely African. On a few occasions on which the author mentioned her birthplace, Rhodesia, to Betty, a sad, meditative expression clouded her face.

Betty is reported to have unacceptable habits not that uncommon among institutionalised women, i.e. she hides her soiled panties and sanitary towels. Although she seems to prefer wearing soiled panties, she is fastidious about outer garments being perfectly clean.

Referred Problems

(1) Unacceptable Level of Personal Hygiene. Betty needed someone telling her to 'soap cloth, wash . . . , rinse . . . , soap cloth'. Some staff thought Betty knew how to bathe, as demonstrated by the fact that she would bathe for some staff but not for others. Other staff felt that she did not know how to bathe and that she did not like bathing. Betty could be particularly smelly and dirty at menstrual times; her soiled panties did not seem to bother her. This unwillingness to be concerned about her personal hygiene meant that Betty was under threat of being 'demoted', i.e. returned to a ward where she would have most things done for her.

(2) Reluctance to Eat a Proper Meal. Despite the fact that she selected foods from a daily menu she would frequently refuse to eat what she had ordered. On some occasions she would eat her food quickly, but mostly she toyed with the food, eating little if any. She could distract staff who were coaxing her to eat by complaining of, for example, toothache. Sometimes she would eat treats (such as sweets) quickly: on other occasions she would store them. Staff were concerned about getting her to eat a balanced diet, and some staff saw her reluctance to eat as having an anorexic quality. This inconsistent reluctance to eat has been a pattern for many years. Apart from a

period about 3 years ago when she was unwell, her weight has remained fairly constant.

Assessment

The purpose of assessment was to find out if Betty actually knew *how* to bathe, i.e. knew the skills of bathing, or if she needed to be taught these skills and to discover whether or not she enjoyed bathing. During this time I had to find a reinforcer that would be effective in Betty's treatment, and it was necessary to build up a rapport with Betty so that she would respond to instruction, praise and verbal reprimands.

(1) Formal and Informal Discussions with Staff. These discussions revealed a variety of descriptions of Betty's bathing and eating problems. The author was given her case file, the 'bath book' rating scales and checklists to study. Because of severe epilepsy, Betty would always require staff to be in attendance when she bathed. During this period, no effective reinforcer for Betty was discovered.

(2) Interview with Patient. The aim here was to introduce myself to Betty, to tell her how I hoped to start teaching her to bathe herself, and to gain her consent to the treatment programme. Betty's manner at first interview typified many of our later encounters. She seemed totally absorbed with other things, looking here and there, pointing, gesturing, speaking in her private language. Attempts to gain her attention did not alter what she was doing. In the end, and in some desperation, with hands in the air I clicked my fingers and thumbs, calling 'Oooeee!' Betty looked directly at me for a few seconds. There appeared little point in prolonging the 'interview'.

(3) Direct Observations. These were aimed at identifying what Betty did (and did not do) in the bath.

First, I observed one of her twice-weekly ward routine baths, using the *running-narrative* method of recording (writing down everything that is observed to occur). Betty spent several minutes 'dilly-dallying' in the dormitory before entering the bathroom. She spent a lot of unnecessary time folding and re-folding her clothes while undressing. When called for her bath, she forgot to take all her toiletries with her. Once in the bath she tended to soap and re-soap the cloth or repeatedly re-washed one area of her body, apparently waiting for the nurse's instruction to 'move on'. Noises appeared to distract her and she would forget what she was doing. During observation I sat behind Betty, some six feet away. When all the nurses left the bathroom Betty sat playing with the bubbles for about 15 minutes until the nurses returned to tell her to get out of the bath.

I also observed Betty in three private or individual bathing sessions. The discovery during earlier observation that, if given no instruction, Betty simply 'did not get a move on' made me decide to investigate whether or not Betty would respond to prompting and praise during these three sessions. She responded to prompting and praise (in the form of saying 'Good girl'), and this made her smile and 'get a move on'. She continued, however, to be extremely prone to be distracted. She appeared to enjoy preparing for the bath and tidying up, and she soon started imitating my behaviour. She seemed to prefer using the sponge to the cloth and, in any case, she made better use of the sponge.

From these four bathing observations, it was clear that Betty knew the actions of bathing and had all the requisite skills, but that she lacked any semblance of order in performing these skills and had no conception of how much time she should spend at any one stage.

(4) The Comparison Group. In order to work out a sequence of steps for Betty and to work out the timing for each stage in the bathing process, I asked a comparison group, comprising five women and two teenage boys, to observe their bathing routines for two baths each. All were asked to bathe at a normal, unhurried rate and to record times for each of the four stages (undressing, bathing, drying, dressing). All seven indicated that they did not keep to any set routine for bathing or drying, i.e. one bath might start with the left arm, another bath might start with the right. Five out of the seven preferred not to use talc, and as Betty had shown great difficulty in manipulating the talc from container to hand, then from hand to foot, it appeared acceptable when drawing up a checklist and bathing programme for Betty to eliminate talc from the procedure. Five out of the seven preferred using the sponge to using the cloth. The same number preferred to wash their face with their hands rather than with the sponge.

(5) Eating Observations. For eating problems I accepted the nursing staff's observations that Betty 'picks at food, spends a long time at the table and seldom completes the middle course of a dinner meal'.

(6) Establishing a Reinforcer. It had already been pointed out that Betty did not understand the principles of token delivery and exchange, and that food reinforcement was ineffective in her case. Further interviews with staff led to the conclusion that finding a potent reinforcer was likely to be an impossible task. However, like the chewing gum that was accidentally found to be a reinforcer in the study with mute psychotics by Isaccs *et al.*, so a reinforcer was accientally discovered in Betty's case.

By chance I visited the ward with my 18-month-old cocker spaniel bitch, Josie. All the patients seemed interested in her, but Betty took over and was totally absorbed for at least 30 minutes in getting Josie to sit and to give a paw, in patting her and in getting others to look at the dog.

To examine her reactions still further, when Betty was on a walk to the hospital farm I joined her group with Josie. Betty took Josie's lead, holding it like an expert and she knew to alternate her hands on the lead before it got tangled round various obstacles. The walk back took considerably longer: Betty made the dog sit every few yards to receive a tickle from her! It seemed that a suitable reinforcer had been found.

Assessment and observation therefore revealed the following:

Low-level assets: Instruction following and attention to task were present but poorly developed.

Absolute deficits: Bathing and menstrual hygiene. Eating a proper meal. Sense of time — 'dilly-dally' behaviour.

Potential assets: Laying tables. Dishwashing. Interest in Josie, the dog.

Targets therefore would be:

(1)   to teach a bathing routine, thereby increasing Betty's instruction-following and task orientation;
(2)   to set time limits for stages of bathing, decreasing 'dilly-dally' behaviour;
(3)   to teach her to discriminate between dirty and clean underwear and to respond appropriately to dirty underwear;
(4)   to increase appropriate eating behaviour.

Preliminary Cost-Benefit Analysis

Benefits of Targets 1-3 for Betty. An increase in social acceptability and possible increase in self-esteem, with a cost to her of effort in training sessions.

Benefits of Targets 1-3 for Staff. They would spend less time prompting personal hygiene habits, with a cost to them of effort in maintaining her programme.

Benefit of Target 4 for Betty. Weight gain and increase in social eating with a cost in effort in training sessions.

Benefit of Target 4 for Staff. They would spend less time prompting her to eat, with a cost in effort in training sessions.

Baseline Data

Bathing Programme

In order to have a measure on which to evaluate any future treatment programme I constructed a checklist of prompts comprising 39 steps in bathing and I recorded the time taken to complete each of the six stages (preparation, undressing, bathing, drying, dressing, and tidying up). Two fellow therapists carried out observations to check (a) the feasibility of implementing the 39 steps, (b) the number of prompts given by myself, and (c) the times Betty took for each stage.

Recordings showed that during Bath 1 she needed 45 prompts and took 9 minutes for the bathing stage and 3½ minutes for the drying stage. For Bath 2 Betty required 71 prompts and took 11 minutes for the bathing stage and 4 minutes for the drying stage. (See Figures 6.1-3.)

As the bathroom where Betty regularly bathed was rather large, it was suggested by ward staff that a smaller bathroom be used for training purposes. This bathroom had three baths in it, with curtains between baths that could be drawn. I encouraged Betty to draw the curtain to be sure of privacy in the event of people walking in.

Eating Programme

I observed six dinner meals using the running-narrative method. A stopwatch was used to check the time Betty took to complete each course. An attempt was made to check the times her three table companions took to complete their meals in order to achieve some form of comparison.

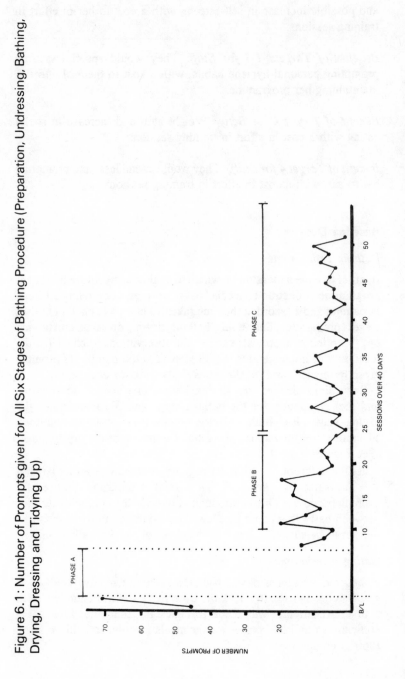

Figure 6.1: Number of Prompts given for All Six Stages of Bathing Procedure (Preparation, Undressing, Bathing, Drying, Dressing and Tidying Up)

Figure 6.2: Number of Prompts for Bathing Stage *only*

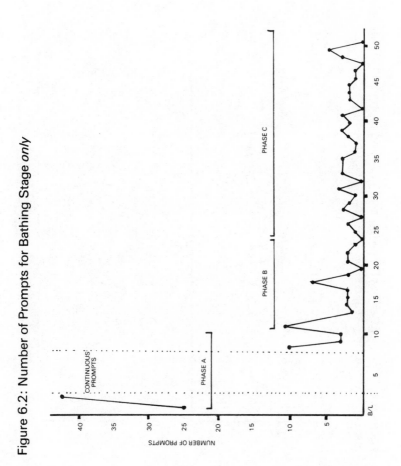

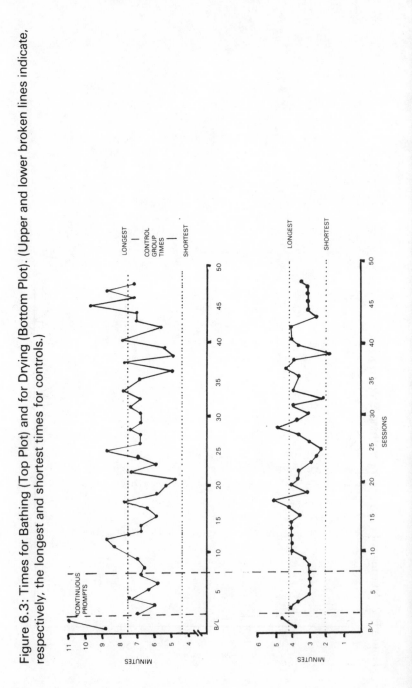

Figure 6.3: Times for Bathing (Top Plot) and for Drying (Bottom Plot). (Upper and lower broken lines indicate, respectively, the longest and shortest times for controls.)

Findings from Observations

The Scene. The dining hall catered for three wards. It featured a lofty ceiling and flagged floors and was equipped with formica-topped tables and metal chairs. Voices echoed loudly within the hall. Serving was done by nurses at a serving hatch and courses were brought on a trolley to the appropriate ward partition. Patients emptied what they did not eat into a slop bucket and assisted in clearing the crockery and cutlery. Betty shared a table with three women and there were 24 women in Betty's dining area.

Information from the Running-narrative Observations. Despite the fact that menu selection was in operation, Betty continued to choose a number of foods which she appeared not to like. She pushed the food around the plate and loaded the fork, but before the forkload reached her mouth she would let it fall back on to her plate. She also tended to gag, complained of toothache and asked the nurses to remove her plate. She would eat up an average portion of some other foods fairly speedily and within the time limits of her peers, and then sit and toy with what was left on her plate. Servings varied (e.g. a portion of shepherd's pie could sometimes have four boiled potatoes and two big spoonfuls of carrots; other servings only had one potato and one spoonful of carrots). Some nurses removed her plate once she had eaten a portion; at other meals the nurses refused to remove the plate, telling her to 'eat up'. The custom was that all women would enter the dining hall together. As soon as individuals had finished their meals, they left the dining hall and the nurses left as well, so when Betty sat for a long time over a meal she was left in the dining hall alone.

Data from Formal Recordings. Figure 6.4 shows the time Betty took for her main course and Figure 6.5 shows the time that she took to consume her soup and pudding over a total of six meals. These data therefore serve as a baseline. It can be seen that she had no time problem with pudding. She could eat soup within 6 to 8½ minutes if there were no vegetables in it (on the two occasions on which she took 10 minutes and 11 minutes, respectively, a lot of the time was spent balancing peas as she removed them from her scotch broth to the side of her plate).

On the three occasions on which she ate the main course within 20 minutes, she smiled when the plate was put in front of her, ate up fairly speedily what she wanted and told the nurse that she had had enough, and the plate was duly removed. At the three other meals the

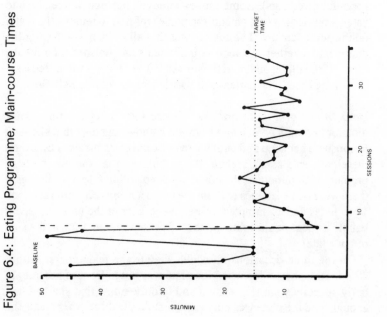

Figure 6.4: Eating Programme, Main-course Times

Figure 6.5: Eating Programme Times for Pudding (Top) and Soup (Bottom)

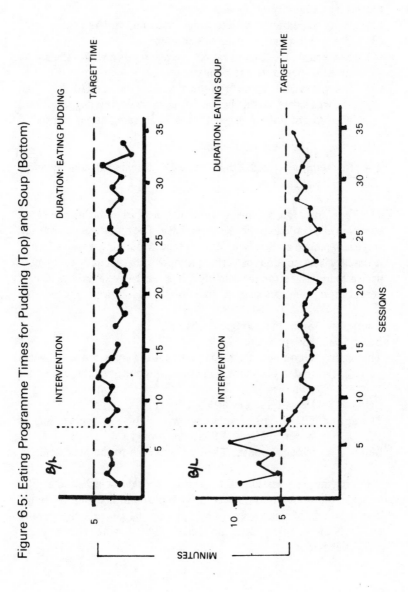

nurses twice refused to remove the plate, and at meal 5 she ate nothing (steamed fish had been served) and then left the dining hall after 45 minutes.

The following points were therefore considered in planning the intervention programme:

(1)   The variability of the servings.
(2)   Betty appeared to dislike some foods and to like others.
(3)   She did not eat the peas in her soup.
(4)   She could on occasion eat an average portion within the eating times of her table companions.
(5)   Betty was often given food she obviously did not like. Although she was asked to state her choice in advance, this suggested that she did not fully understand what was being asked of her.

Operation of the Bathing Programme

The programme consisted of three phases: A, teaching; B, consolidation; and C, generalisation.

(A) Teaching. During the six sessions, the author sat in a position such that she could easily be seen by Betty. The timer was set for each stage and placed so that Betty could see it. Modelling was used when necessary; and continuous verbal prompts were given for every step, praise being given for the completion of each. A sample record of verbal prompting, praise and modelling is as follows.

Therapist	Soap the sponge, Betty.
Betty	[Soaps sponge.]
Therapist	Good girl. That's enough; put the soap down, . . . wash under your arm. [Therapist vigorously rubs under her own arm.]
Betty	[Washes under arm.]
Therapist	Clever girl. That's enough . . . rinse . . . splash lots of water . . . lovely! Soap the sponge.
Betty	[Soaps sponge. Then we move on to the next item.]

During these six sessions, Betty showed considerable distractability, for example pointing to objects in the bathroom, insisting on giving long accounts of some event in her 'private' language and generally wasting time or using 'delaying tactics'. This is what I term 'dilly-dally' behaviour.

In the second and third sessions Betty flatly refused to come to the bathing area. She was reported as being in a 'bad mood' and when I approached her she looked tearful and shook her head. On both occasions I promised her 'time with Josie' if she came for a bath. This brought a smile to her face and she immediately came for the session.

(B) Consolidation. I decided to delay prompting, to give Betty a chance to initiate the step herself. If she did, she was given very enthusiastic praise in the form of 'Good girl!'. If not she was prompted. I sat, with the checklist in front of me, still in such a position that Betty could see me easily. I recorded the steps that she performed independently and those on which she required prompting. (See Figures 6.1-3.)

To control her 'dilly-dallying' behaviour a time-out procedure was introduced. This consisted of the author looking away from Betty for a count of 3 seconds (time out from social reinforcement). Time out invariably had the effect of getting her to 'move on' and to stop 'dilly-dallying'.

For the next three sessions I continued with the first checklist but it was becoming obvious that extra steps should be added. On the fourth and fifth sessions the same two observers checked the reliability of checklist no. 2. On the sixth and seventh sessions the nurse who would be doing sessions while I was away for a 2-week holiday was present during treatment sessions. The following five sessions (sessions 16-20 on Figures 6.1-3) were completed by this nurse.

During the last four sessions of consolidation (sessions 21-24), I sat behind Betty so that she could not see me, and I gave her time to do the steps without prompts and withholding praise if she moved on to the next step of her own accord, thus fading reinforcement to a variable schedule. During the time I was away there was no opportunity for Betty to see Josie but I was told that she frequently asked for her. During the last four sessions of consolidation, she was allowed time with Josie intermittently. I felt that the eating problem could be a more difficult one to tackle, and therefore did not want to swamp or saturate her with Josie during the bathing programme.

(C) Generalisation. By the beginning of the generalisation phase, Betty responded to 'What do you do next?' (a prompt) by standing still, appearing to work it out for herself, then doing what was required. If she had forgotten anything in the preparation or in the

tidying-up stage, a gesture in the general direction of what was required was enough to remind her what to do.

Betty's speech was often more comprehensible than previously; for example, she would frequently say 'Freezing cold' when she tested the water temperature and she was invariably correct. She would often refer to me clearly by name and was heard to call out 'That's *my* dog' when Josie appeared.

As Betty became competent in drying herself and it was time to transfer treatment sessions to the care of ward staff, checklist no. 3 was compiled. During this phase, bathing was transferred to the usual bathroom and was supervised by one of the nurses.

Out of 27 sessions, six were completed by me alone; three by me plus a member of the nursing staff; and 18 by ward staff alone.

Results of Intervention (Bathing)

Out of a total of 43 sessions, she completed seven baths without requiring a prompt (see Figure 6.2). Three of these were supervised by different nurses and four by the author.

During training, Betty completed 34 of the 43 sessions within the comparison group time of between 4½-7½ minutes. Although nine of the sessions were outside the comparison-group time limits, the longest bathtime took only 11 minutes. In the drying stage she completed 40 sessions of the 43 within the comparison-group minimum time of 2 minutes and maximum time of 4 minutes.

The Eating Programme

In view of Betty's distractability and 'dilly-dally' behaviour, she was required to sit at a table away from the other patients in the dining hall. Initially the therapist or a member of ward staff sat at the table with her, and a timer, three photos of Josie, a green card and double-sided sellotape were available for use during the treatment sessions. The therapist planned to record the times she took for each course. Time out from social reinforcement was introduced for any 'dilly-dally' behaviour. I was the therapist for Mondays, Tuesdays and Wednesdays, and on other days of the week, ward nurses carried out the programme. Betty was given the green card to take to the dinner table each Wednesday.

As the soup was placed on the table the therapist set the timer for 5½ minutes, this being the longest time that anybody in the comparison group had taken to eat soup (Betty had eaten her soup once already within the time, during the baseline observations). Once the timer was set, Betty was reminded to finish her soup before the bell sounded. The soup portion was slightly smaller than previously so that she had more chance of being able to consume it within the allotted time. When the soup had vegetables in it, it was strained. Once she became used to eating within the time limit, vegetables were slowly introduced.

If she ate her soup within the allotted time, I gave her praise and stuck photo no. 1 of Josie on the green card as a reinforcer. If she did not finish her soup within the allotted time, I picked up the picture materials and told Betty in as neutral a voice as possible that as she had not eaten her soup within the allotted time she would not be given a photograph of Josie.

As the main course was set in front of her, I set the timer for 15 minutes (the shortest time Betty took during the baseline-observation period and the longest time taken by the comparison group), and reminded her to eat up before the bell sounded. The main course had to be food known to be liked by Betty, and smaller portions were used. I reminded her again during the 15 minutes to 'eat up'. Any 'dilly-dally' behaviour was dealt with by time out from social reinforcement.

If Betty ate her main course within the allotted time, she was given photo no. 2 of Josie, and was praised. If she did not finish within the allotted time, photo no. 1 (for soup) was removed, and no praise was given, her pudding was placed on the table and I picked up the picture materials, explaining why in as neutral a manner as possible.

As her pudding was set in front of her, I set the timer for 5 minutes. On completion of this course (it being generally the case that she would eat her pudding within this time), she was given more praise, and photo no. 3 of Josie was stuck on her card.

When her meal was completed, and if all three Josie photos had been stuck on her card, Betty took the card to the duty room where she was given more praise and she was then able to exchange the three photos for a piece from a Josie jigsaw puzzle. This piece was then stuck on the board above her bed with due ceremony.

There were 36 jigsaw pieces in all, and the occupational therapy department agreed to frame the complete puzzle for Betty to keep.

Results of Eating Programme

Soup. Betty ate within the allotted time in all 28 meals, despite vegetables being introduced in the later sessions. After 16 meals the time allocated was reduced to 4½ minutes. (See Figure 6.5.)

Main Course. Unfortunately there were several unintended variations in the portions provided and it was not possible to guarantee that she be given foods which she liked at each and every meal. However, in only three of the 28 meals was she not able to eat within the time allocated. (See Figure 6.4.)

Puddings. On no occasion did Betty experience any problem in finishing this course within the allotted time. (See Figure 6.5.)

Discussion

The young woman described in this case study has been hospitalised for more than twenty years. As I noted earlier, for many of these years, Betty was the recipient of a 'total care' system, which may have played a large part in fostering the dependence and passivity which were key features in this case. When she was referred for training, she was acknowledged to be very severely handicapped and had proven unresponsive to previous attempts at training in various self-help skills programmes. It should be acknowledged that although personal hygiene problems and the refusal of food are often seen as problems for nursing staff, in this case these were selected for the specific reason that they were noticeably disadvantageous for Betty herself. Staff were concerned about a possible risk to her health through inadequate diet, and the prejudicial effect upon her social relationships of her hygiene problem. It should be noted that from the outset every attempt was made to evaluate both problems objectively: norms for bathing and eating times were established to act as a guide for the intervention phase.

Although both problems were relatively straightforward, the assessment of Betty's bathing and eating performance was rigorous. The careful attention to detail was both time-consuming and demanding for staff, but this rigour may have played a significant part in the achievement of the goals. In particular, it should be noted that the careful analysis of the various stages of bathing undertaken in the assessment provided the basis for the 'training' guide used during the stages of intervention. In a sense, the effort expended in the assessment paid dividends during the treatment phase.

Given that Betty had been involved in a number of other training programmes previously which had shown little success, my own expectations were not high when I first met her. With the accidental discovery of a 'novelty reinforcer' in the form of the dog, we were able to take off in a different direction. This novelty factor was further extended with the use of the 'Josie jigsaw' which was a simple token economy programme translated into a more meaningful format. I was pleased to be able to learn much the same kind of lesson as Isaacs *et al.* (1960) had: that the patient's behaviour is a more important influence on the planning of effective therapy than the therapist's original ideas about the treatment plan.

Given the degree of handicap of the young woman and her length of stay in institutional care, the results of this programme are very encouraging. Although the two programmes required close, individual attention over a 6- to 8-week period, when her 20-year stay is taken into account this training period appears insignificant by comparison. In the case of both problems the goals of 'normal' bathing and eating were realised in the majority of the sessions. In those in which Betty was off target, this was to a minor degree only. Although I have been concerned here only to examine bathing and eating behaviour, it may be that the acquisition of these skills will have other, less specific, psychological benefits for Betty.

References

Ayllon, T. and Azrin, N. (1968) *The Token Economy: a Motivational System for Therapy and Rehabilitation*. Appleton-Century-Crofts, New York

Baer, D.M. 91962) 'Laboratory Control of Thumbsucking by Withdrawal and Re-presentation of Reinforcement', *Journal of the Experimental Analysis of Behaviour, 5*, 525–8

Goffman, E. (1961) *Asylums*, Pelican Books, Harmondsworth

Hemsley, R. and Carr, J. (1980) 'Ways of Increasing Behaviour-reinforcement', in W. Yule and J. Carr (eds), *Behaviour Modification for the Mentally Handicapped*, Croom Helm, London, Ch. 3

Isaacs, W., Thomas, J. and Goldiamond, I. (1960) 'Application of Operant Conditioning to Reinstate Verbal Behaviour in Psychotics', *Journal of Speech and Hearing Disorders, 25*, 8–12

Van Etten, G., Arkell, C. and Van Etten, C. (1980) *The Severely and Profoundly Handicapped*, C.V. Mosby, New York, Ch. 9, p. 308

7 A TIME-LIMITED TREATMENT PROGRAMME FOR PHOBIC AVOIDANCE BEHAVIOUR

Ilse Ablett

Introduction

Is it possible to mistake neurosis for psychosis? *Chambers Twentieth Century Dictionary* defines psychosis as a serious mental disorder, characterised by 'illusions, delusions, hallucinations, mental confusion and a lack of insight into his condition on the part of the patient'. Neurosis, on the other hand, is defined as 'a mental disturbance, usually accompanied by anxiety and obsessional fears'. Hallucinations are usually described as sensory perceptions not founded upon objective reality. In contrast, self-talk is something that we all engage in and is part of the mediational processes of the central nervous system which Mahoney (1974) called 'private events': 'From birth to death, only a very small percentage of a person's behaviours are publicly observable. Our lives are predominantly composed of private responses to private environments . . . ranging from monologues in the shower to senile reveries.' Among the many 'mediational' processes described by Bandura (1969) are *attending* to specific stimuli (the events in our world); labelling or *categorising* such events; and storing such information in a memory. Here Bandura is describing the 'information-processing' model of cognitive psychology. A common feature of such information processing is the kind of self-talk, or self-instruction, which has been closely studied by researchers such as Meichenbaum (1974). The net outcome is that we talk to ourselves in an effort to guide our own behaviour.

Is it possible then to confuse 'self-talk' with hallucinations? Must voices heard inside one's head necessarily be hallucinations? This is one of the issues which was explored in the management of the patient whom I will now describe.

The Subject

Geraldine is about 1.78 m (5 ft 10 in.) tall and of average weight. She

168

is 36 years old, and her eyes are blue and set in an expressive face framed by neatly styled, dark hair. She has a white streak at the front of her hairline of which she is very conscious. She has an elegant posture and is always immaculately dressed, looking as though she had just left a garden party.

Although attractive to others, Geraldine believes that she is very ordinary and that no one would venture a second glance in her direction. She feels vulnerable; she always wears two pairs of tights, and would never wear a short-sleeved garment as she would feel 'too exposed'.

Geraldine is married to a clergyman and the couple have three children, two boys and a little girl. Because her husband practices his profession as an officer in the Navy, the family have to uproot themselves fairly frequently and move to different places. This makes it necessary for Geraldine to be able to socialise with many different poeple.

Geraldine is a trained teacher and, although intelligent, she is inclined to set high standards for herself which at times appear unrealistic.

She was brought up in an upper-middle-class family and has an older brother with whom she does not get on too well. She describes her mother as quiet, warm and tolerant. She had a very close relationship with her until her death. Her father she described as 'the head of the household; his word is law'.

At school Geraldine was bright and always attained good marks. However, she was a nervous child, frightened of the dark, and always eager to please. In her mid-teens she suffered from a variety of ailments and it has been suggested in retrospect that these may have been psychogenic in origin. Her work at school suffered and as a result her 'A' level attainments were poorer than originally expected. As a result, she enrolled at a teachers' training college instead of university, an event which she still sees as her 'big failure'.

While at college, Geraldine became interested in religion and this led to her first meeting with her future husband. They married as soon as she had completed her training and she continued to work part-time as a teacher. Much of the couple's lives centres around the Church and its demanding social activities, making it necessary for Geraldine to be able to entertain and to organise functions.

Geraldine's present problems began in April 1979, six months after her mother's death from cancer of the throat. Her father came on a visit, bringing with him an aunt whom Geraldine had always disliked. They went out for dinner and Geraldine strongly resented the aunt's presence, thinking that it should have been her mother sitting there enjoying herself. During the meal she experienced what she termed detachment from herself for the first time. This was like being 'outside myself — looking on, while my body sat at the dinner table, eating'. From then on, Geraldine developed a range of complaints: claustrophobia, agoraphobia, free-floating anxiety and a variety of physical symptoms. She became progressively more anxious and frightened of this feeling of detachment. To counteract this she took tranquillisers. When she had to attend functions she would sit beside the door so that she could leave quickly. At times she had to sit on the floor for fear that she would faint and fall off the chair. Before any function Geraldine would take diazepam liberally in the belief that this would help her to get her through 'the ordeal'. Instead of coping she became increasingly anxious; she began to shake uncontrollably at the mere thought of meeting people. As a result of this anticipatory anxiety, she experienced palpitations, tremors, cramps, etc. Eventually she felt unable to cope with her commitments and frequently took to her bed as a means of escape. At one stage she believed that she was about to die from a brain tumour, having heard a female voice telling her that she was going to die. She retired to bed completely, as she thought it the most convenient place to 'meet her maker'. She lost 28 lb in weight and was sleeping badly, and her condition continued to deteriorate. She was treated with a variety of drugs, but did not improve. In February 1980 she was diagnosed as 'manic-depressive' and was offered electro-convulsive therapy. After discussion with her husband she refused this and elected to be treated by insight-oriented psychotherapy from a private practitioner. By December 1980 she felt she was incapable of coping with her family, and her cousin had to be asked to come and take care of the household.

By this time Geraldine was unable to go shopping, to meet people, to do her housework or to provide meals for the family. Most of her time was spent in bed, shut away, so that she would not have to face anyone. ECT was offered again and this time she accepted. After completion of eight ECTs there still was no apparent improvement. Geraldine was then prescribed lithium carbonate and amitriptyline, which she takes to this day. She became a day patient, attending the ward three times weekly, and by January 1981 she felt slightly better. Geraldine attributed this to the support which she got from the ward staff. However, she was still unable to go out, to meet people or to cope with her commitments. At the beginning of April 1981, when her anxiety-reducing drugs were discontinued, she went through a particularly 'bad patch' and had to be admitted to hospital for ten days.

During her period as an in-patient on a ward specialising in the treatment of affective disorders she became more aware of what the label 'manic depressive psychosis' implied. She felt very acutely that she was not, and never had been, like some of the patients with whom she shared the ward. Although she was told at a case conference that the general consensus of opinion was that the diagnosis was correct, she refused to believe it. Geraldine expressed feelings of despair. If this diagnosis was correct, she said it meant that her 'condition' was chemical in origin and was totally beyond her control.

Assessment

At the first interview Geraldine presented as an intelligent and energetic woman. She almost fled from the interview room at first when she discovered me there; she had been prepared by nursing staff to meet my supervisor (Philip Barker) only. She displayed marked anxiety at the beginning of the interview, sat facing away from us, with her head and back pressed against the wall and her hand protecting the side of her face. Her free hand was 'flapping' in a marked tremor. She was wide-eyed and appeared highly excited. She complained mainly of numbness all down the side of her body which was facing us. This sensation then turned to pins and needles after approximately ten minutes and the tremor ceased. Then she began to flush, although she was speaking more comfortably by this time. By the end of the interview (45 minutes) she was facing my colleague and me and said she felt no unpleasant somatic sensations of any kind.

She talked a great deal about a feeling of 'detachment', and a variety of somatic sensations (anaesthesia of parts of her body, pins and needles, cramping, etc.). She experienced these sensations only when in company, or when she expected to meet people. These phenomena had been apparent for the past two years.

Geraldine said these problems occurred about ten or twelve times daily. They were relieved slightly by taking diazepam. The 'attacks' lasted either until she, or the other person concerned, left the situation. Adults were more likely to stimulate these 'attacks' than children, although recently, when taking her own children to the cinema in a town near her home, she experienced these sensations all the way there in the car. However, they ceased as soon as she turned to come back *on her own*.

These problems were most evident when she was with people she did not want to be with, or did not like. *Formal* situations she also found highly aversive. Anticipation of any of these venues was enough to bring on an 'attack'. The most common physiological reactions were palpitations and what she referred to as 'shuddering of her internal organs'.

She normally coped with these 'attacks' by leaving (or more likely 'running away' from) the situation. Typically she experienced thoughts of despair as a result. She felt that she would never get over this problem. Usually she would busy herself with some task to occupy her mind. All physiological sensations ceased the moment she ended the social contact.

Geraldine had been very close to her mother. She recalled vividly the first experience of these attacks when her father came to stay with her approximately six months after the funeral. Along with her husband she went out for dinner with her father, who had brought an aunt whom Geraldine did not like. All through dinner she kept thinking 'You are taking my mother's place.' Indeed the aunt was sitting with her father. It is worthy of note that the dining room was one of her key avoidance situations. The social context of that meal in 1979 was also of the *'formal'* nature that she now found unpleasant.

The patient's problem appeared to be that of social anxiety. At a second assessment interview she completed a Fear Survey Schedule which bore out this initial impression. The sensation of 'detachment' of which she complained sounded very like the phenomenon of depersonalisation which is often encountered in cases of severe anxiety. All of her other symptoms are characteristic of intense social anxiety.

Since the night of that formal dinner which took place during a period of extended mourning, her history had been marked by the use of 'escape and avoidance' strategies in increasing abundance and degree. The more she avoided situations, the better she felt; the more she avoided them the more horrendous they appeared in her imaginings.

Problem Summary

Geraldine showed a range of problems, each of which was characterised by anxiety.

(1) She felt extremely anxious (on a psychological level) in any social situation. This varied with the degree of formality; the more formal the occasion, the more likely she would be to feel anxious.

(2) She also experienced anticipatory fear: she was terrified lest she should feel afraid or anxious at an impending social event (in effect a fear of fear).

(3) Her anxiety was also experienced at the physiological level and she reported the following somatic symptoms:

    (a) palpitations
    (b) tremors of all limbs
    (c) flushing
    (d) anaesthesia (of specific parts of her body)
    (e) cramping of various muscle groups
    (f) 'pins and needles'.

(4) In addition to the anxiety features, she had a very poor view of herself. This was apparent in her sensitivity about her height and in her general belief that she was unattractive. This long-standing problem was exacerbated by the attribution of her failure to control her anxiety difficulties to a basic weakness in her own personality.

Intervention

The treatment plan involved two stages, the first dealing with her manifest anxiety, the second with her poor self-image. As Geraldine was shortly to leave the area due to her husband's transfer to another naval base, time was an important issue. In effect the treatment programme would be limited to 30 days.

Stage 1 involved the application of systematic desensitisation and anxiety management techniques.

Systematic Desensitisation

Wolpe (1958) formulated the principle of reciprocal inhibition which stated that if a response antagonistic to anxiety occurred in the presence of anxiety-provoking stimuli, the bond between these stimuli and the anxiety response would be weakened. Adopting Jacobson's (1938) technique of progressive relaxation, Wolpe attempted to inhibit anxiety experienced during exposure to phobic stimuli by teaching the patient to relax. Once mastered, the patient could employ this technique at almost any time, in a variety of situations, both in and outside the therapist's office. It is well known that other measures (e.g. drugs, sexual arousal, expression of anger and eating) can produce the same inhibitory effects as relaxation (Wolpe, 1973).

The anxiety-evoking situations are presented in a hierarchical order, gradually exposing the patient to situations of increasing anxiety-provoking potential. Systematic desensitisation, then, involves two main components: a state that is incompatible with an anxiety response (reciprocal inhibition), and a hierarchy, a series of situations of increasingly higher anxiety-provoking potential. The evidence to support this theory is extensive (Bandura, 1969; Marks, 1969; Goldstein and Chambless, 1977).

Recently it has been suggested that exposure to the fear-evoking stimuli may not really be a necessary condition of fear reduction. De Silva and Rachman (1981) presented evidence quoting seven examples of patients treated by other methods (e.g. assertion training) but also pointed out the need for further research in this direction.

During the first treatment session I explained to Geraldine the overall objective of the programme, which was to reduce anxiety and to help her to live without fear. If successful, this would enable her to take up her responsibilities and become an effective person again.

We also discussed phobias during this session. I explained that a phobia was a persistent fear that frequently led to avoidance of situations which carried no *real* threat. The intensity of her emotional reaction in such situations was out of keeping with the demands of the situation, and by avoidance she gained a feeling of relief which made it less likely that she would face the feared situation in the future. I tried to explain the basis of such fears and how they may be acquired by classical conditioning. We talked about anxiety in more general terms, discussing how difficult it was to separate anxiety and fear; and how anxiety was normal in circumstances which carried real threat. We discussed the different facets of anxiety: (a) cognitive (thinking negatively); (b) behavioural (avoidance patterns); and (c) physiological (muscle tension, increased heart-rate, etc.). I tried to encourage Geraldine by telling her that research had produced a number of effective methods of treatment for such phobic anxiety states.

Desensitisation in Vivo. I explained the rationale of the proposed treatment plan to the patient as follows:

> This treatment is based on the principle that if a response that is antagonistic to anxiety can be made to occur when you are in an "anxiety-provoking" situation, your anxiety is likely to be reduced and ultimately brought under control. To achieve this I am going to teach you how to relax. You will learn how to relax the major muscle groups in your body to achieve a more general state of relaxation. We have also compiled a list of feared situations which we will now rank in order, so that the least feared is first and the most feared situation is last on your list. This is what we call a hierarchy and we will use this list to provide us with the goals for your treatment programme. The overall aim of this part of the programme is to help you to face those specific feared situations. Getting yourself prepared and then going out and facing these situations which until now you have avoided will be the goal of your "therapy".

So far, Geraldine seemed to understand exactly what was required of her and also my role in the programme. She commented, 'It all seems to make sense, what you are saying.'

Anxiety Management

I then proceeded to give a brief explanation of one of the ways in which she might learn to handle her anxiety. I explained that most people suffering from extreme anxiety are sb determined to get the fear-evoking situations out of the way that they rush blindly through them, hoping to succeed by sheer speed and will power. This, of course, simply increases the likelihood of 'panic attacks' occurring. A method of managing is to employ the *WASP procedure*, a cognitive/coping strategy: W, wait; A, absorb; S, slowly; P, proceed. Each letter stands for one basic requirement in the management of anxiety. (cf. Sharpe and Lewis, 1979.) (Further evidence to support the inclusion of coping skills training for anxiety management was produced by Barrios and Shigetomi 1979.)

The important issue of homework was also raised:

'In the sessions we will discuss your next goal and how to approach

achieving it. Between sessions your homework will consist of
exposing yourself to the situation for which we previously prepared
you in the preceding session. Any other problems that may occur will
be dealt with as and when they arise.'

Session I (1 hour). This was the orientation session, the details of
which are described immediately above. At this session Geraldine's
hierarchy of feared situations was also drawn up.

Session II (2 hours). Geraldine was given instruction in relaxation
techniques. The following procedure, which is common to a number
of different relaxation manuals, was adopted. Choose a quiet room,
darken it if the patient finds this more relaxing. Allow your patient to
choose a couch or comfortable chair, whichever is preferred. Get the
patient to settle back as comfortably as possible, and ask the patient to
shut his/her eyes. The therapist begins by telling the patient that he/
she will be asked to relax each group of muscles in turn, covering the
whole of the body. Speaking slowly and deliberately one begins as
follows:
    'Allow yourself to relax to the best of your ability . . . now, as you
relax like that, breathe in and out slowly, notice how, when you
breathe out, you relax a little more. Continue to breathe in and out . . .
taking note of the feeling of relaxation when exhaling. When you are
ready . . . clench your fists, clench your fists tight . . . tighter . . . and
raise your forearms . . . study the tension as you do so . . . study the
tension in your forearms . . . and now let your arms drop and unclench
your fists . . . and relax. Note the difference in the feeling of tension
and relaxation, keeping relaxed all the time, . . . etc.'
    At the end of the session Geraldine was given a pre-recorded
relaxation tape and instructed to practise daily for 15 to 20 minutes
until she became proficient.

Session III (1 hour). Geraldine arrived distressed by intrusive
thoughts (e.g. 'I'm all right now — but how long will it last?').
Intrusion of irrational thoughts is a problem for many patients.
A technique involving snapping a wrist-worn rubber band when the
intrusive thoughts occur has produced good results with cases in
which there are one or two specific intrusive thoughts that occur
regularly at a moderate frequency (Mastellone, 1974). She was
given a rubber band to wear on her wrist and instructed to pull this and
to let go when such thoughts occurred. The reason for this was

explained by pointing out that the short sharp pain would interrupt (stop) this kind of cognitive intrusion. Geraldine reported that she found the relaxation techniques very helpful and was therefore practising them daily.

Session IV (1 hour). Geraldine reported that she had found it difficult to drive across the Tay Bridge as she was frightened that she would hit a lamp post. Arrangements were made for her and the therapist (myself) to drive over the bridge together.

Session V (2 hours). Geraldine drove us across the Tay Bridge and I decided that counting the joints in the concrete road of the bridge would demand sufficient concentration to enable Geraldine to negotiate the bridge. She managed well on the return journey. Geraldine wanted to do some shopping (on her own initiative) but when outside the shop she nearly fled. I managed to persuade her to go in by reminding her to use coping strategies and to relax. Once in the shop, Geraldine coped well. Having visited a shop for the first time in months, she felt extremely pleased.

Session VI (1 hour). Geraldine again successfully completed a homework assignment related to her progress up the hierarchy of feared situations, and I therefore prepared her for the next step in the hierarchy.

Session VII (1 hour). She reported that she had been to church for the first time and had also succeeded in organising a christening party.

Session VIII (1 hour). Geraldine arrived, having had what she called a trying morning. She experienced a 'panic attack' in the bank, but did not flee. She felt very disappointed in herself. We discussed the problem and the need for detailed preparation was again pointed out. Therefore her preparations for a social function which she had to attend with her husband were examined in some detail.

Stage I of the treatment plan had involved 10 hours of therapist-patient contact spread over eight sessions and Geraldine had achieved the first seven items on her hierarchy. Stage II involved the use of a cognitive restructuring procedure and the application of the Premack Principle.

Cognitive Restructuring

The procedures involved in the therapeutic improvement of mediational processes have been variously termed 'cognitive restructuring', 'rational emotive therapy', and 'rational re-evaluation' (Ellis, 1971). The aim is to teach the patient to discriminate, assess and evaluate his thoughts, self-statements and beliefs and then to present realistic alternatives. Mahoney (1974) used the mnemonic aid ADAPT as a cue. Each of the letters in the word represents a cognitive performance element: A, acknowledge; D, discriminate; A, assess; P, present alternatives; T, think praise.

Although the inclusion of cognitive factors is a fairly recent addition to the subject matter of behavioural psychotherapy, there are a number of research studies which provide evidence that mediational processes should not be overlooked, and may indeed play a central role in bringing about therapeutic change (e.g. Ellis, 1962; Beck, 1970; Lazarus, 1971).

The Premack Principle

This is a technique that may be used to increase the occurrence of a low-probability behaviour (e.g. positive self-statements) by pairing it with a high-probability behaviour (e.g. eating, drinking, etc.). This method was widely used in token economy programmes (Ayllon and Azrin, 1968). More recent research has indicated that there is substantial evidence to support the use of this technique (Knapp, 1976).

Session IX (1 hour and 30 minutes). This took the form of a cognitive restructuring session. Through interviewing I identified the following irrational beliefs:

'It is terrible [calamitous] when things don't work out the way I planned.'

'It is necessary to have maximum control over situations.'

'I am indispensible to situations [e.g. social functions]. This makes it essential that I do well and don't break down in such situations.'

'I should cover up my feelings in order to protect myself or to protect others'.

'I must be competent *all the time.*'

Geraldine admitted that she had once believed that her misery was caused by external (or internal) elements which were beyond her control, and that she could not control her emotions. However, she had learned in the past fortnight that these were irrational beliefs and had begun to learn how to stop causing her own misery (e.g. by reducing the frequency of self-defeating statements). By practising relaxation and exposure to feared situations, she was gaining further control over her emotional reactions.

During the session she 'recognised' that her passion for success might be traceable back to her failure at 'O' and 'A' level examinations. She suggested that her 'standards' (in retrospect) might be too high. Two years ago she fell from the pedestal which she had erected for herself. This had become almost as stressful as the 'external' pressure which led to her failure at 'O' and 'A' levels. Although at the beginning of therapy she wanted to 'return to her old self', she now recognised that she might need to aim for a 'new self', one that would be less rigid and one that would be willing to acknowledge that she could be happy and *imperfect*.

I asked her to approach difficult situations by using Mahoney's mnemonic ADAPT as a coping strategy and I offered to discuss her situation with her husband.

Session X. Geraldine was asked to visit my cottage in order to practise calling on someone but she opted out. She had gone to the clinic and had left a message for me to telephone her. I did so and Geraldine apologised and said she would carry out the assignment the following day.

Session XI (1 hour). Geraldine came to the cottage as previously arranged. She coped well, despite the fact that one of my colleagues happened to be there. I discussed her reasons for opting out of accompanying her husband to the social function she had arranged to attend with him. She felt that she had been ready too soon and had too much time on her hands; consequently her anticipatory anxiety became so acute that she forgot her coping strategies and 'just went to pieces'.

Session XII (2 hours). I received a telephone call from Geraldine at 8.30 a.m. She was distressed and felt too frightened to drive across the Tay Bridge. She was asked to wait on her side of the bridge and I promised to meet her as soon as possible in the car park there. I did this and managed to persuade Geraldine to drive across the bridge in her car with me as a passenger, and to give a running commentary of her thoughts and feelings as she drove along. Having done this, we discussed rational responses to her irrational thoughts, and the use of coping strategies. We then agreed to go to the bank and into the shopping centres in Dundee. We visited the bank and a variety of stores. Geraldine felt some anxiety but employed the WASP strategy effectively. She was then persuaded to visit a crowded coffee bar where she did the ordering and spoke to the waitress, and felt that she had coped well. She was very pleased with her achievements. We drove back across the bridge and Geraldine experienced no anxiety in the course of this journey.

Session XIII (1 hour). We discussed her list of positive self-statements as well as her negative thoughts about her height and appearance. The Premack Principle was explained to Geraldine and the positive statements to be transferred to 'cue cards' were decided upon. She was asked to carry them on her person at all times and to make a point of reading them to herself every time she visited the WC and when she took her medication. I explained that both the visits to the WC and the taking of her medication were high-probability behaviours. Making self-positive statements in her case was a low-probability behaviour, and by linking this to the above-mentioned activities the positive self-statements were likely to increase.

Session XIV (1 hour). Geraldine and her husband were seen together. The significance of her husband's constructive support was discussed and we agreed on ways in which he could best help Geraldine to set and achieve her goals.

Session XV (1 hour). This was the final session as Geraldine was due to leave the area the next day. We discussed and prepared her for the forthcoming train journey. She had to travel with the children, her husband having left the previous day to commence his new duties. Geraldine felt that she did not wish to recommence therapy with a different therapist. As she had improved so well with the range of methods I had employed, I decided to carry on treating her by exchanging tape recordings. We said goodbye and I wished her continuing success.

Results and Discussion

This programme involved aiming for fairly simple targets. However, the programme was complicated by my attempts to tailor the programme to suit the patient; doing this largely on a day-to-day basis. As I have noted already, the patient's problems were focused upon anxiety in various social and interpersonal settings. Her attempts to understand 'what was happening' to her gave an added dimension to her free-floating anxiety state.

A number of targets were established at the beginning of treatment. These are summarised in Table 7.1, along with the patient's ratings of *importance*, *experience of anxiety* and present *ability* to handle such situations. The targets listed below showed an interesting mix of specific phobic complaints, e.g. staying in a room with the door closed; various social problems (doing the shopping) and interpersonal ones (receiving visitors at her home). The extent to which these problems undermined her everyday existence can only be appreciated by understanding the demands made upon her as mother, patient and the wife of a naval parson. This latter role carried a heavy responsibility for her to be consistently cheerful, sociable and eminently capable.

As the table shows, before the therapy programme began, Geraldine experienced marked anxiety in all ten situations. By the completion of the short course of therapy, this distress had reduced to zero in four situations; to a level of 2 when meeting someone by chance in the street; with a minimal level of 1 being recorded for the remaining five problems.

During the therapy contact, some brief attention was paid to analysing and modifying Geraldine's negative thinking patterns. When she was asked to describe how she felt, invariably she would offer extreme views about the 'awesomeness' of the task, or of her 'complete inability' to cope. Because of her impending departure, there was not sufficient time available to mount a formal 'cognitive-therapy' programme. However, Geraldine was encouraged to identify her major 'thinking errors' and was helped to challenge these in a simple fashion. The use of the simple mnemonics (WASP and ADAPT) proved particularly useful in this context.

Following her departure from the area, Geraldine maintained contact by means of exchanging tape recordings. She reported her progress and any problems encountered: I offered guidance and reinforced the use of her various coping strategies. She continued to set goals for herself and monitored her own progress. Eight weeks after her departure she reported continued improvement; this despite the stress of having moved into new surroundings and being required to meet a number of new people. During this brief period she reported that she had attended various social functions; was running a Sunday

Table 7.1: Major Targets: Pre- and Post-ratings. ((Importance, anxiety and ability are graded on a scale from 0 (low) to 10 (high))

Targets	Importance		Anxiety		Ability	
	Pre-	Post-	Pre-	Post-	Pre-	Post-
Watching TV with children	8	8	7	0	3	10
Staying in a room with door closed	8	8	9	0	4	10
Chance meeting outside the home	10	10	9	2	1	9
Keeping doctor's appointments	10	10	10	1	2	10
Eating meals with the family	9	9	10	0	0	10
Going shopping alone	9	9	9	1	0	9
Driving (with a passenger)	10	10	9	0	3	10
Receiving visitors at home	10	10	10	1	0	10
Visiting friends and relatives	10	10	10	1	0	10
Attending social functions	10	10	10	1	0	10

School class; felt 'well and energetic'; and was once again able to manage her household unaided. Geraldine was still taking the same medication she had been prescribed in Dundee. However, as she had been taking this for some considerable time prior to her admission to hospital, its role in facilitating her recovery must be seriously questioned. Perhaps the most significant feature of this therapy contact was that a patient who was originally labelled with a psychotic depressive disorder was assisted largely by focusing upon her everyday 'problems of living'. I do not wish to challenge the diagnosis originally proposed for Geraldine. However, as she herself noted at the time, the apparent intractability of such a diagnosis gave her further cause for concern, rather than any kind of reassurance. In conclusion, I thought that it would be appropriate to ask Geraldine to offer he own critical impressions of her experience on the receiving end of therapy. The following comments are included with the full permission of the patient.

My present illness, the first of its kind for me, began in April 1979. It was treated with a variety of drugs until February 1980 when ECT was recommended, although no explanations or reasons were given. I refused it and was treated again with drugs, and with psychotherapy, for which I paid. My condition continued to deteriorate until December 1980 when I accepted ECT out of desperation. There was no apparent improvement and I moved to hospital where I was treated with lithium carbonate and amitriptyline. I am still taking both of these drugs.

Initially, in January 1981, there was an improvement which I felt was due in part to the support I received from the ward staff during the three mornings that I spent there each week. But progress remained slow. After a particularly bad patch in April, when my anxiety-inhibiting medication was discontinued, I was introduced to Phil and Ilse.

Our first conversation was very much a joint one. I was allowed to say as much as I wanted, and my contribution was not dismissed as incorrect or irrelevant. Immediately what they were saying made sense and the clouds on the horizon did not seem so dark. In addition, I was given something to do, something for which I could work, and something which was not beyond my reach. One of my main problems with the manic-depressive diagnosis was that if my condition was chemical in origin, there was nothing I could do about it. And so I sank deeper and deeper into the mud.

Since being introduced to behaviour therapy I have followed an upward path. I am better now than I have been for several years, in spite of moving to a new home 400 miles from Dundee, and being quite unknown when I arrived. I intend to continue with this therapy as long as is necessary. Several reasons spring at once to mind when trying to account for its success: first and most important, it makes sense; the pace and direction are mine; it is constantly supportive, in that I follow at home a code of behaviour worked out at the hospital — I don't feel that I am trying to climb a mountain unaided; it is flexible and can be adjusted to fit new problems as they arise; it is positive and looks forward to health, and so I no longer think of myself as ill. I honestly believe, at the time of writing, that it is behaviour therapy as applied by Phil and Ilse that has prompted my recovery.

[*Editors' Note:* When Geraldine was contacted to request permission to publish a report of her treatment, we found that she had maintained the progress reported here. It is now some four years since the end of her formal therapy contact with Ilse Ablett. She also noted that 'I have been able to pass on something of what I learned to others experiencing similar problems.']

References

Ayllon, T. and Azrin, H.N. (1968) *The Token Economy: a Motivational System for Therapy and Rehabilitation*, Appleton-Century-Crofts, New York

Bandura, A. (1969) *Principles of Behaviour Modification*, Holt, Rinehart & Winston, New York

Barrios, B.A. and Shigetomi, C.C. (1979) 'Coping Skills Training for the Management of Anxiety: a Critical Review', *Behaviour Therapy*, *10*, 491–522

Beck, A.T. (1970) 'Cognitive Therapy: Nature and Relation to Behaviour Therapy', *Behaviour Therapy*, *1*, 184–200

De Silva, P. and Rachman, S. (1981) 'Is Exposure a Necessary Condition for Fear-reduction?', *Behaviour Research and Therapy*, *19*, 227–32

Ellis, A. (1962) *Reason and Emotion in Psychotherapy*, Stuart, New York

Ellis, A. (1971) *Growth through Reason*, Science and Behaviour Books, Palo Alto

Goldstein, A.J. and Chambless, D.L. (1977) 'A Reanalysis of Agoraphobia', *Behaviour Therapy*, *8*, 47–59

Jacobson, E. (1938) *Progressive Relaxation*, University of Chicago Press, Chicago

Knapp, T.J. (1976) 'The Premack Principle in Human Experimental and Applied Settings', *Behaviour Research and Therapy*, *14*, 133–47

Lazarus, A.A. (1971) *Behaviour Therapy and Beyond*, McGraw-Hill, New York

Mahoney, M.J. (1974) Cognition and Behaviour Modification, Ballinger, Cambridge, Mass.

Marks, I.M. (1969) *Fears and Phobias*, Heinemann, London

Mastellone, M. (1974) 'Aversion Therapy: a New Use for the Old Rubber Band', *Journal of Behaviour and Experimental Psychiatry*, 5, 311–12

Meichenbaum, D. (1974) *Cognitive Behaviour Modification*, General Learning Press, New Jersey

Sharpe, R. and Lewis, D. (1979) *Anxiety Antidote*, Souvenir Press, London

Wolpe, J. (1958) *Psychotherapy by Reciprocal Inhibition*, Stanford University Press, Stanford

Wolpe, J. (1973) *The Practice of Behaviour Therapy*, 2nd edn, Pergamon Press, New York

8 INCREASING THE SPEECH OUTPUT OF A MENTALLY HANDICAPPED MAN

Lydia M. Stephenson

Introduction

It is difficult to report accurately the frequency of language deficits in the mentally handicapped population, since both definitions of language handicap and survey methods vary widely. However, it appears that language problems and speech difficulties are exceedingly common. Spreen (1965), in a review of studies on the relationship between IQ and speech and language disorder in adults, reports that the frequency of language handicaps is 100 per cent below an IQ of 20, around 90% in the 21–50 IQ range, and about 45 per cent in the mildly retarded group. Gould (1977) found similar levels of language disability in children. Over 50 per cent of those with an IQ below 70 showed severe language problems, and in children with an IQ below 20, comprehension and spoken language were virtually absent.

Alternatively, Wing and Brown (1970) cite a prevalence rate of poverty of speech as ranging from 23 to 56 per cent in a sample of schizophrenic patients who had been in hospital for more than 2 years and who were aged 60 or less.

Definition

Poverty of speech refers to 'vague, wandering, repetitive or stereotyped speech which renders an interview almost impossible' and to 'muteness or near muteness' (Wing and Brown, 1970). It can be found in individuals who have never learned to speak (e.g. the severely handicapped individual), in individuals who have lost the physical ability to speak (e.g. as a result of brain damage), and in individuals who have lost the motivation to speak. In this latter category fall a proportion of patients resident in institutions for a long period of time. The type of people resident in institutions for longer than 2 years includes those with chronic mental illness, e.g. schizophrenia, people with senile dementia, mentally handicapped individuals, non-demented geriatrics and children in residential care.

186

Institutionalisation

Those who are resident in institutions are, by the very nature of the environment in which they live, at a disadvantage in terms of learning new verbal skills or maintaining any verbal skills they may have. Institutionalisation refers to personal changes brought about by prolonged residence in a relatively closed community. It is not specific only to people resident in long-stay hospitals, but occurs also in other institutions such as prisons. However I wish to concern myself here only with long-stay hospitals. Gruenberg (1967) referred to these personal changes as the 'social breakdown syndrome', comprising behaviours such as loss of initiative, a reduced involvement in recreational activities, neglect of self-care skills and the performance of dangerous and annoying behaviours. In contrast Goffman (1961) mentions behaviours such as dependency, apathy, withdrawal and a lack of responsibility. He also identified several undesirable elements within the institution itself; drawing attention to the distance between staff and patients, with little interaction between the two; to the decisions made by those in authority, with little reference to the individual; to the lack of contact with non-insitutional life; and to the lack of opportunity to practise everyday skills. Although Goffman described these elements in 1961, unfortunately his analysis may be appropriate to many of our long-stay hospitals today.

Later studies looking specifically at nurse-patient interaction (e.g. Paton and Stirling, 1974; Altshul, 1970, 1974) have noticed several features of interest. First, the bulk of conversation from nurses to patients is in the form of instructions, demanding little and receiving little in the way of reply from the patients concerned. Secondly, a genuine attempt at conversation initiated by nurses is infrequent, although patients do respond to this type of interaction on most occasions. Thirdly, patients who have been in hospital longer than eight weeks interact little with nursing staff. Nurses were found to interact more frequently with the less institutionalised patients. Fraser and Cormack (1975) state that 'despite the knowledge that the enrichment of a patient's environment is so important in the treatment of schizophrenic patients, nurse-patient interaction is either not taking place, or is progressing unsystematically'. They argue that nurses should be, but generally are not the principal agents of change in any programme of therapy aimed at reversing institutionalisation.

Possible Causes

Wing and Brown (1970) have demonstrated that a substantial

proportion of the poverty of speech witnessed in the schizophrenic population is caused by their poor social environment. Having nothing to do all day; having no contact with the outside world; having few personal possessions; being regarded pessimistically by nurses; all tend to exacerbate poverty of speech. Altschul (1970, 1974) and Fraser and Cormack (1975) suggested that impoverished styles of nurse-patient interaction taking place within our hospitals are also contributing to the poverty-of-speech syndrome.

At this stage I feel it is important to differentiate between types of speech problem:

(1) Total mutism can be a result of never having learned the skill of speaking, or it may be attributable to lack of motivation or lack of opportunity.

(2) Near-mutism refers to patients who fail to speak spontaneously, but who do have speech abilities since they have been heard to speak in the past. Such individuals do not initiate conversation, though they have been observed replying to other patients or to staff. However, such replies are, characteristically, very brief.

Poverty of speech is the term used for both of the above by Wing and Brown (1970), but in this study it refers to limited non-spontaneous speech as described in (2) above.

Previous Behavioural Treatment Studies

One of the earliest studies to demonstrate the effectiveness of behavioural techniques in reinstating speech was that of Isaacs, Thomas and Goldiamond (1960). They reported some success in the use of a shaping procedure to reinstate speech in a male schizophrenic patient who had a history of 19 years of mutism by using cigarettes and chewing gum as reinforcement, first for lip movements, and later for any form of vocalisation. However, Lovaas, Berberich, Perloff and Schaeffer (1966) found that although children could learn a few words in this manner, i.e. by reinforcing them (usually with bites of food) for random vocalisations, better results were obtained by direct training of imitative responses, rather than by merely reinforcing chance vocalisations. Thomson, Fraser and McDougall (1974) suggest, contrary to the conclusions of Sherman (1965), that it is not sufficient to reinforce only single words and to expect sentence production to emerge spontaneously. Instead they state that it is necessary to design the treatment programme specifically with the aim of sentence production by progressively raising the criteria for the delivery of reinforcement. Lindsay, Taylor and McDonald (1976) taught patients who could answer questions, but who rarely initiated conversation, to ask questions. Patients were instructed to ask questions of the therapist, and later of each other. Money and attention were given contingently on the occurrence of speech. Fraser, Anderson and Grime (1981) report success in reinstating speech in a male schizophrenic patient who had a history of 48 years of total mutism, using a package of behavioural techniques but programming for generalisation of treatment effects across individuals and across settings. In his study, Lindsay (1982) incorporated a method of social comparison. This involved comparing patient performance in conversational skills with the behaviour of peers who were considered competent in the skills being treated. Observation of competent individuals can provide specific behavioural targets for training, and can also establish a normal range of behaviour to assist in the assessment and the effectiveness of treatment. In addition the conversation of patient groups was analysed by Lindsay to determine the extent to which patients' conversation differs from normal patterns of conversation. This was achieved by comparing a group of long-term psychiatric patients with manual workers in employment, both prior to and after the patient group had undergone a period of social skills training.

In the following case study I shall attempt to illustrate how the long-term goal of the development of general conversational skills is achieved. This will include a description of how the intermediate steps taken can contribute towards improving the patient's quality of life.

The treatment package described in this study involves the techniques of instructions, prompting, goal-setting and programming for generalisation across settings and individuals.

Description of Patient

Donald is a small, well-built, single man in his early forties. He lives with 26 other men in a single-sex ward in the local hospital for the mentally handicapped.

He was admitted from his family home at 11 years of age; his mother was reported to be suffering from a heart complaint and his father complained of 'nerves'. His parents felt they could no longer cope with the demands Donald made on them in terms of caring for his everyday needs. The family circumstances were described as fairly impoverished and they lived in a rather deprived area of Dundee. His mother was thought to be of low intelligence. Donald has an older sister who emigrated to Canada in her early twenties. Donald's early childhood development was slow: he did not walk until he was 5 years, he was described as withdrawn, and between the ages of 4 to 8 years he was observed to rock for lengthy periods and he appeared oblivious to his surroundings. His speech development was reported as being slow.

On admission to hospital, Donald was reported to be overactive and troublesome. He would mutilate his skin and he still bears the scars from this period in his life. He was classed as moderately mentally handicapped. However, during his last 30 years in hospital, his diagnoses have differed. In 1973 a differential diagnosis of 'simple schizophrenia' was made, whereas in 1975 he was thought to have 'early infantile autism'.

Donald has never worked in either sheltered or open employment. His day revolves around ward-based therapy which includes him in performing simple tasks such as potato printing, glueing sticks for plant-pot holders, and painting. His other activities include attending keep-fit classes within the hospital twice weekly, visiting the hospital recreational hall when concerts or dances are being held, and going to social functions outside the hospital (supervised by the ward staff), such as bus-trips to places of local interest, or organised holidays. His parents have visited him only twice in the past year. When visiting, the father seldom talks to Donald or indeed anyone, and when his mother takes Donald out for a walk in the grounds, she has been observed to walk several paces behind him. Donald has always been described as a 'loner' throughout his 30 years in hospital.

The Referral

Donald was referred to the psychology department and by the ward team for the following problems: he was rarely heard to speak; he gave poor eye contact; and he appeared to have an extremely short attention span.

Initial Assessment

Assessment of Donald was undertaken in the following manner:

(1) Referral to medical case notes. Objectives:

(a) to become familiar with the patient's past social and medical history;
(b) to record specific information, e.g. date of birth, date of admission to hospital, present address of parents, etc.

(2) Interviews with ward staff. The objectives of the initial interview were:

(a) to introduce myself and explain my goals for the first and subsequent interviews with the staff;
(b) to take a personal history of the patient;
(c) to take a brief history of the development of Donald's problems;
(d) to find out how these problems affected his daily life;
(e) to identify the staff's expectations of any proposed treatment programme;
(f) to outline his assets and deficits;
(g) to complete a motivational analysis of the patient;
(h) to find out why the referred problems were seen as problems and by whom.

(3) Direct observation of the patient. Objectives:

(a) to assist in formulating my own clinical judgement of the patient;
(b) to provide an objective view of Donald's presenting problems.

(4) Global assessment. For this purpose the Everyday Living Skills Inventory (ELSI) was used.

The information gathered from these initial assessments, i.e. from case notes, interviews with ward staff, direct observation and global assessment, revealed the following.

Previous Therapy. Donald had had previous behavioural therapy for the problem of 'lack of social interaction'. This was commenced in June 1981 by a behaviour therapy nursing student. The procedure involved 15-minute sessions provided daily in the therapy room of Donald's ward. The 15-minute sessions were broken up into a 5-minute session of 'physical games', e.g. throwing a ball, clapping hands, etc., to increase physical contact with Donald; a 5-minute session involving attention to task, e.g. colour matching, block building; and a 5-minute session involving tasks with which he was familiar, e.g. jigsaws. Donald was reinforced with praise and sweets for attending to task and for smiling. Unfortunately the programme was discontinued due to an outbreak of salmonella poisoning. Further treatment of Donald's maladaptive behaviour, e.g. rocking and pacing, was commenced by a clinical psychologist in January 1982. This programme involved differential reinforcement of any other behaviour, i.e. the ward nurses would simply approach Donald and give him a sweet on occasions on which he was observed not to be engaged in maladaptive behaviour. This procedure resulted in a slight drop in Donald's maladaptive behaviour but his progress was not maintained when reinforcement was faded out of the programme.

Interviews with Staff. Donald was described by the staff as having a range of problems. He was referred to as a very withdrawn and socially isolated man who sought little contact with either staff or peers in the ward: 'When he is approached by his peers or nursing staff he looks anxious and threatened. He avoids eye contact, darts away and starts mumbling to himself.' They said that very rarely had he been heard to speak spontaneously. On rare occasions he repeated the last word said to him after a few seconds' delay. When spoken to, he often jumped and would hold his hands up to his face. When the nurses were around him, he would speak more to himself, and this was also the case when he was in the ward dining-room and bathroom. He avoided eye contact by turning his head away from the direction of the speaker, or by darting off in the opposite direction. The longest they reported him holding eye-contact for was 3 seconds, although they noticed that he gave more eye contact when in the ward toilet area and on social outings, or when food or drink was being offered.

During the ward-based therapy sessions his attention span was described as being short. 'Donald is easily distracted, he looks out of the window, or looks away from the task in hand or from the person giving him the task, and needs to be verbally prompted to attend to task.' The longest time the ward staff reported that he spent on task was three-quarters of an hour, and the shortest half an hour.

Clinical Impression. Through direct observation of Donald in his natural setting I gained a picture of an extremely threatened and anxious-looking individual. When I entered the ward, Donald was pacing up and down at the far end of the ward, well away from the other residents, who were sitting watching the television in a group. He often stopped to flick imaginary dust off a table and was heard to mumble under his breath. When I walked up to Donald and said hello and gave my name, he immediately turned his head away, plucked at his jersey, started to mumble under his breath, and was heard to say 'You'. He then darted off out of the day room, still mumbling under his breath.

This very aptly demonstrated just how anxious and socially isolated Donald was, and because of this initial impression I felt it inadvisable to pursue any further contact with him that might have served to increase his anxiety.

A summary of the findings from this initial assessment period now follows.

Low-level assets (these are skills which are defined as being present, but which could be increased with further training):

(1) Basic domestic skills, but he requires constant supervision.
(2) He can go to hospital shop, but he requires a written note.
(3) Fork-and-knife usage — requires supervision.
(4) Shaving — requires prompting and supervision.
(5) Group activities — requires constant verbal prompting.

Potential assets (these are skills which are not performed as a result of a lack of opportunity or other restrictions imposed by institutional life):

(1) Basic cooking skills.
(2) Budgeting skills.

Problems defined:

(1) Infrequent speech.
(2) Poor eye contact.
(3) Short attention span.

Additional problems:

(1) *Stereotyped behaviour.* Rocking, pacing, pill-rolling finger movements, flicking imaginary dust from clothes or tables.
(2) *Eating skills.* Eats food too quickly.
(3) *Personal hygiene.* Poor toilet hygiene, smearing toilet seat with faeces and occasionally urinating in public places.

Motivational Analysis. Donald likes sweets, fruit juice and most things that are edible. He also enjoys a pint of lager when on social outings. There are no people in the ward whom he seeks out to be with or whom he appears to dislike more than others. Staff approval is thought to be important to him. He used to enjoy visits from his parents but this was thought by staff to be due to the sweets they brought him.

Problem Analysis. From the information gained from the initial assessments, I hypothesised, first, that Donald's lack of social interaction might be due to the length of time spent living in an institution in which it was not required of him to verbalise frequently; and, secondly, that in his early years he did not come from a family environment which encouraged his speech.

After a discussion with ward staff they informed me that, because of Donald's poor social interaction with themselves and with the residents of his ward and his inability to express his wishes, they could only guess at identifying his needs. This was causing the staff to feel frustrated and sometimes helpless, and it was limiting their provision of care to Donald. They also felt that it would be in Donald's best interests to attempt to increase his social interaction with others as this was limiting Donald's exercise of choice in his life. However, Donald had not expressed a wish for help with this problem.

It was therefore agreed to submit to closer analysis the problems of infrequent speech, and of poor eye contact. As his short attention span was viewed as a less serious problem in the light of the above assessments, no treatment was proposed at this stage. A cost-benefit analysis was compiled and discussed with the ward team (see Appendix 8.1). The object of the cost-benefit analysis was to identify the advantages or benefits which would accrue to the patient, the ward staff and the therapist by implementing a treatment programme for the two problems listed, and to determine the costs or disadvantages of implementing such a programme. In the light of this cost-benefit analysis a decision was made to proceed with treatment.

Baseline Measures

During the initial assessment period the ward staff reported that Donald rarely spoke spontaneously and gave little eye contact. The baseline measures were therefore designed to assess Donald's verbal abilities and his level of eye contact. This involved carrying out, first, ten 15-minute assessment sessions in a quiet room off the ward (known as the therapy room) with few distractions, and then ten 15-minute assessment sessions in the main ward day room, which was a more representative institutional setting with many distractions.

In each session Donald was asked 15 simple questions and each session was structured in the following way. The first six questions required Donald to identify either objects or colours; the next three questions required him to describe the action taking place in pictures; then three further questions were asked about the pictures; and finally, three open-ended questions were chosen to relate to Donald's everyday life (see Appendix 8.2). No prompting, instructions or reinforcement was used during these baseline sessions. Donald was simply asked a question, and after a 10-second delay to allow Donald to answer, the person running the session would move on to the next question. These baseline sessions were carried out by myself and by the permanent staff of the ward.

Donald's replies were measured in terms of word frequency and length of eye contact given. These responses were further divided into incorrect replies and correct replies (see Appendix 8.3).

Results of the Baseline Assessment Sessions

The data from these sessions demonstrated that Donald did have some functional speech. The mean level of correct words spoken in each session was 3, both in the therapy room and in the day room. These responses consisted of one-word answers. The percentage of appropriate eye contact to each question asked was 40 per cent in the therapy room and only 29 per cent in the day room. Appropriate eye contact was judged to be that which was given for at least half of the duration of each question. Only correct replies were considered to be acceptable; however, failures to reply, grunts or mumbles and incorrect replies were recorded. The reason for this was that if no appropriate speech was apparent, then any further treatment programme would have to begin at a much more basic level (cf. Sherman, 1965).

Programme Planning

In developing a programme for Donald, my aim was to develop a behavioural programme that would take into account the fact that my own part in carrying out the programme would be limited as a result of my short-term placement in this ward. Therefore the aim was to produce a behavioural programme which would meet the following criteria:

(a) It could be carried out by the nursing staff in Donald's ward, initially under my supervision.
(b) It would take into account the present nursing resources on the ward.
(c) It would require little in the way of previous behavioral training of the nurses.
(d) It could be planned well into the future, and at a later date it could be carried on by the ward staff under the supervision of the charge nurse on the ward.

From baseline sessions it was shown that Donald did not use speech spontaneously and also that when asked questions he either replied with a one-word answer or by grunting, or gave no reply at all. Therefore the three goals set for treatment were as follows:

Stage I, *short-term goal*: aim to increase Donald's skills in answering questions.
Stage II, *medium-term goal*: aim to increase Donald's verbal skills in answering and asking questions.
Stage III, *long-term goal*: aim to increase Donald's skills in social interaction in a small group setting.

Intervention Stage I. Initially a sub-target was set within the first intervention stage, as we wished Donald to achieve a socially valid change. For this purpose we asked the best speaker in his ward to answer the same 15 questions used during the baseline sessions that we would continue to use throughout the first intervention stage. We used his results as the target for change, and if Donald reached this target (which was 33 words), then the programme would move from the therapy room into the day room.

Intervention was therefore commenced in the therapy room. By introducing the treatment sessions into the day-room setting at a later date, we would be programming for generalisation of the newly acquired behaviours.

Staff Training. As mentioned earlier, it was considered important that the ward staff learn how to administer the treatment programme because of my brief period of placement in this ward. To facilitate this development, three steps were taken:

(1) The staff were given a detailed explanation of the techniques to be

used in the programme.

(2) Each member of staff was given a written handout which described the format of the programme.

(3) All staff were involved in several role-play sessions in which they practised administering the treatment programme.

As we wished Donald to be able to generalise his verbalisations rather than responding solely to one person, we formed a pool of nurses who could administer the programme. This pool included nurses at different stages in training, trained nurses, and nursing assistants.

Procedure. Each session lasted approximately 15 minutes. The nursing staff acted as therapists under the supervision of the author. The same 15 questions and picture cards that were used in the baseline sessions were used in this first stage of intervention. The questions were chosen to give Donald a variety of possible responses, and they were graded in an attempt to elicit phrases and sentences. The techniques of instruction and prompting were used (see Appendix 8.4). Instructions involved explaining to Donald the behaviour that was required of him. Prompting involved eliciting the desired response from Donald.

Each of the 15 questions was asked in each session and if Donald did not respond to a question within 10 seconds, the prompts came into force. For each question, four levels of prompt were used, each giving successively more help in an attempt to elicit an answer. At the first prompt level, the therapist asked the question, e.g. 'What's happening in the picture?'. The kind of response given by Donald determined which of the following three consequences ensued:

(1) He might answer inappropriately, or remain silent, in which case the therapist would go on to the next prompt level.

(2) He might give an appropriate answer, in which case the therapist would go on to the next question.

(3) He might give an appropriate short answer to the last six questions, e.g. 'Floor'. However, for the last six questions, an appropriate reply was judged to be one of at least three words; therefore, if he replied with a one-word answer, the nurse would move on to the next prompt level until a longer reply was given.

Measures. Donald's performance was recorded throughout the programme by the following frequency counts which were taken by the therapist of the following:

(a) the total number of appropriate words spoken in answer to questions asked;
(b) the number of prompts required;
(c) the duration of eye contact given to each question. (see Appendix 8.5.)

Results of Intervention Stage I. Donald is now speaking on average 23 words in each treatment session in the therapy room. He is using single words and short phrases and sentences. His eye contact has increased to 88 per cent over the 15 questions asked. He has not reached the socially valid change target of 33 words. (See Table 8.1.)

Table 8.1: Results of Intervention Stage I

Correct replies	Baseline	Treatment
Words spoken	3	23
% Eye contact	40	88

Some generalisation outside the formal sessions has been reported by the ward staff, although this is not currently being measured, e.g. he has *told* the nurses 'I've got a sore gum', which led to his receiving treatment.

Discussion

The first intervention stage involved the use of the techniques of instructions and prompting. Only instructions and prompts were used during this period as it had been argued in the treatment literature that giving the patient information and instructions and combining this with prompting the desired response is often sufficient (Fraser, 1983). The therapist's verbal interactions with the patient and her demonstration of pleasure at his correct responses through facial expression were thought likely to be reinforcing. As a result, no other form of reinforcement was introduced. However, the nurses found it difficult to withhold verbal praise, and on reflection I feel that the addition of this variable would be likely to help Donald to achieve his target more quickly. The addition of this variable to the treatment programme has, therefore, now been accepted. In attempting to programme for socially significant change, problems were encountered. One of the main difficulties is in choosing whom to select as competent individuals. Several studies have been used to compare children's problem behaviour after treatment with that of their non-deviant peers (Patterson, 1974; Walker and Hops, 1976); to compare mentally handicapped adults' problem eating behaviour after treatment with hospital employees' eating habits (Azrin and Armstrong, 1973), and to assess the outcome of heterosocial skills training programmes (McFall and Twentyman, 1973). This method has several strengths: it can provide upper as well as lower limits of normal functioning. However, as Kazdin (1977) points out, the standard peer group performance may not reflect an optimum level of behaviour. For example, on a ward of long-stay psychiatric patients in which the level of social interaction is generally low, to train the most withdrawn patient to the level of his peers may be to adopt an inadequate criterion. Here it would probably be more appropriate to instigate treatment programmes for the whole ward of patients and to use socially validated criteria from sources outside the ward or hospital area. On the other hand, using the verbose conversation of frequent party-goers would be an over-rigorous criterion for the same population group. Therefore it is important to choose standards that are realistic in relation to the patient.

In Donald's case was it fair to expect him to jump from being the worst speaker in the ward to the level of the best? Using an *average* speaker in the ward would be a more feasible target, and this modification to the programme has now been adopted. However, this does illustrate the need for careful consideration in setting targets for change.

It is felt that Donald's general level of sociability has improved. When approached now, he does not dart away, and he speaks and gives eye contact. There have been many instances of generalisation reported by the staff and they feel that he can exercise more choice now by stating his needs. The programme will continue with the recent alterations made to it, and it is intended that Donald will progress on to his medium- and long-term goals.

Conclusion

In conclusion, I feel that this programme demonstrates to some extent the possibilities for developing the verbal abilities of some mentally handicapped individuals. It also shows that nursing staff can effectively carry out a complicated behavioural programme, given a structured plan of treatment. No extra staffing was required as the programme accounted for only a fraction of the total duties of the nurses who acted as therapists, and it in no way limited their other activities.

Also, given that Donald has been variously described as severely mentally retarded, autistic and schizophrenic, the gains that he has made may have added significance in terms of his future management.

Finally, perhaps if we as nurses were more aware of and made more use of our potential to interact therapeutically with our patients, formal treatment programmes of the type described here might not be required.

References

Altschul, A.T. (1970) 'Go and Talk to the Patients', *Nursing Mirror*, April 10
Altschul, A.T. (1974) 'Relationships between Patients and Nurses in Psychiatric Wards', *International Journal of Nursing Studies*, 8, 179–84
Azrin, N.H. and Armstrong, P.M. (1973) 'The "Mini-meal" — a Method for Teaching Eating Skills to the Profoundly Retarded', *Mental Retardation*, 11, 9–13
Fraser, D. (1983) 'From Token Economy to Social Information System', in E. Karas, (ed.), *Current Issues in Clinical Psychology*, Plenum Press, New York
Fraser, D., Anderson, J. and Grime, J. (1981) 'An Analysis of the Progressive Development of Vocal Responses in a Mute Schizophrenic Patient', *Behavioural Psychotherapy*, 9, 2–12
Fraser, D. and Cormack, D. (1975) 'The Nurse's Role in Psychiatric Institutions', *Nursing Times*, 71, 125–32
Goffman, E. (1961) *Asylums*, Penguin Books, Harmondsworth
Gould, J. (1977) 'Language Development and Non-verbal Skills in Severely Mentally Retarded Children', *Journal of Mental Deficiency Research*, 20, 129–45
Gruenberg, E.G. (1967) 'The Social Breakdown Syndrome — Some Origins', *American Journal of Psychiatry*, 123, 1481–8
Isaacs, W., Thomas, J. and Goldiamond, I. (1966) 'Application of Operant Conditioning to Reinstate Speech in Psychotics', *Journal of Speech and Hearing Disorders*, 25, 8–12
Kazdin, A.E. (1977) 'Assessing the Clinical or Applied Importance of Behavioural Change through Social Validation', *Behavioural Modification*, 1, 427–51
Lindsay, W.R. (1982) 'Some Normative Goals for Conversation Training', *Behavioural Psychotherapy*, 10, 253–72
Lindsay, W.R., Taylor, V. and McDonald, S. (1976) 'A Programme to Increase the

Frequency of Conversation in Long-term Psychiatric Patients', presented to the Annual Conference of the British Psychological Society, Abstract in *BPS Bulletin*, *29*, 206

Lovaas, D.I., Berberich, J.P., Perloff, B.F. and Schaeffer, B. (1966) 'Acquisition of Imitative Speech by Schizophrenic Children', *Science*, *151*, 705–7

McFall, R. and Twentyman, C. (1973) 'Four Experiments on the Relative Contribution of Rehearsal, Modelling and Coaching to Assertion Training', *Journal of Abnormal Psychology*, *91*, 199–218

Paton, X. and Stirling, E. (1974) 'Frequency and Type of Dyadic Nurse-Patient Verbal Interaction in a Mental Subnormality Hospital', *International Journal of Nursing Studies*, *11*, 135–45

Patterson, G.R. (1974) 'Intervention for Boys with Conduct Problems: Multiple Settings, Treatment and Criteria', *Journal of Consulting and Clinical Psychology*, *42*, 471–81

Sherman, J.A. (1965) 'Use of Reinforcement and Imitation to Reinstate Verbal Behaviour in Mute Psychotics', *Journal of Abnormal Psychology*, *70*, 155–64

Spreen, O. (1965) 'Language Functions in Mental Retardation: a Review', *American Journal of Mental Deficiency*, *69*, 482–94

Thomson, N., Fraser, D. and McDougall, A. (1974) 'The Reinstatement of Speech in Near-mute Chronic Schizophrenics by Instructions, Imitative Prompts and Reinforcement', *Journal of Behavioural Therapy and Experimental Psychiatry*, *5*, 835–89

Walker, H.H. and Hops, H. (1976) 'Use of Normative Peer Data as a Standard for Evaluating Classroom Treatment Effects', *Journal of Applied Behaviour Analysis*, *9*, 159–68

Wing, J.K. and Brown, G.W. (1970) '*Institutionalism and Schizophrenia*', Cambridge University Press, London

Appendices

Appendix 8.1: Analysis of Benefit — Cost (A-B-C)

DATE . . . .
REF. BY

. . . .

. . . .

CODE

ANALYSIS OF BENEFIT — COST (A-B-C)

Analyse treatment proposal by comparison of BENEFITS likely to be gained, with COSTS required to be expended by 1, 2 & 3 below. The decision to implement, modify or reject the proposal should be taken by consensus opinion and recorded.

1: Subject . . . DONALD . . . . Resident . . WARD X . . . .
   'Problem' . . . Rarely Speaks, Poor Eye Contact. . . . .
   Proposal . . . Increase Speech, Increase Eye-Contact. . . . .

2: Significant 1 . . . Theresa, Jean, Jim, Tricia . . . . Relationship . . Ward Staff . . . . . .
   Others) 2 . . Isobel . . . . Relationship . . Ward Sister . . . .

3: Programme 1 . . . Ward Sister . . . . Dept . . Ward X . . . .
   Supervisor(s) 2 . . Lydia Stephenson . . . . Dept . . Nurse Therapy Dept . . . .

	BENEFITS	COSTS
SUBJECT	Improve social contact leading to more choice in his daily living and decreasing his dependence on others	1) May find sessions stressful 2) Time consuming for him
SIGNIFICANT OTHERS	Satisfaction of Donald speaking for himself. Staff will know what he wants. Receiving more social interaction from Donald.	1) Learning Sessions 2) Recording Progress 3) Time consuming initially
PROGRAMME SUPERVISOR	Job Satisfaction of doing constructive work with Donald. Seeing programme implemented and effectiveness.	1) Teaching Staff 2) Recording Progress 3) Evaluating Progress
DECISION: Commence Treatment Sessions.		APPROVED BY: Ward Team. DATE 23/8/83 . . . .

ᴸ P BARKER 1978

Appendix 8.2: Donald — Strathmore Villa Guidelines for Staff on Baseline Sessions on Answering Questions

1. *Duration* of each session to be 15 minutes, two sessions per day, one to take place in *THERAPY ROOM*, one to take place in *DAY ROOM*. The sessions may be done at any time during the day-shift period.

2. Give *no* prompts, physical, gestural or verbal, or *any form* of praise or reinforcement during the *baseline sessions*.

3. Allow Donald *10 seconds* to respond to each question asked, if no response, record appropriately and go on to your next question.

4. When recording eye contact, record for *approximate time* Donald spent looking at you for each question, e.g. ½ time, ¾ time etc.

5. *15 Questions* to be asked in each session, *4 sets of 3 questions*, as follows:–

   Object Naming: e.g. Nurse asks Donald 'What is this?' holding up object.
   Question 1.   'What is this?' — using a cup.
   Question 2.   'What is this?' — using a book.
   Question 3.   'What is this?' — using a shoe.

   Colour Naming: e.g. Nurse asks Donald 'What colour is this?' showing Donald a card.
   Question 4.   'What colour is this?' — using blue card.
   Question 5.   'What colour is this?' — using red card.
   Question 6.   'What colour is this?' — using green card.

   Picture Questions: — *Specific* e.g. Nurse asks Donald 'What is the girl doing?' — showing Donald the picture.
   Question 7.   'What is the girl doing?' (Sleeping)
   Question 8.   'What is the girl doing?' (Singing)
   Question 9.   'What is the girl doing?' (Sweeping)

   Picture Questions — General e.g. Nurse asks Donald 'What is happening in the picture?' — showing Donald the picture.
   Question 10. 'What is happening in the picture?' (The boy is having a bath)
   Question 11. 'What is happening in the picture?' (The lady is reading a story)
   Question 12. 'What is happening in the picture?' (The girl is sitting drinking juice)

   Open-Ended Questions: e.g. Nurse asks Donald 'What did you do this morning/afternoon?'
   Question 13. 'What did you do this morning?'
   Question 14. 'What's the weather like today?'
   Question 15. 'What am I wearing today?'

ALWAYS ASK THE QUESTIONS IN THE SAME SEQUENCE EACH SESSION, CARDS ARE NUMBERED ACCORDINGLY.

Appendix 8.3: Sample of Recordings

NAME: DONALD

WARD: Strathmore Villa

	INCORRECT REPLY			CORRECT REPLY				EYE CONTACT DURING QUESTION			
	NO REPLY	GRUNT	WRONG REPLY	REPLY ONE WORD	REPLY TWO WORDS	PHRASE – 3 + WORDS	SENTENCE	¼ OF TIME	½ OF TIME	¾ OF TIME	ALL TIME
Question 1.											
Question 2.											
Question 3.											
Question 4.											
Question 5.											
Question 6.											
Question 7.											
Question 8.											
Question 9.											
Question 10.											
Question 11.											
Question 12.											
Question 13.											
Question 14.											
Question 15.											
TOTAL											

BASELINE:

RECORDER'S NAME:

SESSION NO.:

DATE:

RECORD A TICK FOR EACH RESPONSE IN THE APPROPRIATE BOX.

Appendix 8.4: Instructions for Staff

STAGE 1.–*ANSWERING QUESTIONS. IN THERAPY ROOM, 15 MINUTE SESSION PER DAY, USING FOUR PROMPTS.*

INSTRUCTIONS FOR STAFF:

1. *Inform Donald* at *beginning of each session* that you are going to ask him several questions and you would like him to answer in as many words as he can.

2. Instruct Donald before each question to look at you. Appropriate eye contact is Donald *looking at you* or *at the picture you are showing him*. Record in Box No. 3.

3. Beside each question number score in Box No. 1 his response as follows:
   0 – NO RESPONSE.   1 – GRUNT or MUMBLE.   2 – WRONG REPLY.
   3 – CORRECT REPLY ONE WORD.   4 – CORRECT REPLY TWO WORDS.
   5 – CORRECT REPLY PHRASE 3 + WORDS.   6 – SENTENCE.

4. In Box No. 2. write in no. of prompts given: e.g. 1, 2, 3, or 4.

   4 LEVELS OF PROMPTS AS FOLLOWS: VERBAL ONLY.

Questions 1, 2 & 3. e.g. USING OBJECTS: CUP, BOOK, SHOE.	*1st prompt*:	'WHAT IS THIS?' if no reply or incorrect reply
	2nd prompt:	'IT'S A CUP, WHAT IS IT?' if no reply or incorrect
	3rd prompt:	'IT'S A CUP, SAY CUP' if no reply or incorrect
	4th prompt:	'SAY CUP'
Questions 4, 5 & 6. e.g. USING COLOUR CARDS: BLUE, RED, GREEN	*1st prompt*:	'WHAT COLOUR IS THIS?' if no reply or incorrect
	2nd prompt:	'IT'S BLUE – WHAT COLOUR IS THIS?' if no reply or incorrect
	3rd prompt:	'IT'S BLUE – SAY BLUE' if no reply or incorrect
	4th prompt:	'SAY BLUE'
Questions 7, 8 & 9. e.g. USING PICTURE CARDS SLEEPING, SINGING, SWEEPING	*1st prompt*:	'WHAT IS THE GIRL DOING?' if no reply or incorrect
	2nd prompt:	'SHE'S SLEEPING – WHAT IS SHE DOING?' if no reply or incorrect
	3rd prompt:	'SHE'S SLEEPING – SAY SHE'S SLEEPING' if no reply or incorrect
	4th prompt:	'SAY SHE'S SLEEPING'

Appendix 8.4: *continued*

Questions 10, 11 & 12. e.g. USING PICTURE CARDS	*1st prompt*:	'WHAT IS HAPPENING IN THE PICTURE?' if no reply or incorrect reply
	2nd prompt:	'THE GIRL IS HAVING A BATH – WHAT IS SHE DOING?' if no reply or incorrect
	3rd prompt:	'THE GIRL IS HAVING A BATH – SAY SHE'S HAVING A BATH' if no reply or incorrect
	4th prompt:	'SAY SHE'S HAVING A BATH'

Note for this section appropriate answer is a simple sentence only, either 'having a bath' or 'the girl is having a bath'; go on to prompt Donald if he only gives one or two words.

Questions 13, 14 & 15. eg. OPEN-ENDED QUESTIONS	*1st prompt*:	'WHAT DID YOU DO THIS MORNING?' if no reply or incorrect
	2nd prompt:	'YOU HAD A BATH THIS MORNING – WHAT DID YOU DO?' if no reply or incorrect
	3rd prompt:	'YOU HAD A BATH THIS MORNING – SAY I HAD A BATH' if no reply or incorrect
	4th prompt:	'SAY I HAD A BATH'

Note for this section appropriate answer is a simple sentence only, either 'I had a bath' or 'I had a bath this morning'. Decide before asking the questions what answer you require of Donald.

Appendix 8.5: Recording Form for Intervention I

1. In Box No. 1 record as follows:

0 = NO RESPONSE
1 = GRUNT or MUMBLE
2 = WRONG REPLY
3 = CORRECT REPLY – ONE WORD
4 = CORRECT REPLY – TWO WORDS
5 = CORRECT REPLY – PHRASE 3 + WORDS
6 = SENTENCE

2. In Box No. 2 record as follows:
1 = first prompt needed for
    correct reply
2 = second prompt needed for
    correct reply
3 = third prompt needed for
    correct reply
4 = fourth prompt needed for
    correct reply

3. In Box No. 3 record as follows:

0 = No eye contact
1 = ¼ time
2 = ½ time
3 = ¾ time
4 = all time

QUESTION	BOX 1.	BOX 2.	BOX 3.	COMMENTS
1.				
2.				
3.				
4.				
5.				
6.				
7.				
8.				
9.				
10.				
11.				
12.				
13.				
14.				
15.				

ALL SESSIONS IN
RECORDER'S NAME: ....

15 MINUTES DAILY.
TIME ....

SESSION NO. ....

DATE ....

PLEASE ALWAYS REFER TO INSTRUCTIONS BEFORE SESSION STARTS TO MAKE SURE YOU ARE FAMILIAR WITH THE FORMAT OF THE SESSION.

A TIME-LIMITED THERAPY IN LATE PREGNANCY

Jean Kirby

Introduction

Snakes, more than any other animal, elicit fear and revulsion. Their limblessness and rhythmic movements, their forked tongues and angry hisses seem calculated to produce a reaction of terror in most people. Since the beginning of time, snakes have been surrounded by fanciful stories of evil, mystery and magic. In the Bible they are creatures of ill-omen or symbolise the Devil. In mythology they are used to signify wisdom and healing, and the sloughing of their skin is used as a symbol of rebirth. Within our own times and cultures there are people who still believe that they can regain their youth by eating snakes, or that a snakeskin worn in the crown of a hat will prevent headaches.

Snake fear is shared, approved and commended by a sizeable proportion of the community. It is accepted as a rational, realistic fear and as a consequence is continually reinforced. A fear of snakes is used as a model neurosis for the evaluation of a variety of behavioural treatments. Indeed, much of the present-day knowledge of phobias has been acquired in this way.

Most animal fears are learned in childhood through direct experience or vicariously through the experience of others. Normally these fears are extinguished in a natural way through social learning processes as the child grows up. Exceptions occur when the nature of the phobia permits a consistent pattern of avoidance behaviour to develop, which is what occurred in the case which is described in this chapter.

A phobia is often tolerated and remains untreated until generalisation occurs; when a person transfers his reaction to the original stimuli to stimuli of a similar nature. Then the fear may start intruding into everyday life and involving others.

In terms of treatment, Marks (1969) showed that systematic desensitisation was of value in the treatment of phobias, particularly specific phobias. The technique developed by Wolpe (1958) is based on the principle of reciprocal inhibition, i.e. the inhibition of anxiety by the development of a response that is incompatible with it. The procedure involves graduated exposure to phobic stimuli while the patient simultaneously participates in an anxiety-inhibiting procedure such as relaxation. The patient repeatedly practises entering the feared situation in imagination until anxiety is lowered, then he or she practises entering the same situation in real life until eventually all anxiety related to the situation in real life is substantially reduced.

A trial by Marks, Boulougouris and Marset (1971) showed that another technique, flooding, was equally effective in the treatment of specific phobias. Flooding involves prolonged exposure to the feared object or situation, and high levels of anxiety are often elicited since the feared stimulus is introduced at 'full strength' in contrast to the procedure of graduated exposure.

Watson, Gaind and Marks (1971) suggested that prolonged practice sessions are more effective than shorter sessions, especially when they can be devoted to overcoming avoidance of or escape from the phobic situations. This method produced better results in less time than the alternative treatment methods with which it was compared.

Bandura, Jeffrey and Gajdos (1975) found that treatment that combined modelling with guided participation was highly effective in eliminating avoidance behaviours. The therapist first models the threatening activities in easily mastered steps. The patient can then copy the modelled behaviour with appropriate guidance until he or she can perform it skilfully and fearlessly.

Snake fear in the British Isles is usually regarded as an innate fear. After all, how many people in this country have seen a live snake, far less had a traumatic encounter with one? However the case of the young woman whom I am about to describe represents one of the rare exceptions, in that she has had frequent, direct experience of snakes. She was born in Africa, and the fear-producing incidents occurred before she returned to this country when she was five years old.

The Subject

Megan lives with her 6-year-old daughter, Emma, in a three-bedroomed cottage with a large garden. She is 1.55 m (5 ft 1 in.) tall, has long auburn hair, a fair complexion and freckles. She looks younger than her 30 years. Her slim, neat figure and the brisk manner in which she walks belies her 7 months' pregnancy.

Megan met and married her husband when they were first-year

chemistry students at university. Though she had to discontinue her studies when she became pregnant, she intended resuming her career after Emma's birth. However, the marriage was in difficulties and her plans came to nothing.

Her husband dropped out of university after two years and is now a researcher with an agricultural company. She describes him as very irresponsible but a 'charmer'. The marriage has floundered on for about five years. There have been many separations and reconciliations during this time. The last separation occurred five months prior to my initial assessment of Megan.

The day that the pregnancy was confirmed, Megan's husband left her and went to live with her best friend. Megan could not believe it at first, but when she realised it was likely to be permanent, she felt such hate and anger that it frightened her. She is now awaiting a divorce.

Money has always been short as her husband refused to maintain Megan and Emma when they were separated. Megan supplements her social security allowance by growing her own fruit and vegetables. She preserves or freezes them to provide extras all the year round. She kept bees at one time to provide honey, but found this too time consuming. She is very proud of her prowess as a 'handy' person. She cannot afford to employ outside help when repairs are needed, but over the years she has taught herself how to do repair jobs around the house.

Megan has many good friends who give her things without making it seem like charity, but she would like to be able to give them something instead of always taking from them. She plans to make a career for herself when her children are older. Her parents, now retired, live near Aberdeen. She has a brother who moved to England when he married. Though they all keep in touch, they are not a particularly close family. Megan describes life over the past five years as a battle for survival.

Megan was referred, by a consultant psychiatrist, to Tayside Clinical Psychology Department for treatment of her snake phobia. She had asked for help as it was causing serious problems in her life.

The Assessment

At the first interview, Megan appeared pale, tired and tense. She talked in a fast, clipped and at times breathless voice. She was very apprehensive; several times during the interview she sat on the edge of her seat looking towards the door. If I had produced anything remotely connected with a snake, I am sure she would have fled. She gave a lengthy but precise history of her fear of snakes from its origins to the present day.

She was born in Africa. She lived there until she was 5 years old, when she came to Scotland to go to school. Her parents lived there a further two years before returning to live in Scotland permanently. She had been taught, quite realistically, to be careful about snakes, both inside and outside the house. In particular she had been taught to check in long grass, beds, cupboards and the bathroom.

The first time she can remember being frightened of snakes was when she was about 2½ years old. In two incidents that occurred close together she was hurriedly pulled out of the way of a snake. The next incident was about a year later when her pet kitten was spat at by a cobra and staggered blindly into the house to die at her feet. When she was 5 years old, while sitting in a guava tree eating the fruit, she was frightened by what appeared to be a snake coiled round a branch above her. She found out later that it was only a skin a snake had shed in the tree. However, she can still remember the feeling of utter terror and of being frozen to the spot. She could never eat guavas after that. She was always frightened of snakes after this incident, even after she left Africa and settled in Scotland.

Always an avid reader she would shudder when she read the word 'snake'. She would skip a page or even a chapter if she thought they were going to mention snakes. She would avoid looking at pictures of them and if they appeared on television she would look away or leave the room. She enjoyed going to the zoo but always avoided the reptile house. Dead or alive, she hated snakes. As a keen gardener she has no problems with bees, moths, spiders, caterpillars or other 'creepy-crawlies', though she is not too keen on large fat worms and lizards because they sometimes remind her of snakes, but she is not frightened of them, nor does she avoid them.

During her first pregnancy she had a fear of snakes 'lurking about after dark'. When she wanted to go tc the toilet during the night, her husband had to get up as well to check the way to the bathroom, the bathroom itself, the way back to the bedroom and then the bedroom itself. Sometimes this would happen several times a night. She would feel very ashamed next day when she thought about how she had behaved, but as soon as it was dark the fear returned. This lasted until her daughter, Emma, was about 6 months old, and then gradually faded away.

When her second pregnancy was confirmed, she anticipated that her fear of snakes would return. Her life was in a turmoil at the time as she had finally separated from her husband. She had many financial problems as he would not give her any money, not even for Emma's upkeep. She was sleeping badly and this made her miserable and bad-tempered. As worries about the pregnancy and finances piled up, she began to misinterpret sights and sounds in the house. In half-light she saw the telephone flex, electric cables, belts, etc. as snakes and felt sure that the slithering noise made by fieldmice behind the skirting board was really attributable to snakes. During the day she would see snakes in her peripheral vision and was continually turning round quickly to get a clearer picture of them. Then she started having to check in and under the beds and in the bathroom at night.

At this time she asked her husband if he would return for a short time to help her but he refused saying she was just making it all up to get him to return. Shortly thereafter she was spending most of the day checking and rechecking the home for snakes. She was unable to sleep properly, and if she did, she had violent, terrifying nightmares about snakes. She knew, when she thought about it logically, that there could not be any snakes, but she could not get rid of the feeling that they were lurking in cupboards and corners, and under the bath and the beds.

Emma, who was considered to be a very bright, stable child, became very upset by her mother's checking behaviour. She started bed-wetting and telling lies. The more Megan worried about her daughter's behaviour the more time she spent checking the house. She was very short-tempered with Emma, who was beginning to cause serious problems at school. It was at this stage that Megan felt that things were spiralling out of control. The whole day was monopolised by the thought of snakes; the more she checked, the worse Emma behaved; and eventually Megan began to worry that she might 'batter' the child, such was her hostility towards Emma. The time came when she was too frightened to remain alone with Emma, and if she could not persuade a friend to stay with them, she could not go to bed. She once again asked her husband to help but he did not believe her and refused. She went to see her GP but felt too ashamed to tell her doctor that she was having trouble with Emma. She started to tell her friends but felt they would be disgusted by her behaviour, so she steered off the subject.

The day came when, terrified by her feelings towards Emma, she felt it just was not worth going on and she took an overdose of Panadol. She was seen by a consultant psychiatrist who could find no evidence of psychiatric illness but referred her to the Psychology Department for treatment of her snake phobia. She was frightened by the thought of treatment but more frightened by what was happening to her and Emma. She asked her parents to help and they came to stay until after the baby's birth.

In the month before the first interview, things had settled down a bit. Her sleep improved and although she was still checking the house it was not as often. She still saw snakes in her peripheral vision. Emma's behaviour had improved, especially at school, but her grandparents spoiled her. If Megan kept busy during the day, she could shut out the thoughts of lurking snakes but felt they were there ready to pop back in if she let her guard down.

She asked to start treatment as soon as possible despite her advanced state of pregnancy, her reasons being:

(a) she was 'worn out' by the constant checking and re-checking for snakes;
(b) her behaviour was having an adverse effect on her daughter;
(c) her parents were willing to look after her daughter while she attended for treatment;
(d) she would be unable, as a single parent with two small children, to consider treatment in the future.

At the end of the first interview, because of the apparent strength of the fear and the extent of generalisation, it was decided to offer immediate treatment. We then talked about homework assignments and I stressed the need for practice sessions to be carried out at home of the techniques taught to her during the treatment sessions.

She was asked to keep a record until the next session, a week later, of:

(a) each time she thought the snakes were lurking around, what she was doing and feeling;
(b) what she was doing, thinking and feeling immediately before she thought they were there;
(c) what happened as a result of thinking snakes were present;
(d) how many times she checked and rechecked after such thoughts.

Megan looked very tired and tense and was agitated when she

arrived for the second interview. She was upset that she had been unable to complete the homework assignment of recording her checking behaviour. She had tried for two days but it had caused an increase in the behaviour, she was unable to sleep, and the snakes were dominating her thoughts. She was afraid that if she did not complete the homework, I might be reluctant to start treatment.

Megan completed a Fear Survey Schedule which confirmed that her fear was specific to snakes. She then completed a questionnaire which had been designed to identify the dominant fear regarding snakes. This showed that her greatest fear was of being poisoned.

Megan was also exposed to a variety of objects to measure the extent of generalisation. These had been selected and graded on the basis of the initial assessment. They were presented singly from the least anxiety provoking (the hose) to the most anxiety provoking (the coloured pictures of snakes). This was a long, noisy session which was punctuated by screams, gasps and the pushing back of her chair. However, I managed to prevent her from fleeing, and the results of this session fully confirmed what she had told me in the initial interview (see Figure 9.1).

The next stage of the baseline assessment was designed to measure her anxiety while imagining snakes or scenes with snakes. She sat in a chair and was asked to relax and to close her eyes. She was familiar with the principles of both progressive relaxation and yoga. Then I took her on an imaginary trip to the zoo with Emma, starting at the children's area and working our way to the reptile house, where I presented her with scenes of snakes graded along a hierarchy from a slow worm to a giant boa coiled round a branch. At first there was no anxiety at all because she blocked out the images. Later, when I was able to persuade her to allow them into the scenes, she became very anxious and agitated and blocked them out again.

In the last part of this interview we discussed the merits and demerits of treatment, and drew up a hierarchy of feared objects and a treatment plan. I proposed to Megan that the first part of the treatment plan would consist of graduated exposure along the hierarchy we had drawn up, from the toy snakes to the coloured pictures of snakes. She would remain exposed to the objects until the anxiety related to each particular object had decreased. Only when she was able to handle them fairly comfortably would we move on to the next stage.

The daily sessions at the clinic would last at least 3½ hours, i.e. two treatment sessions of 1½ hours with a lunch-break in the middle. No changes would be made in this plan without joint discussion. There

Figure 9.1: Self-rating of Anxiety during a Baseline Test Designed to Measure the Degree of Fear and the Extent of Generalisation.

Scale: No Anxiety ——————————————————— Avoid
0   10

	Rating										
Hose	0	(1)	2	3	4	5	6	7	8	9	10
Flex	0	(1)	2	3	4	5	6	7	8	9	10
Coiled wire	0	(1)	2	3	4	5	6	7	8	9	10
Patterned belt	0	1	(2)	3	4	5	6	7	8	9	10
Green ribbon	0	(1)	2	3	4	5	6	7	8	9	10
Chinese paper snake	0	1	2	3	4	(5)	6	7	8	9	10
Brown wooden snake	0	1	2	3	4	5	6	7	8	(9)	10
Grey pebble-headed snake	0	1	2	3	4	5	6	7	8	(9)	10
Discussion about snakes	0	1	2	3	(4)	5	6	7	8	9	10
Reptile book	0	1	2	3	4	5	6	7	8	(9)	10
Coloured picture of lizard	0	1	2	(3)	4	5	6	7	8	9	10
Coloured picture of lizard opposite slow worm	0	1	2	3	4	5	(6)	7	8	9	10
Turn page, therapist holding book	0	1	2	3	4	5	6	7	8	9	(10)
Hold book	0	1	2	3	4	5	6	7	8	9	(10)
Touch front of book showing frog's head	0	1	2	3	4	5	6	7	8	9	(10)
Touch back of book with turtle showing	0	1	2	3	4	5	(6)	7	8	9	10
Book 2 ft away	0	1	2	3	(4)	5	6	7	8	9	10
Black-and-white picture of snake	0	1	2	3	4	5	(6)	7	8	9	10
Coloured picture of snake	0	1	2	3	4	5	6	7	8	9	(10)

would be a review session at the end of the first stage, when the second stage of the treatment would be decided. This stage would be based on whatever materials were available but would probably include films of snakes and eventually live snakes.

Pictures of lizards (eight pages):
(a) Black-and-white copies of the coloured pictures from the reptile

book used in the assessment, photocopied to reduce their impact.
(b) Coloured pictures of lizards obtained from the reptile book used in the assessment.

Pictures of snakes (five pages):
(a) Black-and-white copies of the coloured pictures, photocopied to reduce their impact.
(b) Coloured pictures of snakes, which ranged from slow worms to cobras and were mainly African snakes.

Anxiety Self-rating Board: 12 'thermometers' were drawn on 66 x 38 cm (26 x 15 in.) paper and marked with a scale 0–10. This was attached to a piece of polystyrene, and orange-sticks, used as markers, were used to pierce the paper and the polystyrene, thus providing a permanent record of her progress.

The feared objects were presented in the following hierarchical order:

(1) Toy snakes:
    (a) chinese paper snake,
    (b) brown wooden snake,
    (c) grey, pebble-headed snake,
    (d) black rubber snake.
(2) Black-and-white pictures of lizards.
(3) Coloured pictures of lizards.
(4) Black-and-white pictures of snakes.
(5) Coloured pictures of snakes.

Megan accepted this treatment plan with very little hesitation, including the possibility of looking at live snakes. She preferred the prolonged method of exposure to brief sessions of desensitisation. She said that no matter how she did it she knew it would cause her extreme fear so she might as well get it over with by undergoing the more rapid form of treatment.

Treatment Plan

The following treatment plan was agreed at the second session.

(a) Megan was required to attend the clinic daily for at least

3½ hours, i.e. two treatment sessions of 1½ hours with a lunch-break in the middle.

(b) Treatment, including prolonged exposure to the feared objects, would progress along the agreed hierarchy.

(c) Homework was to be completed, as requested, between sessions.

(d) A review session would be arranged after she had reached stage 4 of her hierarchy.

(e) A second stage of treatment (to be implemented after the review sessions) would include films of snakes, and live snakes if available.

(f) No changes would be made to the treatment plan without joint agreement.

The goal of treatment was to extinguish her fear of snakes and the avoidance and checking behaviours which served to maintain this fear.

Materials

A range of materials was used in the first stage of treatment.

Toy snakes:

(a) A Chinese paper snake which writhed when moved.

(b) A brown, segmented wooden snake which writhed when moved.

(c) A grey paper snake with a pebble head which made 'darting' movements when twirled on a stick.

(d) Rubber snakes which were realistic and unpleasant to touch.

Procedure

Treatment consisted of prolonged, graduated exposure to the feared objects. Each session started at step 1 with the Chinese paper snake. The objects were presented to Megan after I had modelled looking at and handling them with minimal anxiety.

At the first treatment Megan arrived tense, apprehensive and very tired. Her sleep had been interrupted by nightmares about snakes but she was determined to start treatment. We discussed the treatment plans for the day and then we began the session. The same procedure was followed each day, preceded by a general discussion about progress, homework, etc., and followed by the setting of homework assignments.

It took 9 minutes for Megan to accept the Chinese paper snake but then it moved, she dropped it and we had to start again from the beginning. This was to become a familiar response pattern during exposure. The time taken from initial exposure to handling the objects comfortably was: the Chinese paper snake, 17 minutes; the brown wooden snake, 24 minutes; the grey paper snake, 18 minutes.

This session lasted 1½ hours and Megan then went to the cafeteria for lunch while I saw another patient. Unfortunately, she came back early, and when I was not there she took her coat and fled, leaving me a note saying that she would come back the next day. However, she returned in half an hour and confirmed her appointment for the next day. I always spent the lunch-breaks with her from this point onwards.

Megan arrived for the second appointment feeling tense, frightened and tired. Her sleep had been disturbed again by nightmares about snakes. We started again with the three toy snakes; with each there was some initial anxiety when they first moved, but this quickly dissipated. Eight minutes elapsed from initial exposure to handling the three snakes.

Then I introduced the black rubber snake and she moved her chair back about 60 cm (2 ft). It was fully 12 minutes before she could touch it with her little finger, a further 5 minutes before she would pick it up, and another 4 minutes before her anxiety decreased. A total of 21 minutes had elapsed from initial exposure to comfortable handling.

After a 30-minute lunch-break we started with the toy snakes again. She picked up the first three snakes without hesitation and was comfortably handling them in a total time of 2 minutes.

It took her 3 minutes to touch the rubber snake, 2 minutes to pick it up, and a further 2 minutes for her anxiety to decrease, a total of 7 minutes from exposure to comfortable handling.

The next step was to introduce her to the black-and-white pictures of lizards. Most pages caused no anxiety but the photographs with close-ups of their snake-like heads and darting tongues caused an initial marked increase in anxiety. It took 30 minutes to work through eight pages of photographs, looking at them and reading the captions. This process was repeated and took a total of 22 minutes.

Homework. As a homework assignment Megan was asked to take home the black-and-white photographs of the lizards and to look at them several times during the evening while sitting relaxed.

Megan arrived for the third session looking somewhat less anxious than had previously been the case. Her sleep was still disturbed but the nightmares had reduced in frequency and intensity. Megan was pleased that she had managed to complete her homework assignment.

The session started with the toy snakes. Only the rubber snake caused her any uneasiness. Then Megan looked through the black-and-white pictures of the lizards: no anxiety was apparent.

Next to be introduced were the coloured photographs of lizards. Megan showed revulsion rather than fear when looking at these lizards, which closely resembled snakes.

After the lunch-break we started looking at the black-and-white pictures of snakes. This was a 'marathon session'. It was 37 minutes before she touched the first page of photographs, for about 2 seconds. This fleeting touch moved the page and the snakes appeared to move. She spent the next 3 minutes with her arms tightly folded and refusing to look at the page. After 5 minutes she agreed to look at the snakes and then to touch the page. It was fully 50 minutes before she could hold the page with both hands and a further 10 minutes before her anxiety decreased. Thus a total of 60 minutes elapsed from the initial exposure to fairly comfortable handling.

Megan was exhausted after this long session so we had a break for a cup of tea. During this break she continued to look at the first page of snakes and to discuss the text on the adjoining page.

After the break Megan picked up page 2 immediately, holding it at the bottom of the page away from the pictures of the snakes. It was 9 minutes before she could hold the sides of the page near to the snakes, and a further 4 minutes before her anxiety reduced. From the initial exposure to comfortable handling, 13 minutes had elapsed.

She was frightened when she first saw the vipers on page 3 but she held the page in both hands in 8 minutes and was fairly comfortable in a further 6 minutes.

Though she was more frightened of the cobras on page 4, she held the side of the page away from the snakes after 9 minutes and both sides after 11 minutes. It was a further 2 minutes before her anxiety reduced.

The last page had pictures of boa constrictors. It was 10 minutes before she held the page in her hand and a further 2 minutes until the anxiety was reduced.

The total time from exposure to comfortable handling of the black-and-white pictures was 112 minutes.

Megan was very tired at the end of this session, which lasted 3½ hours.

Homework. As a homework assignment, Megan was asked to take the black rubber snake home. She was to handle it for as long as possible, during a quiet time in the evening while relaxing. She was to do this several times until she could handle it without discomfort.

When Megan arrived for the fourth session she was smiling and looked relaxed. She said she was not unduly worried about the forthcoming session. She produced the rubber snake from her handbag and sat swinging it by the tail. Megan said that she had held the snake several times during the evening and that her anxiety had dissipated quickly each time, so she had kept the rubber snake on the bedside table all night. Although snakes had been in her thoughts most of the evening, she had slept much better than previously.

The treatment session started with the toy snakes, then the black-and-white pictures of lizards, followed by the coloured pictures of lizards. No anxiety was apparent during exposure to these items.

The next stage involved exposure to the black-and-white pictures of snakes. Page 1, which had caused the sustained bout of anxiety the previous day, produced no anxiety at all. It took 4 minutes' exposure to page 2, 4 minutes to page 3, 6 minutes to page 4, and 4 minutes to page 5, for her anxiety to decrease.

After the lunch-break we moved on to the coloured pictures of snakes. Although it took her 3 minutes to pick up the book, the anxiety each new page produced dissipated fairly quickly, the vipers and cobras taking the longest times of 5 minutes and 6 minutes, respectively. We had a 5-minute break then repeated the exposure. Megan picked up the book straight away and read through it, picking out pieces of text to read.

Megan was very pleased with the day's session and felt that she had achieved a lot in four days, but she was a little apprehensive about an imminent 4-week break in treatment due to holidays. The importance of curbing her avoidance behaviour and the use of positive self-talk as a coping strategy when she was anxious was stressed.

Homework. During the holiday break, Megan was asked to take home the reptile book and the rubber snake. She was to spend a minimum of two sessions per day handling the snake and reading through the book slowly, concentrating on looking at the vipers and cobras, which still caused some uneasiness.

The fifth treatment session took place after the 26-day holiday break. The first part of the session was spent in reviewing the previous treatment and its outcome. Megan was very pleased about the progress she had made thus far.

The snakes had disappeared from her peripheral vision, she had not misinterpreted flex, wire, belts, etc. for about four weeks, and all the checking behaviour had stopped. She had seen a snake on television and shuddered but did not look away. She had been able to watch it all the time it was on the screen. There had been a snake in a book which she was reading and she had been able to look at it and then to read about it without feeling anxious.

Megan found that she had more leisure time since stopping the checking behaviour. During the holiday break she had decorated her kitchen and bedroom and prepared a room for the baby.

In the next part of the interview we discussed the treatment materials available, drew up a revised hierarchy of feared objects and reformulated the treatment plan. This consisted of graduated exposure along the hierarchy we had drawn up from toy snakes to live snakes. It was agreed that she would remain exposed to the feared objects until her anxiety had decreased. Only when she could handle an item fairly comfortably would we move on to the next item in the hierarchy. She accepted this treatment plan without hesitation, including the possibility of looking at and handling live snakes.

A range of different materials was used in this second stage of treatment:

(a) *A snake skin.* this was a 12 ft python skin loaned by Dundee Museum. The head was stuffed and contained sharp teeth and gleaming eyes.

(b) *A stuffed mongoose and cobra.* this was a stylised but realistic representation of a mongoose attacking a cobra.

(c) *A snake film.* This was a video film put together by the Audio-Visual Unit at Dundee University and taken from the BBC's 'Life on Earth' series.

(d) *Live snakes.* We were unable to find any live snakes in Dundee, so a visit to the Reptile House at Edinburgh Zoo was arranged to conclude the programme of treatment.

Revised Hierarchy of Feared Objects

The feared objects were presented in the following hierarchical order:

(1) Four toy snakes

    (a) Chinese paper snake,
    (b) brown snake
    (c) grey snake
    (d) black rubber snake.
(2) Black-and-white pictures of lizards.
(3) Coloured pictures of lizards.
(4) Black-and-white pictures of snakes.
(5) Coloured pictures of snakes.
(6) Snake skin.
(7) Stuffed cobra and mongoose.
(8) Film of snakes.
(9) Live snakes.

The next stage consisted of exposing Megan to the toy snakes, the black-and-white and coloured pictures of lizards, and the black-and-white and coloured pictures of snakes. These did not evoke any anxiety, though the pictures of the vipers and cobras repulsed her.

After the lunch-break the snake skin was introduced. Megan's immediate reaction was to push back her chair and look towards the door. I sat 275 cm (9 ft) away, holding the skin and continually touching the head while I talked to Megan. After 6 minutes I moved it to 180 cm (6 ft), in another 6 minutes to 120 cm (4 ft), in a further 4 minutes to 90 cm (3 ft) and in another 8 minutes to 60 cm (2 ft) away, sitting on the table in front of her. Megan turned the snake's head away from her after 4 minutes, using a paper towel. She was able to touch it with her little finger after a further 6 minutes and with both hands after another 8 minutes. I moved it to 30 cm (1 ft) away; in another 2 minutes she touched the head with both hands and then picked up the skin. Her anxiety kept fluctuating for the next 8 minutes but finally dissipated. A total of 60 minutes had elapsed from the initial exposure to comfortable handling.

It had been a long, exhausting session for Megan so we had a break. She stayed in the room alone with the snake skin while I made a cup of tea.

After the break Megan was willing to go a stage further so we repeated the same procedure using the cobra and mongoose. Starting at 275 cm (9 ft) away, the model was moved to 180 cm (6 ft) in 6 minutes, and 60 cm (2 ft) in a further 6 minutes. She was able to touch the mongoose in another 4 minutes, starting from the tip of its tail. After another 12 minutes she touched the snake's tail where it was wrapped around the mongoose. She moved slowly up the snake and in another 16 minutes was able to touch the head with both hands. It was another 4 minutes before her anxiety dissipated. It took 58 minutes from initial exposure to comfortable handling.

Homework. Megan took the reptile book to read for her homework assignment.

Megan looked pale and tired when she arrived for her sixth session. She was by now more than 8 months pregnant and found the bus journey to the clinic rather arduous.

Initially she was exposed to the toy snakes, to pictures of lizards and to pictures of snakes. These did not evoke any anxiety. Next she was reintroduced to the snake skin. She picked it up straight away and her initial anxiety subsided within 2 minutes. The model of the cobra and mongoose held no fears for her, and though she disliked it, she was able to handle it without anxiety within a minute.

After the lunch-break Megan was repeatedly shown a 12-minute video film of live snakes from the 'Life on Earth' series. This was a noisy session, as all the showings, with the exception of the last, were accompanied by her squeals and gasps.

The colour was eliminated from the television to reduce the impact. After three showings of the black-and-white film, she was able to watch it fairly comfortably. It was next shown slightly coloured and her anxiety remained lowered except when a cobra appeared.

After a tea-break the film was shown twice in full colour. The first time Megan was fairly anxious but there was no anxiety during the second showing, though she shuddered when the cobra appeared — a picture most people considered horrific.

Homework. Megan was to look for books about snakes and to watch programmes on TV if she thought they were likely to be about snakes.

Megan was unable to keep the next two appointments, which had been designed to prepare her for the trip to the Zoo, due to minor problems in her pregnancy. The planned trip was finally cancelled when she went into premature labour. Although it was a false alarm, it was considered too risky to take her to Edinburgh.

Megan was next seen three weeks after her sixth session of treatment. She reported that her fear of snakes and all of the behaviour which had developed from it had disappeared. She thought that treatment had been well worthwhile, although after some of the treatment sessions she had had reservations about returning for the next. She was impressed by the effectiveness of the treatment and by how little time it had taken, considering that her fear of snakes had been a life-long problem. No further appointments were made because of her imminent confinement.

Megan was seen at home 8 weeks later, for a follow-up visit, when her son was 6 weeks old. Eleven weeks had passed since the last treatment session. Her parents had returned to Glasgow and she was living alone with the children. Although many of her personal problems remained, mainly financial problems relating to being a single parent with two small children, she said that she was coping very well. Emma had settled down and her behaviour problems at home and at school had disappeared. Megan happily reported that she remained free of her fear of snakes and of all of the associated problem behaviour.

Discussion

This case study demonstrates the use of prolonged graduated exposure and participant modelling in the treatment of a snake phobic. Relaxation and the use of positive self-talk were used as adjuncts to anxiety management. Homework assignments were given to reinforce the techniques taught in the treatment sessions and to aid generalisation from these sessions to her real-life situation.

Because of the patient's advanced pregnancy, prolonged exposure was considered to be the treatment of choice. Imaginal desensitisation was not employed because of her inability to retain visual images due to extreme fear.

Although the 'marathon' sessions were exhausting for both patient and therapist, they were effective in overcoming the patterns of avoidance behaviour which she had developed over the years. The extreme anxiety which resulted from prolonged exposure was successfully diminished within each treatment session. Once she realised that nothing dreadful would happen if she merely waited for her anxiety to dissipate, the battle was half won.

The success of the programme was aided by the patient's commitment to changing her own behaviour. She travelled 30 miles a day on public transport to reach the clinic. Once the treatment sessions started, she carried out all homework assignments diligently. This aided and probably speeded up generalisation from the treatment sessions to real life. The degree of a patient's compliance to this type of treatment regime is perhaps the main factor influencing outcome.

References

Bandura, A., Jeffrey, R.W. and Gadjos, E. (1975) 'Generalising Change through Participant Modelling with Self-directed Mastery', *Behaviour Research and Therapy*, *13*, 141–52

Marks, I.M. (1969) *Fears and Phobias*, Heinemann, London

Marks, I.M., Boulougouris, J.C. and Marset, P. (1971) 'Flooding versus Desensitisation in Phobic Disorders', *British Journal of Psychiatry*, *119*, 353–75

Watson, J.P., Gaind, R. and Marks, I.M. (1971) 'Prolonged Exposure, a Rapid Treatment of Phobias', *British Medical Journal*, *1*, 13–15

Wolpe, J. (1958) *Psychotherapy by Reciprocal Inhibition*, Stanford University Press, Stanford, Mass.

10 REDUCING THE WEIGHT AND INCREASING THE WORK OUTPUT AND SOCIAL ACTIVITY OF A LONG-STAY PATIENT

Christopher Portues

Introduction

Ayllon and Azrin (1968) in their introduction to *The Token Economy: A Motivational System for Therapy and Rehabilitation* have said:

> Almost every conceivable behavioural difficulty can be seen in a State Mental Hospital. Senile disorders, neurological disorders, adolescent problems, employment problems, sexual difficulties, addiction, alcoholism, intellectual retardation and neuroticism converge and interact in one community. To gaze upon this multiplicity of disorders and problems, is to be overwhelmed by a sense of hopelessness and helplessness. Any simple answer that one might consider for the problems of one patient, seems irrelevant for other patients.

They go on to say:

> Various diagnostic categories have been proposed for creating some order out of this chaos, but the illustrative textbook case is rarely to be found. Who is to know whether the mental state of the young lady is that of paranoid persecution as the case history states, when the young lady has not been heard to utter a word? Consider the gentle, old, motherly lady who has been classified as schizophrenic, but whose only problem seems to be her refusal to be discharged, a refusal strengthened by her family, and society's unwillingness to accept a 70-year-old who has been absent from society for 20 years. Why is she in hospital? How did she ever get here to begin with? The official records give no indication.

Referring to long-stay patients, they continue by saying:

> Even if there were nothing wrong with these patients, it would be

difficult to discharge them into the outside world — since the outside world has no place for them. The longer these patients remain in the mental hospital, the more severe their behavioural problems seem to grow. One currently hears the word 'institutionalisation', which describes a state of apathy and lack of motivation that is acquired by a stay in a mental hospital. The hospital community is usually geared to providing the biological necessities of life and perhaps some minimal level of recreational opportunities, but the overall relationship is a parasitic dependency in which the patient need not function in order to obtain most, if not all, of the activities or privileges that might still be of interest to him.

These words were written in the United States in 1968: yet how aptly the last paragraph describes the present plight of many patients in psychiatric hospitals throughout the British Isles.

Even though many rehabilitation programmes have been initiated in hospitals nationwide, the plight of the long-stay patient remains almost the same. Those people who were rehabilitatable have been discharged into the community. Those that are left are the ones that have been more severely damaged by extended periods of hospitalisation.

Is our task, then, to continue to rehabilitate — with the main aim of treatment being that of discharge into the community? Or would it not be more realistic in some cases to aim for a rehabilitation programme that equipped a patient to lead a more dignified and less dependent life within the hospital?

Kazdin (1972) said that

Although extra-hospital adjustment is, in a social sense, the ultimate criterion by which treatment programmes are evaluated, development of skills within the hospital is also relevant to this end. There is justification for focusing on behaviours adaptive to the hospital setting, at least as long as there are institutions of the sort that presently exist.

It must be emphasised at this point, however, that many of the behaviours adaptive to a hospital setting are of such a nature that they suggest the person is dependent on the institution. It is very important to bear in mind, when teaching patients new behaviours, that we are not doing so just to create a more easily managed institution. We must always ensure that we are developing *independence* and striving to improve the quality of life of our patients.

In the following case study, the author will attempt to illustrate that even though a long-term goal may be one of discharge into the community, any intermediate steps taken can be helpful in improving the patient's quality of life while he or she continues to remain in hospital.

The treatment package described in the study comprises the following techniques: self-monitoring, direct observation, goal-setting, instruction and feedback, conditioned reinforcement, and social approval.

As a therapeutic tool, the reactivity of self-monitoring procedures has proved to be effective in modifying behaviour as diverse as college study habits (Johnson and White, 1971), maternal attention to appropriate child behaviour (Herbert and Baer, 1972), multiple tics (Hutzell, Platzek and Logue, 1974), and smoking (McFall, 1970). To date, however, there is little in the literature which describes the use of self-monitoring with long-stay psychiatric patients, although 'psychotic symptoms', i.e. hallucinations, have been reduced using self-monitoring (Rutner and Bugle, 1969). Kazdin (1974) said that, as a therapeutic strategy, recording one's own behaviour is sometimes reactive, that is, it serves to alter the observed behaviour. Kazdin (1975b) later proposed that providing information about performance can serve as a powerful reinforcer. Feedback can serve as a conditioned reinforcer because it is usually associated with the delivery of other events that are reinforcing. Feedback is implicit in the delivery of any reinforcer because reinforcement serves to indicate which responses are appropriate or desirable from the standpoint of those who provide the reinforcement. Thus, when reinforcers such as food, praise, activities or points are provided, a client receives feedback concerning his or her performance.

Zegiob, Klukas and Junginger (1978) investigated the reactivity of self-monitoring procedures with 'retarded' adolescents, using single case designs. The effects of two variables — social reinforcement and feedback — on the degree of reactivity, were also examined. Both subjects monitored a socially undesirable behaviour and were asked to self-record for extended periods of time. The results indicated that self-monitoring produced reactive decreases in the target behaviours under study. Reinforcement was only effective with one of the subjects.

Much has been written on the use of tokens as conditioned

reinforcers. For example, Ayllon and Azrin (1965, 1968) used token reinforcement with psychiatric patients. Phillips (1968) reported a token programme (using points) for 'pre-delinquent' boys who had committed various offences. Token economies have been implemented by parents in the home to alter child behaviour (Christopherson, Arnold, Hill and Quilitch, 1972), and spouses have used token reinforcement to alleviate marital discord (Stuart, 1969).

However, Nelson, Lipinski and Black (1976), in two experiments with 'retarded' adult subjects of both sexes, found that the magnitude of reactive changes produced by self-monitoring was greater than the changes produced by a token economy.

Description of Patient

Fay is a grossly overweight 51-year-old woman, who can be recognised from a distance by her large, rounded form and her bouncing gait. As she draws near, you may notice that she is quite breathless and that her reddened face is glistening with beads of sweat. When she sees you, depending on her mood, you may be greeted by a beaming smile, or a penetrating stare. Either way, you will notice that her top lip and almost non-existent chin have sparse, spiky growths of dark hair. She may walk up to you with her arms open wide ready to hug you, as if you were her long-lost son come home at last.

Fay was born into a family which over the years has become very well known to the staff of the local psychiatric hospitals. Her father and mother, two of her sisters and her brother have, in the past, all been treated as in-patients. Fay was first admitted when she was 16 years old, suffering from a manic depressive illness. Her second admission, in 1948, has resulted in a 36-year stay in hospital, from then until the present day. She was brought up in Dundee and attended the 'backward class' of a local Catholic school. Before her admission to hospital, she worked for a short time in a jute mill. She became pregnant and gave birth to an illegitimate baby son. Ten days after the birth, she was admitted to hospital and has never lived in the community since.

During her long stay in hospital, Fay's behaviour has varied. There have been many occasions on which she has been very aggressive, voicing bizarre delusional thoughts. On the other hand, she did work for a time doing domestic duties in the hospital. She was even given a job in a local laundry, but only managed to cope with it for a few days. Diagnoses have differed over the years, some doctors deciding she is schizophrenic, others diagnosing a manic-depressive illness. At present, she is considered to be manic depressive.

She has been treated with several courses of ECT and numerous drug combinations. Her behaviour improved considerably when, in 1979, she was prescribed pimozide. She became less impulsive and less aggressive.

Fay's problems now seem to be those that the institution has served to create. She seems to know everyone in the hospital and is often called 'the darling of the hospital'. Unfortunately, this status has not helped her to achieve her discharge from hospital. She has, over the years, built up a repertoire of behaviours which, to some, are quite amusing. She can easily be prompted into fits of inappropriate giggles and laughter. She bounces along, singing and yodelling, and when she speaks, she will often mention that she gave birth to one, two or three babies in the course of the previous night. When she is questioned, she explains, quite happily, that 'the students took them away'. It is difficult to say whether this kind of verbalisation is delusional or not. It is, after all, based on some fact; she has had a baby and there is no doubt that it was taken away from her. What is inappropriate, however, is that she should be saying she had a baby 'last night', but this has been inadvertently reinforced over the years. She has been encouraged by hospital staff to talk like this and to hug and giggle and sing, and generally to perform the 'lunatic role'.

Although she is dependent on the hospital for virtually all of her needs, she does occasionally leave its confines by, for example, taking a bus to the nearby housing estate to visit her cousin. She is well known for her non-compliance, e.g. instead of spending all day in the Occupational Therapy department, she will take her leave halfway through a session and make her way to visit those staff members who she knows are likely to give her a cup of tea or a bun. Or, if she has money, she will spend it on sweet foods and drinks in the hospital shop.

Fay was admitted to the hospital's Intensive Rehabilitation Unit over a year ago, in an attempt to decrease her dependence on the hospital and in an effort to eliminate her inappropriate behaviour. She was assessed by the Unit's multi-disciplinary team and long- and short-term treatment goals were formulated. The most ambitious of these goals is to resettle Fay in a 'halfway house' in the community.

Referral

Fay's case was referred by the clinical psychologist member of the multi-disciplinary team. The problems referred were as follows:

(1) Poor time structuring and lack of participation in recreational activities.
(2) Inappropriate social behaviour.
(3) Poorly developed community skills.
(4) Obesity.
(5) Lack of domestic and everyday living skills.
(6) Difficulties in budgeting.

Assessment: Methods and Materials

An assessment of the patient was undertaken in the following stages:

(1) Interview of Ward Charge Nurse. The objective of this preliminary interview was to:

(a) take a brief history of the present problems;
(b) ascertain how these problems affected Fay's daily life;
(c) clarify the expectations of any treatment programme to be designed by the therapist;
(d) become aware of existing ward rules for patients.

(2) Referral to Medical Case File. The objectives were to:

(a) become familiar with the patient's past medical and social history;
(b) record specific information, for example date of birth, place of birth, etc.

(3) Direct Interview of Patient. The objectives were:

(a) introduction of therapist to patient;
(b) to explain the reason for the first and subsequent interviews;
(c) to take a personal history from the patient's point of view;
(d) to complete a motivational analysis;
(e) to assist in formulating initial clinical impressions of patient.

(4) Interview of Care Co-ordinator (a member of Unit staff

responsible for co-ordinating all ongoing programmes of treatment for Fay). The objectives were:

(a) introduction of therapist to care co-ordinator;
(b) to obtain a further summary of the patient's problems.

(5) Interview of Occupational Therapy Helper. The objectives were:

(a) to get an impression of Fay's performance in the OT department;
(b) to become familiar with patient's daily routine in the OT department.

(6) Global Assessment. The 'Borders Mental Handicap Team — Paton's Assessment Schedule A' (Paton, 1981) was completed by Fay's care co-ordinator. The purpose of this schedule is to give as full a picture of a client's abilities, disabilities and potential for further training as is possible, and although it was designed for mentally handicapped clients, it proved a very useful tool for the assessment of Fay's assets and deficits.

Information Gathered as a Result of the Interviews and Gobal Assessment

Fay's problems were numerous when described by the staff. A picture was drawn of a patient who rarely complied with the rules of the ward or of the OT department. She invariably slept late in the morning (breakfast time was 8.15 a.m.), despite repeated prompts to get up. She retired to bed early on most evenings, well before 7.00 p.m., which resulted in her missing out on any ward- or hospital-based social activity. Although she 'clocked in' at the OT department, she was often late (session times were 9.30-11.30 a.m. and 1.30-3.30 p.m., Monday to Friday); did very little work; and frequently left the department to 'wander around' the hospital. While she was unofficially away from the ward or OT department, she would visit people she knew in the hospital and be supplied with food and drink by them. She would spend all of her money on bottles of Coke, potato crisps and sweets at the hospital shop. She often missed her meals on the ward because of her late arrival. Despite this, she was grossly overweight, probably as a result of her extra-mealtime eating habits.

She was described as being over-friendly, hugging and kissing people she did not know. She could, on occasion, be verbally aggressive and insulting, especially when placed under pressure to comply with instructions. She often laughed and giggled inappropriately, despite attempts by staff to extinguish this behaviour.

Clinical Impression

After I had been introduced to her, Fay escorted me to her room, where the interview was to be carried out. She seemed quite happy to do this and was obviously proud of her very neat and well decorated room. A seat was offered by the dressing table and the interview commenced.

Fay recalled, seemingly without much difficulty, details of her early life. Initially, she answered questions eagerly, but when the subject of her problem behaviour was mentioned, she ignored many questions, or answered by saying 'Don't know'. She began talking about having a baby 'last night'; this is a tactic she used often in subsequent interviews, when she appeared to be having difficulty in answering, or did not want to answer, questions. Because of this, interviews were kept short but frequent. Fay seemed to have a short attention span, and much of the most valuable information was gathered in the first five minutes of an interview.

First impressions were of a patient who did what she pleased and lacked the motivation to change in any way. She did not like being overweight but was not really prepared to change her eating habits: they were too reinforcing. She did not see why she should work in the OT department, or what difference it made to anyone if she went to bed early at night.

Information from the assessments previously described was sub-divided as follows.

Low-level assets (defined as skills that are present but could be improved with further training):

(a) Makes familiar journeys unaccompanied (for example, by bus).
(b) Can shop, but only for simple items like sweets, etc.
(c) Cooks simple meals, but needs supervision.
(d) Can wash and iron, but needs supervision.
(e) Does some work in the OT department, but needs constant prompting and supervision.

Potential assets (defined as skills that are not performed because of lack of opportunity or other organisational restrictions):

(a) Road crossing.
(b) Using a public telephone.

Problems

(1) Patient grossly overweight.
    (a) Spends all of her money on sweet foods and drink.
    (b) Begs for food and is given it by hospital staff.
(2) Does not comply with routine daily timetable.
    (a) Late in rising every morning.
    (b) Regularly late for OT.
    (c) Often leaves OT department early.
    (d) Sometimes leaves hospital when she should be attending OT.
    (e) Regularly goes to bed before 7.00 p.m.
(3) Rarely participates in social/recreational activities.
    (a) Opts out of evening-time social activities by going to bed.
    (b) Unable to concentrate for more than a short time.
    (c) Takes little active part in organised activities on the ward.
(4) Poor work rate in OT.
(5) Inappropriate social behaviour.
    (a) Frequently giggles and smiles inappropriately during conversations with staff.
    (b) Sometimes expresses delusional ideas, e.g. 'I had a baby last night'.
(6) Verbal aggression: occasionally verbally aggressive when under pressure to comply.
(7) Poor budgeting skills.
(8) Poor community skills.

Targets

After discussion with staff, the following targets were set:

(1) Reduce her weight.
(2) Increase her participation in recreational and social activities.
(3) Increase her work output.

Baseline measures

During the initial period of assessment, ward staff had reported that

Fay was frequently late in rising and late in arriving at the OT department, and that she went to bed very early. In addition she spent very little time actually in the OT department, as she would leave mid-session to wander around the hospital grounds with total disregard for the daily timetable that had been drawn up for her.

The first baseline measure was designed to ascertain exactly how far Fay strayed from her prescribed daily routine. This measure comprised a record sheet which Fay carried on her person throughout the day. On the record sheet were 20 instructions and 24 times of the day. The nursing and OT staff were instructed to sign opposite the times laid out on the sheet, recording, for example, whether Fay was present in the OT department at 11.00 a.m.

However, because of the design of the measure and the fact that Fay called it 'her programme', instead of it having little effect on her behaviour, as anticipated, it appeared to be an effective form of intervention. She began going to OT (although still arriving very late) and she stayed there for most of the prescribed period. Because of this 'reactive' effect of observations and monitoring, the information gathered by using this technique was regarded as inadequate for purposes of obtaining a baseline measure of her behaviour. However, it proved useful in two respects: it demonstrated that Fay was willing to participate in her own treatment programme by carrying a record sheet with her; and it seemed to indicate that 'obtrusive' observation might be an effective behaviour change technique in the treatment of this particular patient. The recording technique was discontinued and Fay was informed that she had been taken 'off her programme'. Despite this, her time-keeping never deteriorated to the level reported by staff before this measure was used.

Baseline Measure One. This measure was designed such that Fay would be unaware that observations were being carried out. Ward and OT staff were given instructions to keep their observations as unobtrusive as possible. The period of observation ran over five days, Monday to Friday. Again, it was designed to measure her time-keeping. The measure was broken down in the following manner:

(1) *Observations made by ward staff* (see Appendix 10.1). This phase of observation involved the staff in recording

    (a) The time Fay arrived upstairs after rising (her bedroom is situated on the lower floor). This was considered to be important because breakfast was only served until 8.15 a.m., and if Fay arrived any later than this, she missed her breakfast. Missing her breakfast may have been one reason for her eating while she was supposed to be working.

(b) The number of prompts required to get Fay out of bed. Despite her having an alarm clock, it was reported that she rarely got up when it went off. Staff were instructed not to prompt her on days 4 and 5.

(c) The time she left the ward to go to OT, mornings and afternoons.

(d) The time she arrived on the ward from OT, mornings and afternoons.

(e) The time she went to bed.

(2) *Observations made by OT staff* (see Appendix 10.2). OT staff were instructed to observe Fay on a half-hourly basis to record exactly what she was doing at the time of observation, for example eating, working, wandering around. They were instructed to record nothing if Fay was not present. They were also asked to record Fay's work output in each session.

(3) *Times of arrival and departure from OT.* This recording was taken from the OT clocking card system, which Fay used competently.

Results. The results of the 'time-keeping' measure have been tabulated for easy comparison with the result of intervention (see Tables 10.2-4 in the 'Results' section of this chapter). They show that, despite the lingering effects of the first recording measure, Fay was a very poor time-keeper in all aspects of her daily routine. Of special interest was the time at which she was retiring to bed; on only one occasion did she stay up until 7.00 p.m.; her average time of retiring was 6.00 p.m. This early retiring time was obviously preventing her from participating in any ward-based social or recreational activity. She got up in time for breakfast only once in the five-day observation period.

The results of the OT staff's observations are depicted in Figure 10.1. The histogram shows that Fay was absent from OT on ten occasions, because of ward-based activities and that recordings had not been carried out by OT staff on another ten occasions. With these twenty observations omitted, the following pattern was observed:

Unofficially absent — on 46 per cent of observations
Working — on 26 per cent of observations
Eating — on 15 per cent of observations
Wandering around — on 11 per cent of observations

Figure 10.1: Histogram Showing Results of OT Staff's Baseline Observations

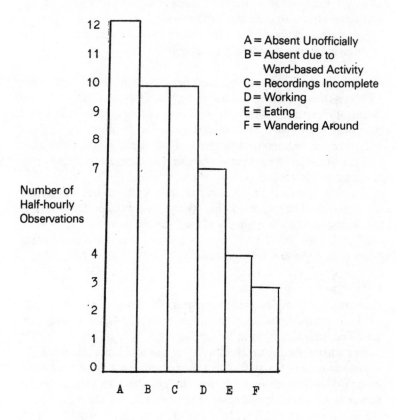

Baseline Measure Two. As the first priority of treatment was for the patient to reduce weight, it was decided that her between-meals food intake should be monitored. Because of Fay's wandering, it would

have been extremely difficult for an observer to record this, as it would have been necessary for him to follow her wherever she went. Besides being very time consuming, another difficulty was that Fay was, despite her size, quite elusive and often managed to 'disappear' quite effectively.

Fay was approached and asked if she would be willing to write down what she ate between meals. By this time, I had established a working relationship with her and it was not a difficult task to persuade her to do this. A small pocket notebook with a short pencil attached (see Appendix 10.3) was made ready and, on Fay's request, was decorated with drawings of flowers.

Her weight was being recorded weekly by ward staff and there was no reason to alter this during baseline.

Results.   Fay consistently recorded her 'between-meals' food intake for eleven days and then suddenly stopped. Despite all efforts by the therapist and ward staff to persuade and encourage her to continue recording, she did not. She would start the day by promising to do it, but when her notebook was checked at night, she had recorded nothing. Attempts were made throughout treatment to persuade Fay to recommence recording, but with no success.

However, the recordings she had made over this eleven-day period were useful. They showed that every day without fail she had consumed substantial amounts of food and drink outside her regular mealtimes (see Table 10.1). It was obvious that she was spending every penny she had on food and drink.

Intervention I

A record sheet was designed in the form of a 'day plan' (see Appendix 10.4). It comprised a list of instructions and the times at which the specified activities were to be carried out.

Fay carried the record sheet with her and was instructed to hand it to the nurses or to OT staff so that they could sign it. Staff were asked to give Fay praise for good time-keeping and to give a neutral response for poor time-keeping. Fay was asked if she would mind wearing her wrist-watch and she agreed to do so. She could read the time quite competently; I tested her ability by turning the pointers of her alarm clock and asking her to read out the time displayed. She did this with a haphazard mixture of words and figures, but consistently recorded the correct time.

She was then given a drawing of two alarm clocks, one with the

Table 10.1: Fay's Self-monitoring of Between-Meals Eating

Day	Food and drink consumed between meals (morning)	Food and drink consumed between meals (afternoon)
1	1 large bottle of lemonade 1 packet of crisps 2 packets of chewing gum	1 can of Tab Cola 1 cup of coffee
2	1 packet of crisps 1 Snowball 1 glass of milk	1 large bottle of Pola Cola 1 packet of crisps 1 packet of chewing gum
3	—	2 packets of chewing gum 2 Snowballs 1 glass of orange juice
4	3 Snowballs	2 peanut chews
5	1 chocolate biscuit	4 penny sweets 1 large bottle of lemonade 1 glass of milk
6	1 large bottle of lemonade 1 Mars bar 2 Bounty bars 1 plain cake	2 glasses of Pepsi 2 grapefruits 1 cup of milk
7	—	2 glasses of Pepsi
8	—	2 cups of Cola 1 packet of chewing gum
9	2 fruit pastries	1 bottle of lemonade 1 packet of Polo Mints
10	—	1 large bottle of Pola Cola 1 Snowball
11	—	1 large bottle of lemonade 1 can of beer 1 Milky Way

pointers set at 7.30 a.m. with instructions to get up and the other with the pointers set at 8.00 p.m. with the instructions that she should not be going to bed before this time. Below the drawings was a record sheet and Fay was asked to record the time she got up and the time she went to bed.

Obtrusive observation was used along with self-recording because of its apparent effectiveness in changing Fay's behaviour in the pre-baseline phase. This phase of intervention was designed to attempt to change Fay's time-keeping. The anticipated effects of her success-fully carrying out this plan were as follows:

(1) By being upstairs in time for breakfast, she might not be hungry during the morning session at OT and would therefore be expected to eat fewer sweet foods.
(2) Being up earlier might help her to get to work on time and thereby assist in increasing her work output.
(3) Knowing she was being observed while in OT might have an effect on whether she stayed there throughout a session.
(4) Presenting the staff with her recording sheet gave them an opportunity to give her social praise for appropriate behaviour.
(5) Providing her with a target time for going to bed and getting her to record her bedtimes might serve to increase the amount of time available for participating in social activities during the evening.
(6) Being awake and active for much more of the day might assist, to some extent, in weight reduction.

This stage of intervention ran from Monday to Friday for eight weeks.

Intervention II

In an attempt to improve upon the results of Intervention I, a motivational system was designed. Points were used as conditioned reinforcement. Fay earned points according to how close she came to her targets. A new day plan was designed which contained instructions, e.g. 'Be upstairs at 8.15 a.m.'; 'Leave OT at 3.30 p.m.'. Adjacent to the instructions were the number of points which she could earn if she carried out the instructions. The next three columns were used for nurses to record their signatures, the time at which Fay, for example, 'arrived upstairs' and the points she earned for doing so. A sliding scale of times and points was constructed (see Appendix 10.5). Each behaviour on the record sheet had a points value. The points values were calculated after analysing the results of the baseline period and of Intervention I.

Those behaviours that rarely occurred, e.g. going to bed at or after 8.00 p.m., were weighted with considerably more points than those behaviours that occurred frequently. Forty per cent of the maximum possible daily points total would be earned if Fay lost any weight. As well as being designed to improve her time-keeping and reduce her weight, the programme was also designed to increase her work output in OT.

In order to set a work-output target, Fay's work rate was compared with that of two other patients in the OT department. One of these patients was described by OT staff as a 'good worker', the other a 'poor worker'. A continuous recording of Fay and the other two patients' outputs was made and the amount of work done by each patient, every five minutes, was recorded. The observations were carried out in a two-hour morning session in the OT department. The work being performed involved attaching strings to clothing labels; this had been the regular work of the three patients for some time before the recordings were made. The patients were aware of the observer's presence, but not of his intent. The results are shown in Figure 10.2.

From the results, it can be seen that Fay did considerably less work than either of the other two patients, completing only 46 units of work in two hours compared with 104 for the 'poor worker' and 176 for the 'good worker'.

Back-up Reinforcers

It was necessary for the back-up reinforcers which were being employed in this treatment phase to be more powerful than the reinforcement Fay was getting from, for example, going to bed early. She obviously enjoyed fizzy drinks and she appreciated a 'long lie in bed'.

In the search for potent back-up reinforcers it was discovered that she frequently expressed a wish to visit the town to do some shopping. In order to see how much she valued the town, I accompanied Fay on a shopping trip. She appeared to enjoy this excursion enormously. As well as using the trip as an opportunity for Fay to sample a potential back-up reinforcer, it also provided an opportunity to assess her community skills. The following behaviours were observed:

(a) Use of public transport.
(b) Ability to cross roads safely.
(c) Behaviour in shops.
(d) Behaviour in cafés.
(e) Ability to use money.
(f) Behaviour in the street.
(g) Use of public telephone.

It was found that Fay was deficient in the performance of all these skills. If a weekly trip to town was to be used as a back-up reinforcer, it

Figure 10.2: Graph showing Work units Completed by Fay, by a 'Poor Worker', and by a 'Good Worker'

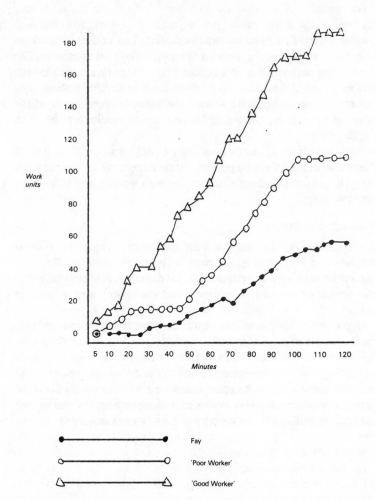

would also be an excellent opportunity for Fay to practise and to improve upon these skills.

After discussion with ward staff, it was decided to use as back-up reinforcers: a weekly trip to town; a can of Diet Pepsi daily (which she had previously enjoyed while on her first town visit); and a long lie in bed at the weekend. It was decided that I would accompany Fay to the town in order to instruct her in appropriate community skills. While in town, she would buy her weekly supply of Diet Pepsi. Bus fares to and from town were to be taken from ward funds for this purpose. The programme was drawn up and a copy given to ward and OT staff. I explained each step of the programme to the staff. A copy of the programme follows.

Behaviour Therapy Programme

the programme is designed to attempt to achieve the following:

(1) Reduce weight.
(2) Increase participation in recreation and social activity.
(3) Increase work output/attention to task in OT.

The programme will operate as follows. Fay will earn points for achieving daily targets of which there are eleven each day. The targets are weighted with points according to their importance and relevance to the above. The programme is designed as a structured day and the patient has been following very similar instructions during the baseline recording period.

How Will it Work to Reduce Weight? Fay will be given 40 per cent of the potential points available for any one day for losing weight. Any weight loss will be reinforced this way irrespective of the amount lost. As well as the points the patient will receive praise for weight lost. Even if Fay does not lose weight over the period of a week, i.e. if she loses 1 lb on day 1 but gains 2 lb on day 2 and stays the same on days 3, 4 and 5, the emphasis of the programme will be on the weight she lost on day 1 and she will be reinforced for this; the weight gains will be emphasised as little as possible. For example, I have set a target of 400 points for the first five days of the programme. To achieve this, Fay will only have to lose weight on one day to earn the points and thus increase the likelihood of earning the major reinforcer. The points target will gradually increase according to the patient's progress.

The structured day may also help with weight reduction in the following way:

(a) by increasing the amount of time in any one day during which the patient is active and thus expending energy;
(b) by eating set meals, e.g. breakfast: this may reduce her intake of sweet foods while in the OT department.

How Will it Work to Increase Participation in Recreation and Social Activity? Fay is rarely available for any form of social activity, particularly in the evening as she invariably retires to her bed very early. I have weighted her bedtime target with a large number of points so as to make it more attractive for her to stay up.

In addition to this, I would like to introduce a programme that will increase her attention to task in recreation.

How Will it Work to Increase Work Output/Attention to Task in OT? From my observations the majority of Fay's time in the OT department is spent wandering around, eating and drinking. By setting a target of work output per session in the OT department, I hope to decrease the time spent in non-production, and increase that in production. This work rate is fairly heavily weighted with points as compared with some other aspects of the plan.

Reinforcement. On reaching a pre-set weekly target of points, Fay will be eligible to receive the following reinforcers: a can of Diet Pepsi every evening if she reaches her daily target; she will be allowed to stay in bed at the weekend if she meets the target set for this; and she will be taken on a shopping trip to the town on Tuesday or Wednesday of the following week if she meets her major target requirement of points.

Points. Fay can potentially earn 1000 points per day but as this would be unlikely to be achieved if I were to set this as a first target, the points will be staggered to how near Fay gets to her targets. For example, the targets for plan 1 will be no more than Fay has achieved over the past four weeks of baseline recording. They will gradually be raised as Fay finds it easier to achieve them, and we will work towards the desired target in this way.

Maximum points for each target are as follows:

(1) *Time of arrival upstairs.* Target: to be upstairs, washed and fully dressed at 8.15 a.m. (breakfast time). Her alarm is set for 7.30 a.m. This gives her three-quarters of an hour to achieve her target. Points value for arriving upstairs at 8.15 a.m., **120**.

(2) *Time of arrival at OT department (morning session).* Target: the starting time at the OT department in the morning is 9.30 a.m. It will help Fay to achieve her work-output target if she is there at or near 9.30 a.m. But as it seems that hardly anyone else adheres to this starting time, it would be unfair to expect Fay to. This is, therefore, weighted fairly lightly. Points value for arriving at OT at 9.30 a.m., **20**.

(3) *Work rate/attention to task in OT.* Fay's work rate has proven to be very inconsistent over the weeks I have been observing her (work units range from 0 to 70 per day). During a period of continuous observation she completed 46 work units in a 2-hour period (during this period she was 20 minutes late and left 20 minutes early). If she had been present for the full 2-hour period, I calculate she could have achieved 69 work units. She was aware, however, that she was being observed, and this may have influenced her to do more. Therefore, for the first stage of the programme, I will set her target at 35 work units per work period which, although it is half her assessed potential, should help her to achieve success during the first stage. Work-rate target, first stage: 35 work units. Points value for achieving 35 work units, **60**.

(4) *Time leaving OT department (morning session).* Target: the work period finishes at 11.30 a.m. but again the majority of patients do not adhere to this time, so it would be unfair to expect Fay to do so. Therefore, this is weighted fairly low. Points value for leaving OT at 11.30 a.m., **20**.

(5) *Time arriving on the ward.* From recordings over the past week, Fay has shown that she can reach the ward from the OT department in 10 minutes or less. This gives her very little time to go to the hospital shop to buy food. However, as my recordings have shown, she rarely seems to do this in the morning anyway, so this again is weighted fairly low. Points value for arriving on the ward at 11.40 a.m., **20**.

(6) *Time of arrival at OT department (afternoon).* Target: the starting time for the afternoon session at the OT department is 1.30 p.m. For the reasons stated above for the morning session, this is again weighted fairly low. Points value for arriving at OT

department at 1.30 p.m., **20**.

(7)   Work rate/attention to task. The afternoon period will have a points weighting the same as that of the morning session, and again this will increase in stages. Work rate target, first stage: 35 work units. Points value for achieving 35 work units, **60**.

(8)   Time leaving OT department (afternoon). The afternoon work period finishes at 3.30 p.m. Fay has invariably left before this time, but again so have many other patients, so this period is lightly weighted. Points value for leaving OT at 3.30 p.m., **20**.

(9)   Time arriving on the ward (afternoon). Fay has shown that she often takes much longer to return to the ward from the OT department after work in the afternoon. She has occasionally taken 45 minutes to return. I can only speculate as to what she does with this time as it would be very difficult to observe her, but on her own admission she visits the hospital shop and buys food and drink, and she has occasionally, in the past, visited other wards in the hospital to ask for food. In order to give her an incentive to take less time to get back to the ward, and thus hopefully to curtail her food intake, I have weighted this period relatively heavily. Points value for arriving on the ward at 3.40 p.m., **40**.

(10)   Time of going to bed. Fay often goes to bed well before 7.00 p.m. and occasionally as early as 5.30 p.m. By doing this she is opting out of any social and recreational activity. In an attempt to keep her in circulation at least until 8.00 p.m., this section has been heavily weighted with points. Points value for going to bed at or after 8.00 p.m. **120**.

(11)   Weight loss. If Fay loses any weight during the day she will be awarded **400** points. She should be weighed at the same time each day and a graph kept on her bedroom wall as a record. I also intend to keep a record of my own weight to introduce an element of competition, and to be weighed at the same time as Fay.

The staff agreed that the programme was easy to follow, but raised the point, 'What happens if Fay is officially absent from work for any reason?' It was decided that if this happened, she would be awarded half of the points she could have earned in the normal course of events. This would prevent her daily points total from being in jeopardy because she was unable, through no fault of her own, to carry out her programme. The staff were given a weekly record sheet on which to record points and times (see Appendix 10.6).

Fay was asked if she would like to visit the town every week. She was delighted at the idea, but when it was suggested that she would have to work a little harder to achieve this she was, to say the least, somewhat lacking in enthusiasm. The points system was explained to her and she was told that the closer she got to her target times and the more weight she lost, the more points she would earn and this would enable her to go into town. She came around to the idea after considering it for two days, and the programme commenced.

As well as incorporating a motivational system, the programme also involved obtrusive observation by staff. Again, Fay took an active part by carrying her own record sheet and by presenting it to staff for signing as in Intervention I.

The programme ran over a 7-week period. It was reviewed regularly in discussions with ward staff. During these review meetings, the importance of social approval as a variable in the day-to-day running of the programme was emphasised. The programme was evaluated during a meeting of all the people concerned with its implementation, and certain aspects of the programme were subsequently altered.

Intervention Stage III

From the results of Intervention II (see Tables 10.2 and 10.3) it can be seen that Fay's performance at OT had deteriorated in two important respects: she was leaving earlier and doing less work.

It was felt that perhaps the back-up reinforcement was too far removed in time from the behaviour which it was intended to control. It was decided to concentrate on her behaviour during the morning sessions and to offer her an afternoon off if she completed a whole morning's session in OT. However, she would be given bonus points if she attended OT in the afternoon when she had been allowed the afternoon off.

In addition to reinforcing weight loss, it was also decided to award Fay points for maintaining a steady weight. She would now be weighed at night and, immediately afterwards, given her can of Diet Pepsi if she had earned her points for performing the other required activities during the course of the day. The record sheet and points scale were redesigned to accommodate these changes. The redesigned programme was intended to run from bedtime until the time at which she was weighed the following day (approximately

Table 10.2: Mean Number of Minutes 'Off Target' per Programme Stage

	Baseline	Intervention I	Intervention II	Intervention III
Up in time for breakfast	27	43	22	2
Arrive at OT on time (a.m.)	16	10	7	4
Leave OT on time (a.m.)	16	11	20	4
Arrive at OT on time (p.m.)	17	16	8	5.5
Leave OT on time (p.m.)	17	14	46	14
Go to bed at or after 8.00 p.m.	120	42	31	+7

Table 10.3: Results of Treatment in Terms of Work Rate

	Mean no. of work units performed per session per programme stage
Baseline	23
Intervention I	25
Intervention II	18
Intervention III	33

7.00 p.m.). This arrangement was agreed upon as it meant that Fay's daily total would be added up at the time at which she was weighed, and there was therefore no need to wait to see how long she stayed up before she was given her Diet Pepsi.

The redesigned programme was explained to Fay and she appeared delighted with the changes, especially with the idea of an afternoon off. Her wall chart was altered, giving her new visual instructions and points targets. She was also moved to another bedroom, next to a patient who regularly arose in time for breakfast. It was felt that if Fay had a model to copy, she might improve her own rising time.

This stage of intervention is ongoing. Results have been calculated from the first 5 weeks of recording.

Results

The results have been calculated in terms of means taken during the baseline period and during Interventions I, II and III. You will recall that the target behaviours were:

(1) Rising in time for breakfast.
(2) Arriving in OT on time (morning).
(3) Leaving OT on time (morning).
(4) Time taken to walk from OT to ward (morning).
(5) Arriving at OT on time (afternoon).
(6) Leaving OT on time (afternoon).
(7) Time taken to walk from OT to ward (afternoon).
(8) Going to bed at 8.00 p.m. or after.
(9) Participation in recreational and social activities.
(10) Increasing her work output.
(11) Weight reduction.

Many of the results were calculated in terms of the average number of minutes by which Fay was 'off target' or late (see Table 10.2). For the time taken to walk from OT to the ward, the results were calculated as an average of the number of minutes she took per programme stage (see Table 10.4). Fay's work-rate output was calculated as an average of the amount of units of work completed per programme stage. Her weight was calculated as an average over each of the three separate intervention periods and compared with the average for the baseline period.

Table 10.4: Time Taken to Walk from OT to the Ward

| | Average time taken per programme stage (minutes) | |
	Mornings	Afternoons
Baseline	24	38
Intervention I	8	35
Intervention II	33	30
Intervention III	20	17

Summary of Results

(1) *Rising in time for breakfast* (see Table 10.2). The target time set was 8.15 a.m. (breakfast time on the ward); Fay had to be up and dressed before this time.
Intervention I: Fay in fact arrived upstairs 16 minutes later on average in this stage of treatment, as compared with baseline.
Intervention II: This shows an average improvement on baseline of 5 minutes.
Intervention III: There is an average improvement of 25 minutes on baseline. It should be noted that another patient modelled the appropriate behaviour at this stage. Fay arose in time for breakfast 14 times out of 25 recordings taken.

(2) *Arriving in OT on time, morning session* (see Table 10.2). Morning OT sessions commenced at 9.30 a.m.
Intervention I: Shows an average improvement of 6 minutes on baseline, that is, she was arriving 6 minutes earlier.
Intervention II: Shows an average improvement of 9 minutes on baseline, that is, she was arriving 9 minutes earlier.
Intervention III: Shows an average improvement of 12 minutes on baseline, that is, she was arriving 12 minutes earlier. Recordings show that she arrived in time for work 13 times out of 21 sessions held during Intervention III.

(3) *Leaving OT on time, morning session* (see Table 10.2). The morning session in OT ended at 11.30 a.m.
Intervention I: Shows an average improvement of 5 minutes on baseline, that is, she was leaving OT 5 minutes later.
Intervention II: Shows an average deterioration of 4 minutes on baseline, that is, she was leaving OT 4 minutes earlier than during baseline.
Intervention III: Shows an average improvement of 12 minutes on baseline, that is, she was leaving OT 12 minutes later. Recordings show that she left work on time (at 11.30 a.m.) 13 times out of 21 sessions held during Intervention III.

(4) *Time taken to walk from OT to ward, after morning session* (see Table 10.4).
Intervention I: Shows an average improvement of 16 minutes on baseline, that is, the time taken for her to reach the ward was

16 minutes less than the baseline.

Intervention II: Shows an average deterioration of 9 minutes on baseline, that is, it took her 9 minutes longer to walk from OT to the ward.

Intervention III: Shows an average improvement of 4 minutes on baseline, that is, the time taken for her to reach the ward was 4 minutes less than the baseline. She reached the ward 8 times in 10 minutes or less out of 21 sessions held during Intervention III.

(5) *Arriving in OT on time, afternoon session* (see Table 10.2). Afternoon OT sessions commenced at 1.30 p.m.

Intervention I: Shows an average improvement of 1 minute on baseline, that is, she was arriving 1 minute earlier.

Intervention II: Shows an average improvement of 9 minutes on baseline, that is, she was arriving 9 minutes earlier.

Intervention III: Shows an average improvement of 3 minutes on baseline, that is, she was arriving 3 minutes earlier. What should be taken into consideration with this result is that, in terms of the revised programme which was in operation in Intervention III, Fay need not have attended 11 of the 21 sessions held.

(6) *Leaving OT on time, afternoon session* (see Table 10.2). The afternoon session in OT ended at 3.30 p.m.

Intervention I: Shows an average improvement of 3 minutes on baseline, that is, she was leaving OT 3 minutes later.

Intervention II: Shows an average deterioration of 29 minutes on baseline, that is, she was leaving OT 29 minutes earlier than on baseline.

Intervention III: Shows an average improvement of 3 minutes on baseline, that is, she was leaving OT 3 minutes later. Again it must be considered that Fay need not have attended 11 out of the 21 sessions held.

(7) *Time taken to walk from OT to ward after afternoon session* (see Table 10.4).

Intervention I: Shows an average improvement of 3 minutes on baseline, that is, she was taking 3 minutes less to walk from OT to the ward.

Intervention II: Shows an average improvement of 7½ minutes on baseline, that is, she was taking 7½ minutes less to walk from OT to the ward.

Intervention III: Shows an average improvement of 20 minutes on baseline, that is, she was taking 20 minutes less to walk from OT to the ward. She reached the ward eight times in 10 minutes or less out of 21 sessions held during Intervention III.

(8) *Going to bed at or after 8.00 p.m.* (see Table 10.2).
Intervention I: On average, Fay was going to bed at 7.18 p.m.; this was a 58-minute improvement upon baseline.
Intervention II: On average, she was going to bed at 7.29 p.m.; this was an 89-minute improvement upon baseline.
Intervention III: On average, she was going to bed at 8.07 p.m; this was a 127-minute improvement upon baseline. Of the 25 recordings made, Fay went to bed on five occasions after 9.00 p.m.

(9) *Participation in recreational/social activities.* the programme had the effect of keeping Fay 'in circulation' and therefore available for social activities for an average daily increase time of 127 minutes by intervention stage III (when compared with baseline levels).

(10) *Work rate* (see Table 10.3). This improved on average by ten units per session when her baseline performance and her performance during intervention III are compared.

(11) *Weight* (see Table 10.5). In the course of the programme there was an overall reduction in weight of 2.7 kg (6 lb).

Table 10.5: Results of Treatment in Terms of Weight Reduction

	Mean weight per programme stage
Baseline	88 kg (13 st 12 lb)
Intervention I	87 kg (13 st 9 lb)
Intervention II	86 kg (13 st 8 lb)
Intervention III	85 kg (13 st 6 lb)

Discussion

The results of the treatment programme demonstrate that, in some respects, the patient's behaviour changed considerably over a relatively short time. The patient had been hospitalised for 36 years and it may have taken many of these years to develop the style of life which she was leading prior to treatment.

The intervention package involved several techniques: self-monitoring, obtrusive observation, goal-setting and instructions, conditioned reinforcement, social approval and feedback. There was also a great deal of individual therapist contact. The results suggest that Intervention III was the most effective and this phase included all of the treatment techniques listed above.

The results suggest that offering Fay 'the afternoon off' for working a full morning had the desired effect of increasing her work output during both the morning and the afternoon sessions. She was actually 'volunteering' to go to work when she need not have done so (she might easily have spent her free time wandering around the hospital: no one could have objected). The decreased amount of time she took to walk from OT to the ward also suggests that she was spending less time 'wandering'. The results of Intervention II were disappointing. However, at that time Fay's 'mental state' had deteriorated somewhat. Staff reported an increase in her delusional speech and that she was frequently verbally aggressive. She was prescribed chlorpromazine 50 mg p.r.n.; this, however, was only administered once. The effects of the programme might, at this stage, have been reversed, but this was not the case. After a lengthy process of evaluation, the programme was adjusted and the effects of this can be seen in the results of Intervention III, during the course of which improvement can be seen in all Fay's target behaviours.

If a similar programme were to be attempted on another patient, several alterations would be made to the treatment procedures. For instance, a suitable model would be brought in at an earlier stage of the programme. Tangible conditioned reinforcers (e.g. tokens) might be more effective than points, as they can be 'spent and saved' like money. On review, the points system certainly seems a little cumbersome and complex.

It is generally agreed that Fay's quality of life has improved enormously. Her active day has been lengthened by over two hours on average. She is visiting town very regularly now and these excursions have been beneficial in a way that was unforeseen during assessment.

Many of her community skills have improved considerably, even though she will need more practice and training in some of these skills. She is attending OT for longer periods, is doing more when she is there, and she appears to be getting something out of it. It is no longer a boring, repetitive job offering very little reward.

The effect of the programme on her weight is not by any means substantial but the results suggest a slight downward trend, and as the programme is still ongoing this may continue.

In terms of cost-effectiveness, the programme was labour intensive, but when the complexity of the problems tackled are matched with the encouraging results, it might be said that the effort was justified. Three entirely different behaviours were effectively improved at the same time by using one (admittedly complex) treatment package. Costly it might have been, but when the cost of this relatively short programme (which, if continued, could possibly lead to a community placement) is compared with the cost of keeping a patient in hospital for 36 years, there is ample justification, in the author's opinion, for offering this type of individualised treatment to other long-stay patients.

References

Ayllon, T. and Azrin, N.H. (1965) 'Reinforcement and Instructions with Mental Patients', *Journal of the Experimental Analysis of Behaviour, 9,* 327–31

Ayllon, T. and Azrin, N.H. (1968) *The Token Economy: a Motivational System for Therapy and Rehabilitation,* Appleton–Century–Crofts, New York

Christopherson, E.R., Arnold, C.M., Hill, D.W. and Quilitch, H.R. (1972) 'The Home Point System: Token Reinforcement Procedures for Application by Parents of Children with Behaviour Problems', *Journal of Applied Behaviour Analysis, 5,* 485–97

Herbert, E.W. and Baer, D.M. (1972) 'Training Parents as Behaviour Modifiers: Self-recording of Contingent Attention', *Journal of Applied Behaviour Analysis, 5,* 139–49

Hutzell, R., Platzek, D. and Logue, P. (1974) 'Control of Symptoms of Gilles de la Tourett's Syndrome by Self-Monitoring, *Journal of Behaviour Therapy and Experimental Psychiatry, 5,* 71–6

Johnson, S.M. and White, G. (1971) 'Self-observation as an Agent of Behavioural Change', *Behaviour Therapy, 2,* 488–97

Kazdin, A.E. (1972) 'Nonresponsiveness of Patients to Token Economies', *Behaviour Research and Therapy, 10,* 417–18

Kazdin, A.E. (1974) 'Reactive Self-monitoring: the Effects of Response Desirability, Goal Setting and Feedback', *Journal of Consulting and Clinical Psychology, 42,* 704–16

Kazdin, A.E. (1975a) *Behaviour Modification in Applied Settings,* The Dorsey Press, Homewood, Illinois

Kazdin, A.E. (1975b) 'Recent Advances in Token Economy Research', in M. Mersen, R.M. Eisler and P.M. Miller (eds), *Progess in Behaviour Modification,* Volume I,

Academic Press, New York

McFall, R.M. (1970) 'Effects of Self-monitoring on Normal Smoking Behaviour', *Journal of Consulting and Clinical Psychology, 35*, 135–42

Nelson, O.R., Lipinski, D.P. and Black, J.L. 'The Reactivity of Adult Retardates' Self-Monitoring: a Comparison among Behaviours of Different Valences, and a Comparison with Token Reinforcement', *The Psychological Record, 26*, 189–201

Paton, X. (1981) 'The Borders Schedule', in *Care and Training of the Mentally Handicapped*, C. Hallas, W. Fraser and R. McGillivray (eds), Wright, Bristol

Phillips, E.L. (1968) 'Achievement Place: Token Reinforcement Procedures in a Home-style Rehabilitation Setting for "Pre-Delinquent" Boys', *Journal of Applied Behaviour Analysis, 1*, 213–23

Rutner, I.T. and Bugle, C. (1969) 'An Experimental Procedure for the Modification of Psychotic Behaviour', *Journal of Consulting and Clinical Psychology, 33*, 651–3

Stuart, R.B. (1969) 'Operant Interpersonal Treatment for Marital Discord', *Journal of Consulting and Clinical Psychology, 33*, 675–82

Zegiob, L., Klukas, N and Junginger, J. (1978) 'Reactivity of Self-monitoring Procedures with Retarded Adults', *American Journal of Mental Deficiency, 83* (2), 156–63

Appendices

Appendix 10.1: Record Sheet for Staff's Observations during Baseline

PLEASE RECORD:
1. Time patient arrives upstairs
2. Time patient leaves Ward for O.T.
3. Time patient arrives on Ward from O.T. (a.m. and p.m.)
4. Time patient goes to bed.

N.B. It is important that the patient is unaware of recording.

DAY	Time Up	Prompt	Time to O.T.	Time from O.T.	Time to O.T.	Time from O.T.	Time to bed
1							
2							
3							
4							
5							
6							
7							
8							
9							

Appendix 10.2: Record Sheet for Staff's Observations during Baseline

N.B. It is important that the patient is unaware of recording.

DAY .... DATE ....

TIME	WHAT IS THE PATIENT DOING?	SIGNATURE
9.30		
10.00		
10.30		
11.00		
11.30		

TIME	WHAT IS THE PATIENT DOING?	SIGNATURE
1.30		
2.00		
2.30		
3.00		
	Please record what the patient is doing at the times stated, e.g. working, eating, talking, wandering around. RECORD NOTHING IF SHE IS ABSENT	

Appendix 10.3: What Do I Eat at Work and in My Free Time?
(Example of First Two Pages from the Patient's Food Recording
Booklet.)

I would be very happy if you
could help me in the following
way. Please write down in this
little book everything you have
to eat at the Therapy and in
your free time.

THANK YOU VERY MUCH !

Christopher Portues

Monday - 10th March

MORNING

AFTERNOON

Appendix 10.4: A Planned Day for ....

TODAY IS:

F A Y - Ask the Nurse or O.T. to Sign here
          At these times

Nurse or O.T. please
record time when you
sign.

Time	A L A R M !! Time to Get Up!	Time	Signature
8.15	Arrive Upstairs ————————	____	_____
9.20	Time to Leave for O.T. ————	____	_____
9.30	Arrive at O.T. ————————	____	_____
10.00	Tea Break ————————————	____	_____
10.30	Still in O.T. ? —————————	____	_____
11.00	Still in O.T. ? ————————	____	_____
11.30	Leave O.T. to go back to Ward. ———	____	_____
11.40	Arrive on the Ward. —————	____	_____
1.20	Time to Leave for O.T. ————	____	_____
1.30	Arrive at O.T. ————————	____	_____
2.00	Tea Break ————————————	____	_____
2.30	Still in O.T. ? ———— ————	____	_____
3.00	Still in O.T. ? ————————	____	_____
3.30	Leave O.T. to go back to Ward. ———	____	_____
3.40	Arrive on the Ward.————————	____	_____
4.30	Still on the Ward. —————	____	_____
5.30		____	_____
6.00	Nurse only to	____	_____
6.30	sign if Fay is	____	_____
7.00	<u>NOT</u> in bed!	____	_____
7.30		____	_____
8.00		____	_____

Appendix 10.5: Sliding Scale of Points Values

POINTS TABLE

1)   **Time of Arrival Upstairs.**

Time	Points
· 8.15	120
8.20	110
8.25	100
8.30	90
8.35	80
8.40	70
8.45	60
8.50	40
8.55	20
9.00	10
9.05	0

2)   **Time of Arrival at O.T. Department** (morning session)

Time	Points
9.30	20
9.35	18
9.40	14
9.45	8
9.50	2
9.55	0

3)   <u>Work Rate</u> (morning session)

Work Units	Points
35	60
30	30
25	25
20	20
15	15
10	10
Less than 10	0

4)   <u>Time Leaving O.T. Department</u> (morning session)

Time	Points
11.30	20
11.25	15
11.20	5
11.15	0

5)   <u>Time Arriving on Ward</u> (morning)

Time	Points
11.40	20
11.45	10
After 11.45	0

Appendix 10.5: *continued*

6) <u>Time of Arrival at O.T. Department</u> (afternoon)

Time	Points
1.30	20
1.35	18
1.40	14
1.45	8
1.50	2
1.55	0

7) <u>Work Rate</u> (afternoon session)

Work Units	Points
35	60
30	30
25	25
20	20
15	15
10	10
Less than 10	0

8) <u>Time Leaving O.T. Department</u> (afternoon session)

Time	Points
3.30	20
3.25	15
3.20	5
3.15	0

9) <u>Time Arriving on the Ward</u> (afternoon)

Time	Points
3.40	40
3.45	30
3.50	20
3.55	10
After 3.55	0

10) <u>Time of Going to Bed</u>

Time	Points
8.00 or after	120
7.45 "	100
7.40 "	90
7.35 "	80
7.30 "	70
7.30 or before	0

11) <u>Weight Loss</u>

Any weight loss = 400 points

Appendix 10.6: Weekly Record Sheet

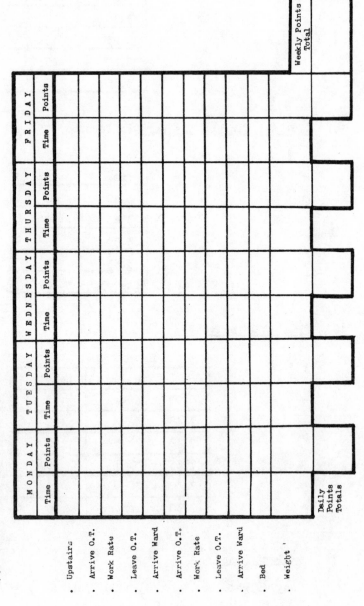

	MONDAY		TUESDAY		WEDNESDAY		THURSDAY		FRIDAY		Weekly Points Total
	Time	Points	Time	Points	Time	Points	Time	Points	Time	Points	
Upstairs											
Arrive O.T.											
Work Rate											
Leave O.T.											
Arrive Ward											
Arrive O.T.											
Work Rate											
Leave O.T.											
Arrive Ward											
Bed											
Weight											
Daily Points Totals											

11 THE MANAGEMENT OF CHRONIC PAIN

William Harkin

Introduction

For most of us pain serves the useful purpose of warning us of something wrong and prompts us to seek assistance. However, when pain persists for some time, it imposes severe emotional, physical, and economic stresses on the individual, and on the family. Data from a variety of sources suggest that chronic pain states cost billions of pounds annually (Bond, 1984). Even more important is the cost in terms of human suffering. Many chronic pain sufferers, in search of pain relief, are referred from specialist to specialist, becoming increasingly despondent as they realise that they present seemingly insoluble problems to the health service (Linton, 1982).

Two Concepts of Pain

Since the beginning of this century, the transmission of pain information was thought to be along a direct path from peripheral pain receptors to a pain centre in the brain. This 'reductionist' view of the pain experience suggested that pain was a specific sensation with a single quality, namely intensity. The complaint of pain was viewed from the perspective of a medical model — a symptom of some underlying pathology. The strategy of treatment was to modify the underlying pathology in order that the symptom would disappear. Where the underlying pathology could not be influenced significantly, medical management focused on symptomatic relief using palliative medication or surgery (Fordyce, Fowler, Lehmann and de Lateur, 1968).

In 1965 the 'gate control theory' of pain was proposed (Melzack and Wall, 1965). This suggests that the information arising as the result of noxious stimulation is modified in its passage from the peripheral nerve fibres to those in the spinal cord by a specialised 'gate' mechanism situated in the posterior horns of the spinal cord. When the 'gate' is open, the pain information passes to the brain, but if partially or completely closed, less information or no information will reach the brain. The gate can be closed by the activity of fibres derived from the periphery and by the influence of control centres in the brain. Thus, previous learning and the state of arousal can influence the setting of the gate (Melzack, 1980). In contrast to the one-cause, one-effect concept of pain in the reductionist model, the 'gate control' theory suggests multiple interactions that determine the experience of pain. Moreover, pain is viewed not as a specific sensation that can vary only in intensity, but as a variety of qualities categorised under a single linguistic label (Melzack and Torgerson, 1971). As the pain arises from the complex interaction of sensory and psychological factors, the strategy of treatment is widened to include psychological interventions.

The Measurement of Pain

Assessing and understanding the nature of a patient's pain complaints are important but difficult clinical tasks. Rating scales that measure intensity remain in common use in spite of evidence that they fail to reflect the complexity of the pain experience (Frederiksen, Sterling, Lynd and Ross, 1978). They supply limited information to the clinician faced with the challenge of understanding a patient's pain. Misconceptions about the effectiveness of treatment can occur when clinicians use measurement techniques that measure only pain intensity to evaluate therapeutic strategies that attempt to modify psychological reactions to pain. Attempts at measurement should consider the nature of pain, a complex subjective experience that involves variations on several dimensions (Sternbach, 1978). Moreover, because pain relief for a substantial proportion of patients is seldom total, one task of measurement may be to identify the degree and nature of the change that is brought about by treatment. This is important in the behavioural approach when therapeutic intervention is often designed to increase the patient's ability to cope with pain.

An important advance in the assessment of pain reports was achieved with the development of the McGill Pain Questionnaire (MPQ: Melzack, 1975). This was produced in an attempt to measure multi-dimensional aspects of pain. Melzack and Torgerson (1971) found subjects were able to classify reliably a wide range of pain descriptors into three basic groups, which represented different dimensions of pain. These were:

(a) a sensory dimension, which described pain in terms of its spatial,

temporal, pressure and thermal properties;
(b) an affective dimension, which described pain in terms of its associated tension, fear and autonomic properties;
(c) an evaluative dimension, which described the subjective aspects of the total pain experience.

The three main measures on the MPQ are: a pain rating index: this is based on numerical values that can be assigned to each word descriptor; the number of words chosen; and the present pain intensity: this is based on an intensity scale from 1 to 5. The MPQ has been widely employed and its effectiveness as an evaluative instrument has been demonstrated. The validity of the affective dimension against other independent measures of affect has been confirmed by Kremer and Atkinson (1981). Gracely, McGrath and Dubner (1978) have demonstrated that the three dimensions (i.e. affective, sensory and evaluative) do operate independently.

Aspects of Chronic Pain

Chronic pain usually refers to the complaint of pain over at least a six-month period, although most patients have suffered much longer (Linton, 1982). Fordyce (1978) has suggested that the time period has significance for the behaviour of the chronic pain sufferer. Actions that express pain he terms 'pain behaviours'. These include grimacing, moaning, verbalising the pain experience, asking to be helped, taking medication. Thee pain behaviours are subject to influence by conditioning effects. Given time, they can be learned by operant methods and can then be elicited independent of the original cause, and can persist after the lesion that initially gave rise to the pain has healed. Moreover, the 'chronicity' of the pain means that the patient and those around him will modify their social, vocational and household activities to accommodate the demands of the patient's pain. Many of their 'pre-pain' activities will be curtailed, and the longer the duration of the pain the greater will be the disuse of these activities as pain behaviours replace them. The effective treatment of chronic pain must, therefore, address both the task of reducing pain behaviours and that of re-establishing healthy behaviour.

Sternbach (1978) has described patients who demand pain relief, insisting that their pain is unbearable and even excruciating, but who sit calmly as they describe it, and can even be led into a joking conversation. Careful measurement of their pain indicated it to be slight to moderate in severity, and their persuasiveness was part of their expressive style. Szasz (1968) has drawn attention to a pain-prone type of individual. This person complains of chronic unbearable pain in the absence of an identifiable cause. The subject adopts a role of 'a professional in pain' and engages in 'painmanship' which is characterised by the presence of undiagnosed pain and unrelieved suffering. The patient demands frequent medical and sometimes surgical interventions. This appears to give meaning or purpose to life. The lifestyle is that of a pain sufferer whose conversation is monopolised by pain complaints and his experiences in trying to obtain relief. The initial sympathy that he draws from others is gradually replaced by antagonism as they realise that they are being manipulated by the pain sufferer. Such a patient is resistant to the conventional methods of pain treatment.

Almost all pain sufferers are believed to have some emotional disturbance. Psychological testing usually shows chronic pain patients to be depressed (Sternbach, 1978). Viewed from the behavioural perspective, depression is considered as a deprivation of reinforcers (Lewinsohn, Weinstein and Shaw, 1969) or as a state of learned helplessness (Seligman, 1975). In either event, the person verbalises negative thoughts which commonly take the form of a devaluation of self, a negative view of life experiences and a pessimistic view of the future (Beck, 1970). Although the person is clinically depressed, he may not experience the depressed mood as he becomes increasingly absorbed in his somatic symptoms (Sternbach, 1974). Reduction or abolition of the pain reverses the depression associated with it (Bond, 1973).

Conventional Treatments for Chronic Pain

A wide range of physical treatments has been developed to relieve pain, and the number and range of these treatments reflect the nature of the problem.

Drug Treatments

Analgesic Drugs. These reduce or abolish pain without affecting consciousness. A very wide range of analgesics, which vary in their potency and mode of action, are available. However, as Bond (1979) has indicated, the ideal analgesic has not yet been produced.

Analgesics are usually divided into the narcotic and antipyretic groups. The narcotic analgesics produce analgesia and depress activity of the nervous system by acting centrally on the brain. They are used to relieve severe pain and have the added property of producing mental tranquillity. However, this latter quality is linked with their tendency to produce drug dependency. It is for this reason that many medical practitioners will not prescribe these drugs for patients with chronic pain other than those with malignant disease (Lipton, 1979).

The antipyretic analgesics interfere with the metabolism of peripheral pain-producing substances in the tissues, such as the kinins and prostaglandins. They are generally used to relieve mild to moderate pain.

Psychotropic Drugs. These influence the patient's emotional state through their action on the brain. They are divided into groups which reflect their actions. The major tranquillisers, especially chlorpromazine, are frequently used to produce emotional tranquillity and to potentiate the effect of analgesic drugs. A minor tranquilliser, diazepam, is often used to relieve tension in voluntary muscles, either alone or in combination with an analgesic drug.

There are problems associated with the use of drugs in chronic pain treatment. Each drug has side-effects which may or may not be withstood by the patient. Tolerance is an additional problem that arises commonly in the drug treatment of chronic pain. This means that when the drug is taken repeatedly it becomes less effective unless the dose is steadily increased. Not infrequently, the point is reached when further increases in the dose fail to maintain the desired effect.

Nerve Blocking

This is the injection of a neurolytic agent, commonly alcohol or phenol, around the appropriate sensory nerve or ganglion. The neurolytic agent can, alternatively, be injected inside the spinal column to exert its effect on the nerve root. When accurately injected, this can give relief from pain for a period of up to several years, and can be repeated with further relief. However, the resultant numbness is troublesome to some patients (Bond, 1979).

Transcutaneous Electrical Stimulation

This involves stimulating the skin area over the site of the pain, using an electrical stimulator. The electrodes from the stimulator are placed on the skin area and a current of about 65 V is passed into the skin for a few minutes. The pain is replaced by a tingling sensation. When the current is switched off, the pain is usually found to be reduced or abolished. The duration of pain relief varies from a few minutes in some instances, to 8 or 10 hours in others (Long, 1973).

Surgical Treatment

The surgical division of nerve pathways has been performed but there are very few conditions, and very few techniques, with high long-term success rates (Sternbach, 1978). Over a period of time the nerve tissue regenerates and sensation returns. During the period of recovery there is a peculiar, unpleasant quality to the sensation in the area until full sensation returns. Often it does not return and the patient continues to experience various kinds of abnormal sensation. Patients with a normal expectation of life should not have any portion of their central nervous system damaged or destroyed because the end result to the patient may be a much more unpleasant and uncomfortable life than the initial one (Lipton, 1979).

Behavioural Approaches to Chronic Pain

Behavioural methods were first applied to the problem of chronic pain by Fordyce and colleagues (Fordyce *et al.*, 1968). Since then, the original 'operant package' has been used on many occasions with equal success. Other methods have also been developed with varied results. Cognitive strategies have been tried, but with little success (Linton, 1982). The three main approaches that have had some success are the 'operant approach', the 'respondent approach' and 'multi-modal' interventions.

The Operant Approach

The operant model views pain as a set of overt responses or pain behaviours. The patient may verbalise complaints, moan audibly, assume a particular posture, seek distraction or request medication. When pain behaviour occurs, people in the patient's environment are likely to respond. Their responses are commonly of a supportive or solicitous nature, or consist of some kind of action designed to relieve the patient's pain. Such responses may function as favourable consequences to the pain behaviour. They may do this by reducing the pain, by distracting the patient from his pain, or by evoking pleasant feelings associated with the attention and concern expressed. Such responses serve as reinforcers, increasing the probability of the occurrence of the pain behaviours in the future.

Fordyce *et al.* (1968) developed a treatment package based on operant techniques. Initially, the activity levels of the patient are developed by systematically reinforcing gradual increases with social reinforcement and the opportunity to rest. Medication is gradually decreased by giving the patient progressively smaller doses in a pain 'cocktail' given on a fixed-time rather than on a pain basis. Later, the patient's family are trained not to reinforce pain behaviours by providing, for example, sympathy or a reduction in domestic work contingent on pain as was previously the case. Increases in activity levels and large reductions in medication intake were achieved. However, subjective ratings of pain were lowered by moderate amounts which, although statistically significant, were clinically unimpressive (Linton, 1982). Modified versions of this programme have since been used widely with rather similar results.

The major drawback to this operant approach has been the high rate of drop-outs. Only a minority of the populations seemed to complete the programme. Moreover, White and Donovan (1980) reported problems in gaining control over important reinforcers when treating out-patients.

The Respondent Approach

This approach assumes that the muscles at the site of the pain tend to tense, thereby protecting the site from further trauma. When the muscles are chronically tensed, the tension itself produces more pain, which in turn causes greater local tension. Thus, a pain-tension cycle is created (Turner and Chapman, 1982). Support for this model is limited, but therapeutic intervention to break the cycle has shown that many patients benefit. Two main techniques have been described.

One respondent approach makes use of electromyographic feedback. Electrodes are placed on the skin over the appropriate muscles and these detect the state of muscle tension. This information is fed back to the electromyograph instrument, which provides visual and/or auditory feedback to the patient. The patient is directed to try to reduce the degree of muscle tension at the site of the pain. Relaxation exercises are commonly employed with the electromyogram. The successful outcome is that the patient reduces the degree of muscle tension to relaxation levels and, after training, is able

She was referred to the Medical Clinic in August 1980, with complaints of tiredness and lethargy. She was found to be losing blood in her stools. She was admitted, and 4 units of blood were administered. The loss of blood was thought to be due to the effects of aspirin taken by Mary, in proprietary analgesics, for the relief of her abdominal pain. A follow-up barium enema examination indicated 'sigmoid diverticular disease' for which 2 dessertspoons of unprocessed bran daily were prescribed.

In August 1981, she was referred to the Rheumatology Clinic due to the 'stomach muscles going into spasm'. She was discharged with the recommendation that she undertake exercises for her back.

Mary has also sought treatment outside the National Health Service. She attended a physiotherapist privately. He administered exercises and massage which, Mary said, 'loosened my back'. She gained a little benefit from this. She also sought assistance from an acupuncturist. This had little effect.

In June 1982, she was referred again to the Psychiatric Clinic and was transferred to this department to 'see if the behavioral approach could be of value'.

Assessment

The initial interview provided the opportunity for the patient to meet and get to know something about me. At this initial interview I attempted to obtain a statement of the problem and a history which would provide a background to the problem. In subsequent assessment interviews attempts would be made to clarify the problem and enable me to consider the treatment options available.

Initial Interview. At the initial interview, Mary was seen to be a small, lean woman, approximately, 1.47 m (4 ft 10 in.) tall. She walked with rapid, small steps and waddled slightly. She was neatly dressed in a skirt and cardigan under a light coat. She smiled only fleetingly when introductions were made, and when seated she fidgeted with a coat button for about 20 minutes.

She very freely related her experiences associated with her attempts to obtain pain relief. She said she preferred an upright chair as this did not bring on the pain. However, she sat throughout the interview, of about one hour's duration, in an easy chair without showing evidence of pain.

Although facial evidence of depression was not noted, she dwelt upon and frequently returned to the problems she had encountered in obtaining treatment for the pain. She said, 'The pain has got me down. I can't do the things I used to enjoy.' She indicated that her husband, Matt, had driven her in the car to the clinic. 'We go everywhere together now', she said. However, she went on to indicate that she did not get out and about as much as she did in the past. 'I can't remember the last time I trailed the shops in Dundee', she said. She also said she had put off doing many things that in the past she would have done 'without thinking about it'.

Problem History. Mary described the pain as 'constant — like toothache', with remissions when doing housework or when she was in bed. It extended from the mid-axillary line towards the anterior abdominal wall, following the line of the lower ribs. She experienced it on both sides, but the right side was much more troublesome. It had gradually developed about 3 years ago. Matt had undergone surgery for a lump on his breast a few months previously. He was undergoing investigations for a tumour in his throat. Her older daughter, Linda, was having marital difficulties. Her marriage later ended in divorce. Her younger son, Billy, who lived in London, had just told Mary he was receiving treatment for a 'drinking problem'. Mary decided at this time to follow Matt into retirement, although she was only 56 years old.

She listed the various medications she had taken for the relief of the pain. These included a variety of proprietary analgesics, DF 118, Fortral, Naprosyn and Sedapam. A few of these medications had given some relief, but for a short time only. Her sleep and appetite were unaffected by the pain.

Mary described the one episode of severe abdominal pain she had experienced. This occurred when she was in hospital for a blood transfusion about 2 years previously. 'It went right into spasm', she said, 'and I got out of bed. The nurse was not pleased and made me get back into bed.' Neither the medical nor nursing notes for this period had any reference to this incident. Since this episode of severe pain, Mary said she had a fear that it would recur. This fear increased when she sat in the car or an 'uncomfortable' chair. However, she does continue to travel by car. Mary had no previous problems with pain. She rarely experienced even headaches. 'Matt', she said, 'has had a lot of pain. He can bear it.'

At the end of the initial interview, Mary was asked for her expectations of her visits to me. She said she was 'not sure — I just want to get rid of this pain so I can be the way I was 2½ years ago.'

Second and Third Assessment Interviews. During these two interviews, the analysis of Mary's problem was completed. However, she frequently returned to the difficulties and problems she had encountered in trying to obtain pain relief. She frequently entered into long narratives about her experiences with health-care staff. She frequently said, 'I can't understand why they can't take this pain away.'

Problem Analysis of Pain Behaviours

A problem analysis was conducted to determine the antecedents and the consequences of her pain behaviours. Information obtained might show a relationship between these contingencies which could be helpful in selecting intervention techniques.

Physical Antecedents. Mary stated that the pain was experienced almost anywhere, but rarely in bed. She thought it most troublesome in other people's homes.

Social Antecedents. She said her husband was usually with her at the time of onset of the pain. However, she agreed that he was almost always with her in any event. She noted that it often came on when she was with her grandchildren. She did not approve of their behaviour at times although her daughter seemed unconcerned.

Behavioural Antecedents. The pain, she said, was worse when she was sitting as opposed to standing or lying. She preferred an upright chair in which she could keep her back straight. Easy chairs and car seats were uncomfortable, in that they induced the pain.

Cognitive Antecedents. Mary revealed that every morning when she awoke she 'expected the pain to be there'. It became worse when she talked to others about it. She said she often felt 'hopeless' and 'helpless'. Some of the thoughts expressed included: 'The pain has got me down'; 'I can't do the things I used to enjoy'; I don't enjoy my grandchildren any more.'

She said she usually talked about the pain when she met people in the shops or on the street. 'They all say I'm looking well. I think half the time they think I'm daft', she said, 'They don't seem to understand.' This made her feel 'hopeless' and the pain became troublesome.

Physical Consequences. Mary said she sometimes stayed in bed in the mornings or lay down for a few hours in the afternoon. This relieved the pain and she 'felt better'. When the pain was experienced while she was visiting others, she 'just wanted to get back home'.

Social Consequences When she stayed in bed, Matt did the housework. He would not cook or shop but would do everything else. He was sympathetic and advised Mary to 'do as the doctor says'. 'He is very good about it', Mary added.

Her general level of activity had reduced over the previous 3 years. She no longer shopped in Dundee and had cancelled several appointments and visits to relatives and friends because, she said, 'I just didn't feel like going'. She no longer attended church and had put off doing many things about the house. She said she rarely went out without Matt, who drove her everywhere. She described him as 'a quiet man', who 'is happy with his paper and the television'. 'He has never been interested in going out much', she added.

Cognitive Consequences. With the onset of pain, Mary said she felt 'helpless' and 'hopeless' and did not know what to do. She asked, 'What have I done to deserve this?'

Physiological Consequences. When the pain persisted, Mary said, 'I feel weak and tired'.

Motivational Analysis. A brief analysis of Mary's likes and dislikes was undertaken to find potential reinforcers that might be used in operant intervention. This revealed that she smoked 15 cigarettes each day. This had remained fairly constant over many years. She said she enjoyed watching television with her husband and spent most evenings doing this. She liked going for an evening walk through the village with Matt. Mary said she took alcohol only occasionally.

Analysis of Self-control Potential. As self-control techniques were thought to be potentially very useful for Mary's problems, a brief analysis of her self-control potential was undertaken. She said when she lay on her bed she sometimes promised herself that she would undertake certain activities later. However, she rarely carried through these promises. She had persisted in trying to obtain pain relief. However, this appeared to be instigated by members of her family. Her older daughter, Linda, and Linda's husband had made many treatment suggestions. These included acupuncture, manipulation and hypnosis. Mary had been asked to continue with the back exercises prescribed by the rheumatologist and taught by the physiotherapist. She had not done this as she thought that they did not help. She said she wanted 'someone to wave a magic wand' over her to take away the pain.

Social Relationships. The most significant people in Mary's life were thought to be Matt and her older daughter, Linda. Matt is Mary's constant companion: 'We go everywhere together', she said. He has been much involved with the health services in recent years and his attitude appears to be reflected in his advice to Mary to 'do as the doctor says'.

Mary visits Linda and her two children at least weekly. Linda told her mother on one occasion, 'You must learn to live with it', referring to the pain. She has made several treatment suggestions to Mary and drew to Mary's attention a series of television programmes on alternative medicine. Linda appears to have some influence on her mother's behaviour.

Summary of Behavioural Analysis

The behavioural analysis revealed three main interrelated pain behaviours which were regarded as indicative of Mary's inability to cope with the pain. These were: the complaints of pain; the reduced level of activity; and the presence of negative thoughts.

Complaints of Pain. Mary's main complaint was of the constancy of the pain, and consideration was given to the measurement of this. It was decided that the inverse (namely 'pain-free periods') should be measured.

She was asked to observe and record the time and duration of each occasion on which she was free from the abdominal pain. She was asked also to record *where* she was at the time, *who* she was with, and *what* she was doing at the time. It was thought that these additional observations might be of value in the selection of intervention techniques. The value of the recordings as a concrete record of her pain-free periods and its later use in the evaluation of intervention were explained to Mary.

There was discussion of which sensations constituted pain for the purposes of her recordings. It was agreed that if a sensation at the appropriate site was 'unpleasant', this would be regarded as pain. As

Mary was usually free from pain when in bed, it was agreed that the recordings should be made between 7.30 a.m. and 11 p.m., the usual period of her time out of bed. Mary's secretarial experience was thought likely to be an asset to her recording.

A second measure of Mary's pain complaints was taken in the form of the McGill Pain Questionnaire. This was completed by me at the clinic. Mary held a copy of the questionnaire and I read aloud the questions and entered the answers. I explained to Mary that information from the questionnaire provided details of the quality and intensity of the pain, and that this would later help me to evaluate the effectiveness of treatment. She expressed some difficulty in selecting appropriate words to describe the pain from the word descriptor lists provided in the questionnaire. However, she did manage to complete it satisfactorily.

Reduced Level of Activity. Mary's activity level was thought to be an appropriate behaviour to measure as she had expressed dissatisfaction with the reduction in her activity that had occurred. A self-monitoring approach was attempted at first, but Mary experienced difficulty in determining which activities were appropriate for recording purposes as there were 'so many of them'. Finally, it was decided to draw up a list of activities which she thought she should have performed.

(1) Clean out wardrobe units.
(2) Organise kitchen cupboards.
(3) Take shopping trips to Dundee.
(4) Attend church.
(5) Clear out personal papers.
(6) Go swimming at swimming pool.
(7) Visit elderly lady friends.

It was noted that some of the activities demanded only a single performance (activities 1, 2 and 5), whereas others could be performed regularly (activities 3, 4, 6 and 7).

Presence of Negative Thoughts. Mary had expressed feelings of 'weakness', 'tiredness' and 'hopelessness' and these were thought to be associated with negative thoughts. Attempts were made to measure their frequency but Mary met with difficulty in determining whether or not many of her thoughts were negative. It was decided to use an indirect approach to the measurement of her negative thoughts using the Beck Depression Inventory (Beck, Ward, Mendelson, Mock and Ehrbaugh, 1961). The inventory was completed at the clinic. Mary held a copy of the inventory and I read the statements aloud and recorded her responses.

Baseline Measures of Behaviour

It was decided to use the measures of pain behaviour described above as baseline measures. These behaviours would be measured again after intervention and the two sets of results would be compared to indicate the effectiveness of treatment.

Preparation for Intervention

The aim of intervention was to increase Mary's ability to cope with the pain by providing her with pain coping skills. Objectives were prepared to reflect this aim. These were:

(a) to increase the duration of pain-free periods;
(b) to increase the level of activity;
(c) to reduce negative thoughts.

Intervention Techniques

A multi-modal approach was considered to be appropriate in light of the pain behaviours. No attempt was made to determine the effectiveness of any of the components, the principal concern being effective treatment.

Eight major techniques were selected for intervention:

to increase the duration of pain-free periods
(1) reactive self-monitoring;
(2) progressive muscle relaxation;
(3) distraction methods;
(4) active measures to oppose pain and overcome passivity;

to increase level of activity
(5) activity scheduling;
(6) positive reinforcement;

to reduce negative thoughts
(7) cognitive restructuring;
(8) distraction methods.

The intervention was planned to allow a gradual introduction of the techniques in the above order.

Explanation to Patient

At the third assessment interview, the objectives of treatment and the intervention techniques were described to Mary. She expressed reservations about the objectives. She indicated her desire to be free from pain, which was not a stated objective of the programme. I explained again to her that the aim of the programme was to help her *cope* better with the pain. I said I expected the duration of her pain-free periods to increase but it was likely that some pain would persist. She was not satisfied with this aim but said that she would discuss it with her family in the forthcoming week and we agreed to discuss it again on her next visit.

Intervention

First Treatment Session

The following week Mary attended the clinic with her husband and stated her agreement to undertake the programme. Indeed, she had already started it. She said she had been lying in bed one evening and promised herself that she would clean and tidy the bedroom wardrobe units. The following day she spent one hour with Matt cleaning and tidying a wardrobe. The remaining bedroom units were tidied the following day, Matt again assisting. She had also spent half an hour shopping alone in the village for the first time in some weeks.

Mary was praised for her efforts by both Matt and me. Matt said, 'She did well'. A marked increase in the pain-free periods was noted during that week.

Matt was given an outline of his role in Mary's programme. He agreed to witness target activities set by Mary, to encourage her towards completion of them and to praise her efforts to meet the targets. A description of the initial interventions was given to Mary.

Activity Schedule. Mary was asked to set activity targets she thought she could attain. She was warned against setting difficult targets. She agreed to set simple targets initially, and to develop them gradually. When she had set a target she was then to set the day and time to perform the activity, and to inform Matt of this. At the predetermined time she was to take the necessary action to complete the activity. She was asked to record the activity in the 'Remarks' column of her recording sheet.

Progressive Muscle Relaxation. Mary was asked if she had any joint or muscle disorders prior to initiating progressive muscle relaxation. Mary expressed some reservations regarding the effect it might have on her abdominal muscles where she experienced the pain. She agreed to proceed with the technique.

Mary was directed to lie comfortably on the examination couch. This proved difficult as the limited range of adjustment of the clinic couch prevented Mary from adopting a comfortable position. In addition, as Mary was wearing a dress, she found it difficult to preserve her dignity. Arrangements were made for subsequent sessions to be held in another room where a recliner chair was available. On subsequent visits to the clinic, Mary wore a trouser suit.

She was asked to close her eyes, relax her arms by her sides and uncross her legs. She was told not to try too hard but to let relaxation happen at its own pace. She was then given a series of exercises for each of the major muscle groups of the upper limbs, shoulders and neck to help her differentiate between contraction and relaxation in these muscles. Instructions were given in a clear, quiet and non-modulated voice to promote relaxation.

Mary was asked to contract as tightly as possible a named muscle group. She was encouraged to concentrate on the sensations of tension in the muscles while maintaining them in the contracted state. She was then directed to relax the muscle group and to concentrate on the changing sensations as the muscle group relaxed. She was asked to identify any sensations such as warmth or tingling, commonly experienced by subjects, and to concentrate on these while slowly repeating the word 'relax' to herself. After first warning Mary, I checked for evidence of relaxation by raising an upper limb and noting the degree of limpness in the muscles.

Mary appeared to relax the muscles of the upper limbs, shoulders and neck without difficulty despite the unsuitability of the examination couch.

Homework. In the forthcoming week, Mary was asked to: self-monitor her pain-free periods; schedule her activities; and practise relaxation exercises.

Second and Third Treatment Sessions

At the beginning of each treatment session, Mary recounted the main points of her week. This enabled problems to be examined and provided an opportunity for me to praise her efforts. Then each of the components of therapy was reviewed and developed.

Self-monitoring. Mary's self-monitoring of pain-free periods continued. The daily average of the total duration of her pain-free periods was computed each week. This was illustrated on a graph and presented to Mary as feedback on her performance.

Activity Scheduling. Mary gradually developed a pattern of shopping alone in the village. She shopped, also, in Dundee for the first time in many months. She attended church on the Sunday of the third week of treatment. This was her first attendance at church in several months. She also sorted out letters and personal documents, a task she had intended doing some months ago.

Progressive Muscle Relaxation. Mary said she had practised the progressive muscle relaxation at home. She was unsure as to whether or not she was successfully relaxing her muscles. She was reassured that, with practice, she would learn to differentiate between tension and relaxation.

Instruction in relaxation was extended to the muscles of her face, to breathing, to her abdominal muscles and to the muscles of her back, hips and lower limbs. She expressed difficulty in relaxing the muscles in her throat as she found it difficult to perform the exercise. She was asked to leave out this exercise as the emphasis was on the muscles of her breathing, abdominal muscles and back muscles, all of which might influence the pain. Difficulty was also found with the muscles of breathing, her breathing being 'jerky' on exhalation. Mary was encouraged to continue practising breathing at home, concentrating on a smooth exhalation.

Abdominal relaxation proved to be most difficult. Mary was apprehensive about performing this exercise as she feared it would induce an episode of severe pain. However, she did succeed in increasing the degree of contraction. Mary was given a cassette tape recording of the relaxation procedures for use at home.

Measures to Reduce Passivity. Mary was encouraged to perform daily the exercises taught to her by the physiotherapist to mobilise her back. This was to encourage her to actively oppose the pain rather than passively accept it. This she agreed to do.

Homework. Mary was asked to: monitor pain-free periods; practice 'back exercises' and record these practice sessions; practise relaxation and record these practice sessions; continue activity scheduling.

Fourth Treatment Session

Mary was rather despondent at the beginning of the fourth treatment session. She said she had visited her general practitioner during the week and he had replaced her Naprosyn with a 'coated aspirin'. She found no difference in the effect. She said also that she had asked him to refer her again to the orthopaedic surgeon. She spoke of seeking hypnotherapy in Perth. She said she was 'never really free from pain — there is always a niggle there to remind me'.

Activity Scheduling. She had not shopped alone in the past week and had not attended church as she 'did not feel up to it'. No activity targets had been set in the past week.

Progressive Muscle Relaxation. Mary said she had practised muscle relaxation during the past week. She had tried it in the car but 'it did not help'. She expressed difficulty with abdominal relaxation and further instruction was given. She appeared to contract the muscle fairly well and afterwards said she thought the muscles were 'easier'.

Self-monitoring. Mary's monitoring of her pain-free periods demonstrated that the increased level of freedom from pain had been maintained. She had practised her back exercises and relaxation.

As the session progressed, Mary's negative statements declined. The Beck Depression Inventory was completed.

Homework. Mary was asked to: monitor pain-free periods; practise and record back exercises; practise and record relaxation; continue activity scheduling.

Fifth to Ninth Treatment Sessions

Self-monitoring. This was carried out only intermittently and showed a steady increase in the duration of pain-free periods. The pain was gradually becoming less troublesome and on one occasion Mary said, 'It couldn't really be called acute pain — more like aches'.

Activity Scheduling. Mary maintained her attendance at church and she joined the Women's Guild which she attended weekly. She developed a pattern of weekly shopping trips to Dundee. On these trips she travelled by bus. During this period she rearranged her kitchen cupboards, 'a job I've been putting off for months — since we moved into this house', she said. She also went to see two elderly friends whom she had intended visiting some time ago.

Distraction. This was introduced during this period when Mary was encouraged to change her activity at the onset of her pain. This she did and reported that it sometimes helped.

Progressive Muscle Relaxation. Mary continued to practise relaxation and reported that abdominal muscle relaxation sometimes helped to reduce the pain.

Action against Negative Thoughts. This was initiated by Mary. She mentioned one day 'the struggle that Douglas Bader had' in overcoming his injuries. She spoke also of Jean Johnstone, a local woman who had been a 'thalidomide baby'. Mary had worked with Jean and had been impressed by her ability to cope in spite of being without upper limbs. She suggested that her problems were minor when compared to those of Douglas Bader and Jean. Mary was encouraged to think further about this when she experienced thoughts of hopelessness and self-pity. Mary reported at a later session the reduction of negative thoughts. She felt that thinking about Jean Johnstone helped her control these negative thoughts.

As Mary was gradually progressing via the use of these therapeutic techniques, it was decided not to introduce additional methods. She was asked to continue with the present treatment programme and to return to the clinic in 3 weeks' time.

Final Treatment Session

Mary appeared much more alert at this session. Self-recording of pain-free periods showed a further increase in periods of relative freedom from pain. She said she was never really free from pain but that 'it does not bother me much'. She indicated that she continued with the back exercises each day.

She said that she continued to experience fear when sitting in the car. However, she continued to travel by car. She expressed the view that it was her position in the car that was the problem.

Mary said that the level of her activity had been maintained. She regularly shopped in Dundee using public transport, and attended church and the Women's Guild weekly. She had visited her elderly friends on two occasions in the past fortnight and expressed concern about their welfare. Negative thoughts were not in evidence. Mary said she rarely experienced them now. She indicated also that she was now taking more interest in her grandchildren.

Mary agreed that the pain was less troublesome, she felt better and was leading a fuller life. However, she continued to hope that her general practitioner would refer her again to the orthopaedic surgeon in an attempt to obtain 'freedom from pain'. Mary was asked to continue with the current methods of treatment and was discharged.

Results

Pain-free Periods

Figure 11.1 shows the average daily sum of pain-free periods in each week during which observations were recorded. There was an immediate increase following intervention, rising from 1 hour 34 minutes daily before treatment to 9 hours 2 minutes by the fifth week of treatment. After 4 further weeks, during which no recordings were made, there was a further increase to 12 hours 38 minutes at the end of treatment. This represents a sixfold increase in daytime pain freedom.

Activity

Mary completed six of the seven activities listed on page 279. Activities 3, 4 and 7 were being regularly performed on completion of treatment. Activity 6 was not performed.

Beck Depression Inventory

The scores before and after treatment were 29 and 11 respectively. It will be noted from Table 11.1 that the 'before treatment' score of 29 is in the upper limits of 'moderate depression'. The 'after treatment' score of 11 is the lowest limit of 'mild mood disturbance' and below the limits of clinical depression.

McGill Pain Questionnaire

Table 11.2 shows the scores before and after treatment on each of the scales of the McGill Pain Questionnaire. There was a reduction in all but one of the scales. However, the greatest reductions are in the affective and evaluative components of the Pain Rating Index.

Figure 11.1: Average Daily Sum of Pain-free Periods per Week
(7.30 a.m. to 11.00 p.m.)

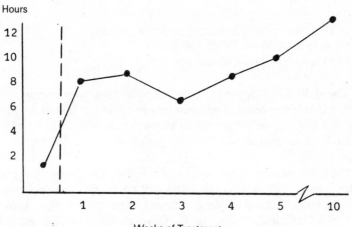

Weeks of Treatment

Table 11.1: Interpretation of Scores on the Beck Depression
Inventory (Burns, 1980)

1-10	These ups and downs considered normal
11-16	Mild mood disturbance
17-20	Borderline clinical depression
21-30	Moderate depression
31-40	Severe depression
Over 40	Extreme depression

Table 11.2: Scores on McGill Pain Questionnaire

Pain rating index	Before treatment	After treatment	Percentage difference
Sensory	11	15	+36.36
Affective	7	0	−100.00
Evaluative	5	3	−40.00
Miscellaneous	7	0	−100.00
Total	30	18	
Number of words chosen	12	7	−41.66
Present pain intensity	3	2	−33.33

Discussion

The aim of intervention was to help Mary cope better with the pain. Three objectives were prepared to reflect this aim. These were:

(1) to increase the duration of pain-free periods;
(2) to increase her level of activity;
(3) to reduce negative thoughts.

The sixfold increase in the duration of daytime pain-free periods after treatment meets the requirements of objective 1. It should be noted that at the end of treatment Mary was pain-free for 21 hours of each 24-hour period (12½ hours during daytime, 8½ hours at night).

Mary attained six of the seven activities listed at the beginning of intervention. However, in the absence of an acceptable measure of Mary's level of activity before treatment, there are insufficient data available to satisfy objective 2. Consequently, the success of intervention has not been clearly demonstrated. However, Mary was regularly performing activities 3, 4 and 7 (page 279) at the end of treatment, and these activities she had not performed for several months prior to intervention. This offers some support to the view that she had increased her activity levels.

The third objective, to reduce negative thoughts, cannot be clearly demonstrated in the absence of a measure of Mary's negative thoughts before intervention. However, although the Beck Depression Inventory cannot be regarded as being a measure of negative thoughts, negative thoughts such as those described by Mary are commonly associated with depression (Beck *et al.*, 1961). A significant reduction in negative thoughts would be expected to follow a reduction in the score on the Beck Depression Inventory of the order seen in Mary's ratings. Moreover, Mary stated at the end of treatment that she rarely experienced negative thoughts.

The reduction in the Pain Rating Index of the McGill Pain Questionnaire was due to changes in the affective, evaluative and miscellaneous components. I am unable to offer any explanation for the alterations in the sensory and miscellaneous components. The reductions in the affective and evaluative components of the Pain Rating Index are consistent with the findings of Wolff (1978) who found high correlations between tolerance of pain and affective and evaluative variables. The aim of intervention was to increase Mary's ability to cope with or tolerate the pain she was experiencing. Such reductions in the affective and evaluative components would, therefore, be expected after successful intervention. Similarly, the reduction from 3 to 2 in the 'present pain intensity' score is consistent with the aim of intervention, to help Mary cope better with the pain rather than to relieve pain.

Discussion of Techniques

The relative contribution of each of the components of intervention cannot be determined. This was envisaged when intervention was planned. The literature on the behavioural treatment of chronic pain reveals that almost all interventions employ several techniques simulataneously, making it impossible to determine the effectiveness of any one component. However, I will comment on some of the techniques as applied to Mary.

Intervention in the form of cognitive restructuring and distraction was planned for the latter stages of treatment. However, Mary progressed to the point that such intervention was considered unnecessary. Mary took a step in this direction on her own initiative when she found that when she thought of the plight of others 'less fortunate' than herself, namely Douglas Bader and Jean Johnstone, she felt better. The pain, she found, persisted, but 'it did not ache as much'. She dwelt on this subject for several weeks and found that directing her thoughts to these people not only reduced the ache but also reduced her negative thoughts, allowing her to 'feel better'. At one level this might be considered as 'distraction', these thoughts replacing 'pain thoughts'. At another level it might be considered a cognitive change in which Mary's attitudes towards her pain were modified when seen in the light of the problems of the other people.

Claims have been made in the literature (see, for example, Varni, Bessman, Russo and Cataldo, 1980) that muscle relaxation can achieve significant reductions in pain. Mary did appear to gain some reduction in the pain from this technique, although this effect was not consistent.

Discussion of Problems Encountered

Many problems were encountered in both the assessment and intervention stages but only a few are discussed here. As part of the assessment of her level of activity, Mary was asked to record her daily activities. I explained the use of the information and we discussed what constituted relevant activities, for example, washing or drying dishes, making the bed, shopping in the village, visiting her daughter Linda, etc. At the end of the discussion, I was satisfied that she could identify and record relevant activities. However, the following week Mary returned to the clinic and calmly stated that she was unable to determine which of her activities were appropriate for recording purposes. I tried again to define relevant activities, but Mary stated determinedly that she had tried and could not do it.

Another similar incident took place the following week when she was asked to count the number of negative thoughts that she experienced. Again, I was satisfied that Mary could recognise negative thoughts. However, she returned the following week and expressed her inability to recognise negative thoughts. Encouragement to try again was unsuccessful. Later in treatment she did identify many such thoughts.

In the early stages of treatment when there was a marked increase in the duration of her pain-free periods, I became excited at this response. However, Mary, troubled by negative thoughts, brought me back to reality when she said, 'but I'm never really free from pain — there is always a niggle there to remind me'. I understood at this point how Szasz might have been motivated to write of 'painmanship' and 'pain careers'.

The greatest problem encountered was in relation to Mary's desire to be free from pain. She had pursued pain relief through a series of medical practitioners, a long list of analgesics and private treatment, at some expense, from a physiotherapist and an acupuncturist. She had been advised to obtain assistance from a hypnotherapist and was giving consideration to doing so. Her objective was 'freedom from pain'. However, I could not offer this. At best, I would try to help her cope better with the pain. The pain would be less troublesome, but would probably persist. When treatment to help her cope with the pain was offered, she was initially unwilling to accept. However, she discussed it with her family and returned the following week having already started treatment.

It would have given immense satisfaction to be able to say that after behavioural intervention Mary had terminated her quest for 'freedom from pain'. This was not the case. At the conclusion of treatment she agreed that the pain was much less troublesome, that she rarely experienced negative thoughts and that her level of activity had increased. However, in spite of this, Mary expressed her intention of asking her general practitioner to refer her again to the orthopaedic surgeon.

Mary's objective and my objective were at variance.

Postscript

At the time when Mary was discharged, she was given an appointment for a follow-up visit to the clinic for 6 weeks later. However, on the arranged day she telephoned to say that she was unable to attend due to influenza. She was eventually seen 9 weeks after discharge.

Mary appeared bright and alert when seen at the clinic and said she was feeling very much better. Her husband, Matt, who attended with her agreed that she was now 'back to her old self'.

Pain-free Periods

During the previous week Mary had recorded each occurrence of pain as these she thought easier to record than the almost constant pain-free periods. A summary of the average sum of pain-free periods per week is illustrated in Figure 11.2. In the week prior to her follow-up visit (week 19), Mary had on average 15 hours 8 minutes of freedom from pain per day (7.30 a.m. to 11.00 p.m.), and as she remained pain-free overnight, she was free from pain on average 23 hours 38 minutes per day. Moreover, she had three consecutive days without pain.

Beck Depression Inventory

The Beck Depression Inventory was completed. The follow-up score was 6 (before treatment 29; after treatment 11). The score of 6 at her follow-up visit is comfortably within normal limits (see Table 11.1).

McGill Pain Questionnaire

This was completed and a summary of scores is provided in Table 11.3. Further reductions are noted in all three scales of the questionnaire. Of the present pain intensity score of 1, Mary said, 'It's hardly a pain at all but I've called it that because 1 can still feel something there.'

Discussion

The results show further reductions in the frequency and intensity of pain and in the frequency of negative thoughts. Mary indicated also

Figure 11.2: Average Daily Sum of Pain-free Periods per Week
(7.30 a.m. to 11.00 p.m.)

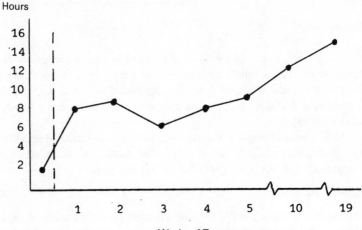

Table 11.3: Scores on McGill Pain Questionnaire

Pain rating index	Before treatment	After treatment	Follow-up	Percentage Difference
Sensory	11	15	1	−90.90
Affective	7	0	0	−100.00
Evaluative	5	3	1	−80.00
Miscellaneous	7	0	0	−100.00
Total	30	18	2	−93.33
Number of words chosen	12	7	2	−83.33
Present pain intensity	3	2	1	−66.66

that she was functioning at her former level of activity. She expressed
satisfaction with her state and said she had abandoned all thoughts of
further referral to the orthopaedic surgeon. Mary's objective and my
objective were reconciled by a satisfactory outcome.

References

Azrin, N.H. (1977) 'A Strategy for Applied Research: Learning based but Outcome
Orientated', *American Psychologist*, *32*, 140–9

Beck, A.T. (1970) *Depression: Causes and Treatment*, University of Pennsylvania Press, Philadelphia

Beck, A.T., Ward, C.M., Mendelson, M., Mock, J. and Ehrbaugh, J. (1961) 'An Inventory for Measuring Depression', *Archives of General Psychology*, 4, 53–63

Bond, M.R. (1973) 'Personality Studies in Patients with Pain Secondary to Organic Disease', *Journal of Psychosomatic Research*, 17, 258–63

Bond, M.R. (1979) *Pain: its Nature, Analysis and Treatment*, 2nd edn, Churchill Livingstone, Edinburgh

Burns, D.D. (1980) *Feeling Good*, Morrow, New York

Fordyce, W.E. (1978) 'Learning Processes in Pain', in R.A. Sternbach (ed.), *The Psychology of Pain*, Raven Press, New York

Fordyce, W.E., Fowler, R.S. Jr, Lehmann, J.F. and de Lateur, B.J. (1968) 'Application of Behaviour Modification Techniques to Problems of Chronic Pain', *Behaviour Research and Therapy*, 6, 105–7

Frederiksen, L.W., Sterling, M.A., Lynd, R.S. and Ross, J. (1978) 'Methodology in Measurement of Pain', *Behaviour Therapy*, 9, 486–8

Gracely, R.H., McGrath, P. and Dubner, R. (1978) 'Ratio Scales of Sensory and Affective Verbal Pain Descriptors', *Pain*, 5, 5–18

Herman, E. and Baptiste, S. (1981) 'Pain Control: Mastery through Group Experience', *Pain*, 10, 79–86

Kanfer, F.H. and Karoly, P. (1972) 'Self-control: a Behaviouristic Excursion into the Lion's Den', *Behaviour Therapy*, 3, 398–416

Kazdin, A.E. (1974) 'Reactivity of Self-monitoring. The Effect of Response Desirability, Goal Setting and Feedback', *Journal of Consulting and Clinical Psychology*, 42(5), 704–16

Kremer, E. and Atkinson, J.H., Jr (1982) 'Pain Measurement: Construct Validity of the Affective Dimension of the McGill Pain Questionnaire with Chronic Benign Pain Patients', *Pain*, 11, 93–100

Lewinsohn, P.M., Weinstein, M.S. and Shaw, D.A. (1969) 'Depression: a Clinical-research Approach', in R.D. Rubin and C.M. Franks (eds), *Advances in Behaviour Therapy*, Academic Press, New York

Linton, S.J. (1982) 'A Critical Review of Behavioural Treatments for Chronic Benign Pain Other than Headache', *British Journal of Clinical Psychology*, 21, 321–37

Lipton, S. (1979) *The Control of Chronic Pain*, Academic Press, London

Long, D.M. (1973) 'Externally Applied Stimulation for the Relief of Chronic Pain', in J. Bonica (ed.), *Proceedings of the International Symposium on Pain*, Raven Press, New York

Melzack, R. (1975) 'The McGill Pain Questionnaire: Major Properties and Scoring Methods', *Pain*, 1, 277–99

Melzack, R. (1980) 'Psychological Aspects of Pain', in J. Bonica (ed.), *Pain*, Raven Press, New York

Melzack, R. and Torgerson, W.S. (1971) 'On the Language of Pain', *Anesthesiology*, 34(1), 50–9

Melzack, R. and Wall, P.D. (1965) 'Pain Mechanisms: a New Theory', *Science*, 150, 971

Seligman, M.E.P. (1975) *Helplessness: on Depression, Development and Death*, W.H. Freeman, San Francisco

Seres, J. and Newman, R. (1976) 'Results of Chronic Low Back Pain at the Portland Pain Centre', *Journal of Neurosurgery*, 45, 32–6

Sternbach, R. (1974) *Pain Patients: Traits and People*, Academic Press, London

Sternbach, R. (1978) 'Clinical Aspects of Pain', in R. Sternbach (ed.), *The Psychology of Pain*, Raven Press, New York

Szasz, T.S. (1968) 'The Psychology of Persistent Pain. A Portrait of L'Homme

Douloureux', in A. Soulairac, J. Cahn and J. Charpentier (eds), *Pain, Proceedings of an International Symposium on Pain*, Academic Press, New York

Turner, J. and Chapman, C. (1982) 'Psychological Intervention for Chronic Pain: a Critical Review (I, II)', *Pain, 12*, 1–46

Varni, J., Bessman, C.A., Russo, D.C. and Cataldo, M.F. (1980) 'Behavioural Management of Chronic Pain in Children', *Archives of Physical Medicine and Rehabilitation, 61*, 375–8

White, B. and Donovan, A. (1980) 'A Comprehensive Programme for the Assessment and Treatment of Low Back Pain in Western Australia', in C. Peck and M. Wallace (eds), *Problems in Pain*, Pergamon, New York

Wolff, B.B. (1978) 'Behavioural Measurement of Human Pain', in R. Sternbach (ed.), *The Psychology of Pain*, Raven Press, New York

AUTHOR INDEX

AABT Task Force 81, 86
Ackner B. 3, 14
Agras W.S. 62, 91, 102, 112
Albee G. 74, 86
Alberti R.E. 99, 112
Alleridge P. 10, 14
Altschul 44, 52, 86, 187, 188, 200
ANA 8, 14
Anderson J. 58, 88, 189, 200
Argyle M. 99, 114
Arkell C. 148, 167
Armstrong P.M. 199, 200
Arnkoff D. 137, 139
Arnold G.M. 229, 254
Ascione F.R. 77, 90
Atkinson J.H. 293
Atthowe J.M. 54, 86
Ayllon T. 21, 35, 37, 43, 44, 58, 60,
    61, 65, 86, 148, 167, 178, 184,
    226, 254
Azrin N. 58, 65, 75, 76, 79, 80, 86,
    87, 88, 101, 112, 148, 167, 178,
    184, 199, 200, 226, 254, 272,
    292

Bach P. 78, 87
Baer D.M. 78, 90, 148, 167, 228,
    254
Baker R. 54, 67, 86, 117, 127, 140
Bales R. 9, 15
Bandura A. 28–30, 35, 40, 44, 53,
    86, 168, 174, 184, 209, 225
Baptiste S. 272, 293
Barker P. 13, 14, 44, 45, 150
Barrerra F. 64, 87
Barrios B.A. 175, 184
Barrman B. 81, 86, 87
Barton R. 9, 14, 48, 87, 120, 139
Beck A.T. 41, 45, 99, 112, 135, 139,
    178, 184, 268, 288, 293
Beck C.M. 41, 45
Begg J. 54, 88
Bella D.A. 127, 139
Bellack A. 73, 87, 117, 140
Bennett D.H. 130, 141
Berberich J.P. 188, 201
Berke R. 54, 90
Berry I. 81, 87

Bessman C.A. 289, 294
Bijou S.W. 74, 87
Birnbrauer J. 74, 87
Black D. 63, 64, 88
Black J.L. 229, 255
Blewitt E. 75, 90
Blunden R. 75, 90
Bobbitt W.E. 66, 88
Bond M.R. 265, 269, 293
Borgerson M. 94, 113
Borkowski J. 35, 45
Bornstein P. 78, 87
Boskind-Lodahl M. 100, 112
Boulougouris J.C. 209, 225
Broen W.E. 64, 90
Brown G.W. 48, 50, 87, 91, 125,
    137, 139, 141, 186, 187, 188,
    201
Bryant B. 99, 114
Buckley N.K. 63, 90
Buehler R.E. 52, 87
Bugle C. 228, 255
Burchard J. 64, 87
Burns D. 293
Burrish T. 78, 91, 102, 112
Buss A. 64, 87
Butterfield E. 37, 45
Butterworth C.A. 111, 112

Campbell A. 72, 87
Canter D. 120, 139
Canter S. 120, 139
Capie A. 77, 90
Carr J. 77, 91, 111, 167
Carr P. 112
Carstairs C. 50, 90
Cataldo M.F. 289, 294
Cavanaugh J. 35, 45
Chambless D.L. 97, 112, 174, 184
Chapman C. 294
Charbonnea M. 99, 114
Cherniss C. 136, 138, 139
Christopherson E. 229, 254
Cockram L. 57, 63, 64, 88, 89
Collins C. 78, 91
Connolly 13, 14, 39, 45, 93, 113
Cormack D. 88, 187, 188, 200
Crisp A. 75, 87

295

Dallison B. 87
Davis P. 54, 88
Dawson M. 81, 90
De Kock U. 77, 87
De Lateur B. 265, 293
Denny D.R. 102, 112
Dobson N.R. 45
Dobson W.R. 88
Donovan A. 271, 294
Dubner R. 293
Durham R. 48, 116, 119, 139

Ellis A. 45, 178, 184
Ellis N.R. 75, 87
Emery G. 99, 112
Emmons M.L. 99, 112
Eysenck H. 11, 14, 25, 26, 39, 45

Fairweather G.W. 137, 139
Faulkner G.E. 52, 90
Felce D. 77, 87
Fernandez J. 68, 87
Figueroa J.L. 102, 112
Fischer I. 68, 87
Fleming I. 101, 112
Foa E.B. 97, 112
Forbank J.A. 98, 112
Fordyce W.E. 265, 267, 270, 271, 293
Fowler R.S. 265, 293
Foxen T. 81, 89
Foxx R.M. 76, 79, 80, 86, 87, 88
Frame C.L. 97, 112
Fraser D. 45, 52, 54, 57, 58, 63, 64, 66, 88, 89, 90, 119, 139, 187, 188, 189, 198, 200
Frederickson L.W. 266, 293
Friman P. 78, 87
Fuller P.R. 21, 45
Fuller W.B. 53, 89
Furniss J.M. 52, 87

Gardner W. 74, 88
Garland M. 137, 139
Gelder M. 98, 113
Gelfand D.M. 36, 45, 52, 88
Gelfand S. 36, 45, 52, 88
Georgiades N. 137, 139
Gershaw N.J. 119, 140
Ginsberg G. 94, 112
Glass C. 137, 139
Glenn W. 119, 141
Glickman H. 54, 88
Goffman E. 6, 14, 115, 119, 124,

147, 167, 187, 200
Goldfried M. 135, 139
Goldiamond I. 77, 88, 148, 167, 188, 200
Goldin J. 99, 114
Goldstein A.J. 97, 112, 174, 184
Goldstein A.P. 119, 140
Gordon W.L. 70, 89
Gottlieb L. 80, 86
Gould J. 186, 200
Graceley R. 267, 293
Grant G. 75, 88
Graves G. 97, 112
Greaves S. 54, 90
Grey S. 97, 113
Grime J. 57, 58, 88, 89, 189, 200
Gripp R.F. 66, 88
Grubb A.B. 55, 90
Gruenberg E. 47, 99, 187, 200
Grunewald K. 71, 88
Guralnick M. 81, 88
Guthrie D. 102, 112
Guthrie R. 112

Halford K. 99, 113
Hall J. 67, 86, 117, 127, 140
Hallam R.S. 13, 14, 39, 45, 93, 113
Harris T. 139
Haughton E. 60, 61, 86
Hauser M.J. 34, 45
Hawks D. 50, 88
Hawthorne J.H. 54, 88
Heather N. 101, 113
Hemsley D. 65, 89
Henderson S. 124, 137, 140
Herbert E.W. 228, 254
Herman E. 272, 293
Hersen M. 73, 87, 117, 140
Higgins J. 94, 113
Hill D.W. 229, 254
Hodges B. 111, 112
Hogg J. 81, 89
Holland J. 75, 89
Holley J. 89
Holmgren S. 100, 113
Hopkins B. 56, 89
Hops H. 199, 201
Hord J.E. 66, 88
Horne D.J. 94, 113
Hughart L. 80, 86
Hughes D.D. 59, 90
Hunter M. 45
Hunter P. 113
Hutchinson K. 67, 86

Hutzell R. 228, 254

Insell P. 120, 140
Isaacs W. 154, 167, 188, 200

Jacobsen E. 174, 184
Jenkins J. 77, 87
Johnson S.M. 228, 254
Johnston D.W. 98, 113
Johnston M.B. 81, 91
Jones M. 34, 45, 124, 140
Jones R. 98, 101, 112, 114
Junginger J. 228, 255

Kale R.J. 56, 89
Kanfer F.H. 272, 293
Karoly 272, 293
Katz R.C. 101, 113
Kaye J.H. 56, 89
Kazdin A. 33, 45, 52, 64, 89, 199,
    200, 227, 228, 254, 272, 293
Keefe F.J. 102, 113
Keene T.M. 98, 112
Kelly B. 75, 89
Kennard D. 124, 128, 140
Kiernan C. 77, 89
King R.P. 71, 90, 119, 125, 140
Klaber M. 37, 45
Klukas N. 228, 255
Knapp T. 178, 184
Kornbluth S. 99, 113
Krasner L. 54, 86
Kratz C. 133, 140
Kremer E. 267, 293

Lacks P. 101, 113
Lader M. 10, 14
Lamont J. 59, 90
Lang P.J. 64, 87
Latimer P. 94, 113
Launier R. 135, 140
Lazarus R.S. 135, 140, 178, 184
Leck I. 70, 89
Lehmann J.F. 265, 293
Leitenberg H. 62, 91, 97, 113
Lentz R.J. 52, 90, 119, 140
Levis D. 97, 114
Lewinsohn P.M. 99, 113, 268, 293
Lewis A. 3, 5, 14
Lewis D. 175, 185
Liberman R. 56, 89
Liddell H.S. 23, 45
Lindsay W.R. 189, 200
Lindsley O.R. 24, 45

Linton S.J. 265, 267, 270, 271, 292,
    293
Lipinski D.P. 229, 255
Lipton S. 269, 270, 293
Logue P. 228, 254
Long D.M. 270, 293
Lovaas O.I. 37, 45, 188, 201
Lutzker J.R. 81, 89
Lynd R.S. 266, 293
Lyons P. 78, 87

McBrien J. 81, 89
Mcdonald S. 188, 200
McDougall 57, 90
McFall M. 78, 87
McFall R. 199, 201, 228, 255
McGowan H. 94, 113
McGrath P. 267, 293
McKeown T. 70, 89
Mcleod W. 54, 88
McPherson F.M. 43, 45, 57, 89,
    119, 140
McTiernan G. 94, 113
Macmillan P. 41, 45
Magaro P. 66, 88
Mahoney M. 30, 45, 105, 113, 178,
    184
Malott R. 77, 91
Mansell J. 77, 87
Marks I.M. 13, 14, 39, 40, 45, 93,
    94, 111, 112, 113, 174, 185,
    208, 209, 225
Martin E.D. 88
Martin P.L. 54, 90
Masserman J. 23, 25, 45
Mastellone M. 176, 185
Masters J. 117, 140
Mathews A. 98, 113
Matson J. 78, 81, 89
Maughan B. 125, 140
Mayer A. 6, 15
Meichenbaum D. 30, 45, 168, 185
Meldrum M. 94, 113
Mellow J. 7, 15
Melzack R. 265, 266, 293
Mendelson M. 293
Mertens G. 53, 89
Michael J. 21, 35, 37, 44
Milby J. 56, 89
Milne D. 133, 140
Mitchell W. 52, 90
Moeller T. 102, 112
Monck E. 50, 91
Moore C.H. 66, 88

Moores B. 75, 88
Moos R. 120, 140
Morris B. 49, 50, 79, 91
Morris P. 70, 89
Mortimore P. 140
Mowrer O.H. 26, 45
Murray W. 81, 86

Naster B.J. 101, 112
Nelson O.R. 229, 255
Newman R. 272, 293
Nomellinin S. 101, 113

O'Donoghue F.P. 94, 113
Ognjanov V. 59, 90
Orford J. 124, 140
Oswin M. 70, 89
Ouston J. 125, 140

Panyan M. 77, 90
Parsons T. 9, 15
Paton X. 52, 90, 187, 201, 232, 255
Patterson G.R. 52, 87, 199, 201
Paul G.L. 52, 90, 119, 140
Pavlov I.P. 18, 20, 25, 35, 45
Pearlin L.I. 140
Peck D.F. 37, 46, 94, 113
Peplau H. 7, 15
Perkins E.A. 77, 90
Phillimore L. 137, 139
Phillips E.L. 229, 255
Philpott R. 13, 14, 39, 45, 93, 113
Piercy F.P. 101, 113
Platzek D. 228, 254
Plutchik R. 54, 88
Porterfield J. 75, 90
Pratt M. 126, 140
Presly A.S. 55, 57, 89, 90

Quiltich H.R. 229, 254

Rachman S. 97, 113, 174
Rahn T. 80, 86
Rapoport R. 124, 140
Rayner R. 22, 46
Raynes N. 71, 90, 119, 126, 140
Rees T. 8, 15
Rehm L.P. 99, 113
Richardson A. 120, 141
Rimm D.C. 117, 140
Risley T.R. 37, 46
Robertson I. 94, 101, 113
Rose M.J. 102, 113
Rosenthal T. 28, 46

Ross J. 266, 293
Rupert P. 102, 113
Rush A.J. 99, 112
Russo D.C. 289, 294
Rutner I.T. 228, 255
Rutter M. 125, 140
Ryan E. 58, 87

Sanders D. 137, 139
Sanok R. 77, 90
Sartory G. 97, 113
Schaeffer H.H. 54, 90
Schaller D. 94, 113
Schneider J. 102, 112
Schroeder F. 80, 88
Seligman M. 268, 293
Seres J. 272, 293
Shapiro M.B. 12, 15
Sharpe R. 175, 185
Shaw B.F. 99, 112
Shaw D. 268, 293
Shepherd G. 119, 120, 140, 141
Sherman J. 55, 90, 188, 195, 201
Shigetomi C.C. 175, 184
Silverstein L. 102, 113
Sims A. 133, 141
Singh N. 81, 90
Sirlin J. 100, 112
Skinner B.F. 18, 20, 22, 35, 45, 46
Slade P. 100, 114
Sletten I. 59, 90
Smith A. 125, 140
Sprafkin R.P. 119, 140
Spreen O. 186, 201
Stampfl T. 97, 114
Stecker H. 54, 90
Stein L. 119, 141
Stephens R.M. 78, 89
Sterling M. 266, 293
Sternbach R. 266, 267, 268, 269,
  270, 293, 294
Stirling E. 52, 90
Stoffelmayer B. 52, 90
Storms L. 64, 90
Stranynski A. 99, 114
Strauss N. 94, 113
Stuart R. 229, 255
Sturmey P. 75, 87
Suchotliff L. 54, 90
Sullivan H. 7, 15
Sutton G. 127, 141
Szasz T.S. 268, 293

Taylor C.B. 102, 112

Taylor J.W. 101, 114
Taylor P.D. 77, 90
Test M. 119, 141
Thomas J. 148, 167, 188, 200 ·
Thompson N. 57, 90, 188, 201
Thorndike E.L. 17, 20, 27, 46
Tierney A. 13, 15
Tizard J. 119, 140
Torgerson W. 266, 293
Tosh M. 150
Towell D. 10, 15
Trower P. 99, 114
Turner S.M. 97, 112
Twardosz S. 78, 90
Twentyman C. 199, 201

Van Etten C. 148, 167
Van Etten G. 148, 167
Varni J. 289, 294
Vitali D.L. 81, 87

Walk A. 3, 10, 15
Walker H.H. 199, 201
Walker H.M. 63, 90
Walker L.G. 60, 90
Wall P.D. 265, 293
Watson J.B. 22, 46, 209, 225
Watts F. 130, 141

Webster J. 75, 89
Weinstein M.S. 268, 293
Wesolowski M. 80, 86, 90
Whaley D. 77, 91
Whelan P. 56, 89
White B. 271, 294
White G. 228, 254
Whitman, T.L. 81, 91
Wilson G.T. 33, 45, 52, 89, 114
Wilson P.H. 99, 114
Wilson-Barnett, J. 39, 46
Wincze J. 62, 91
Wing J.K. 48, 49, 50, 65, 87, 91,
    125, 141, 186, 187, 188, 201
Winkler R.C. 54, 91
Winton A.S. 81, 90
Wolfensberger W. 119, 141
Wolff B. 288, 294
Wolpe, J. 23, 24, 46, 97, 114, 174,
    185, 208, 225
Wood J. 81, 87
Woodward R. 98, 114

Yule, W. 77, 91

Zawlocki R.J. 80, 90
Zegiob L. 228, 255
Zigler E. 73, 91

SUBJECT INDEX

Activity schedule 279, 280, 283
Adjunct therapy 98
Aggressive behaviour 79, 115
Agoraphobic syndrome 95
Alcohol abuse 100
Anorexia 99
Antecedents 72, 276
Anxiety 25, 34, 96, 171
  generalised 98
  management 173, 175, 224
Apathy 54
Assessment 14, 39, 42, 72, 105, 116,
  152, 166, 171, 190, 193, 210,
  231, 233, 274
  see also Baseline
Atmosphere 123
Attention 28
Attitudes 128
Autism 12
Aversion therapies 13
Avoidance behaviour 26

Baseline 12, 64, 66, 76, 155, 159,
  165, 194, 215, 234, 280
  see also Assessment
Bathing 147, 155
Behaviour
  analysis 76
  behavioural psychotherapy 40, 42
  modification 26, 42
  therapy 24, 26, 31, 39, 43, 44,
    54; applications of behaviour
    therapy 32–3
  therapy nursing 44
Behaviourism 25
Bethlem Royal Hospital 40
Biofeedback 102, 272
Bulimarexia 100

Carpal tunnel syndrome 102
Change agents 11
  see also nurse's role
Checking 212
Chronic pain 265
Classical conditioning 16, 18, 27, 30
Clinical poverty syndrome 49
Cognitive restructuring 99, 178, 280,
  289

Cognitive therapy 31, 35, 43, 272
Community care 3, 50, 60, 71
  psychiatric nursing 92
  resources 50
Compulsive rituals 96
Conjoint therapy 101
Consequences 72, 277
Constructional approach 77
Controlled drinking 100
Coping strategies 134
Cost-benefit analysis 154, 194
Curriculum planning 82
Custodial
  care 10
  role of nurses 34

Delusions 52, 65
Dental anxiety 102
Depression 34, 268, 274
Desensitisation 25, 96, 272
Diabetes mellitus 102
Differential reinforcement of other
  behaviour 80
Distraction 280
Disturbed behaviour 47, 79
Drugs 268
Dysfunctional beliefs 30

Eating
  disorders 99
  skills 76, 147, 155, 193
Educational activities 82
Elderly 35
Environment 62, 70, 71, 74, 115,
  188
Escape behaviour 20
Ethics 13
Expectations 119
Exposure 96
Extinction 18, 20, 61
Eye contact 192

Facial screening 81
Fears 25, 28, 208
  see also Phobias
  Fear Survey Schedule 172, 214
  Feedback 119, 228
  Flooding 97, 209

Frequency count 198
Functional analysis of behaviour 13

Gate-control theory 265
Generalisation 19, 23, 163, 198, 213
Generalised phobias 95
    see also Fears and Agoraphobic
    syndrome
Goals 196, 217
Graded exposure 96
    see also desensitisation
Group therapy 34

Hallucinations 168
Homework assignments 282

Imitation 29, 40, 188
In-service training 133
Individualised care 14, 121
Information
    feedback 54
    overload 65
    processing 30
Insomnia 101
Institutionalisation 36, 115, 187
Institutional neurosis 48, 120
Institutions 7, 14, 48, 49, 50, 71, 72
    see also Environments
Instructions 68
    see also Prompts
Instrumental learning theory 16
    see also Operant Conditioning
Intensive treatment units 83
Interpersonal
    problems 101
    relationships 34
    skills 78
Interview 152, 210, 231

Job performance 52, 58

Labelling 3
Lack of initiative 48
    see also Institutional neurosis
Language deficits 186
Law of effect 17
Learning theories 16
    see also Operant conditioning and
        Classical conditioning
    Little Albert 22
    Little Peter 25

Manic depressive psychosis 171,
    183

Marital discord 101
Maudsley Group 39
Mediational processes 128, 168
    see also Information processing
Medical model 74
Milieu therapy 9, 34, 36
Modelling 30, 79, 162, 209
Motivation 29
    analysis 277
    system 247
Multi-modal approaches 272
Mutism 188

Negative thoughts 285
Neurosis 39, 168
Normalisation 119
Nurse–patient interaction 68
Nurse's role 35
    as therapist 22, 40

Obesity 100
Observations 4, 153, 159, 191
    see also Assessment
Obsessional disorder 96
Operant
    approach 270
    conditioning 20, 30, 59
    see also Instrumental learning
Overcorrection 80

Pain
    behaviour 267
    chronic pain 102
    management 102
    painmanship 290
    Pain Rating Index 288
Panic attack 177
Passivity 48
    see also Institutional neurosis
Patient centred care 11
Patient–nurse interaction 61
    see also Nurse–patient interaction
'Penny game' 101
Personal hygiene 54, 151, 193
    see also Self-care
Personal scientist model 105
Phobias 39, 95, 168, 208
    see also Fears and Anxiety
Poverty of speech 49, 186
    see also Institutionalisation
Primary handicaps 48
Primary therapist role 93, 132
Private events 168

Problem
 analysis 194
 problems of living 42, 183
 problem solving skills 81
Progressive relaxation 174
Prompting 68, 78, 162, 198
 see also Instructions
Psychoanalysis 26, 30, 34
Psychologists 11, 12, 35, 43, 94,
 149, 192, 231
Psychotic patients 24, 30, 47, 55, 60
Psychosexual disorders 96

Quality of care 71
Quality of life 116

Rating scales 105, 266
Rational Emotive Therpay 30, 178
Reciprocal determinism 28
Reciprocal inhibition 25, 174, 208
 see also systematic desensitisation
Reciprocity counselling 101
Record keeping 133
Rehabilitation 52, 55, 58
Reinforcement 20, 27, 61, 154, 188,
 228, 241, 280
 schedules 24
 social 68
 verbal 66, 68
 vicarious 40
 see also Modelling
Relationships 103
Relaxation training 20, 27, 61, 154,
 188, 228, 241, 280
Required relaxation 80
 see also Overcorrection
Respondent approach 271
 see also Classical conditioning
Response cost 64, 79
Restitution 80
Ritualistic behaviour 52, 60
Role of the psychiatric·nurse 8, 9, 34,
 38, 82, 119
 see also Nurse's role
Room management 75
Running narrative 159

Secondary handicaps 48
Self-care 12, 47, 52, 54, 55, 66, 75,
 82
 see also Eating and Personal
 hygiene
Self control 99, 277
Self esteem 36

Self help group 98
Self injurious behaviour 80
Self instruction 30, 168
Self monitoring 228, 239, 272, 280,
 283
Self rating 216
Self reinforcement 99
Self relaxation 102
 see also Relaxation training
Self talk 98, 224
 see also Self instruction
Senile dementia 186
Smoking 228
Social
 anxiety 98, 172
 behaviour 47, 68, 82
 breakdown syndrome 47, 187
 interaction 82
 reinforcement 60, 79
 see also Verbal reinforcement
 relationships 278
 skills training 47, 58, 77, 79, 99,
 115, 189
 withdrawal 48, 49, 52, 55, 65
Speech, delusional 60
Spontaneous remission 26
Staff training 197
Stereotyped behaviour 193
Systematic desensitisation 25, 173
 see also Desensitisation, exposure
 and Reciprocal Inhibition

Targets 154, 234
Tender loving care 37
Therapeutic community 9, 128
Therapeutic role 44
 see also Nurse's role
Thinking errors 30
Thought disorder 30
Tics 228
Time out 79
Toilet training 75
Token economy 13, 53, 54, 59, 62,
 65, 82, 226
Total institutions 6
 see also Institutions
Traditional nursing role 40
Trichotillomania 101
Two-factor theory 27

Unassertiveness 101

Videotape, use of 79

Ward functions 132

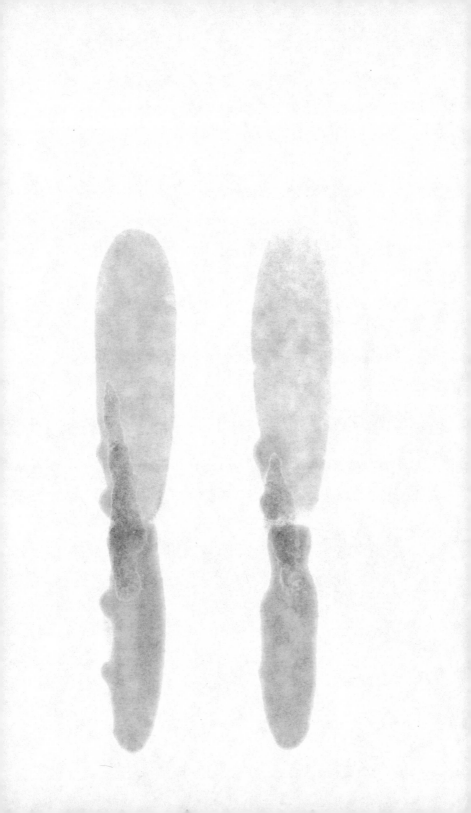

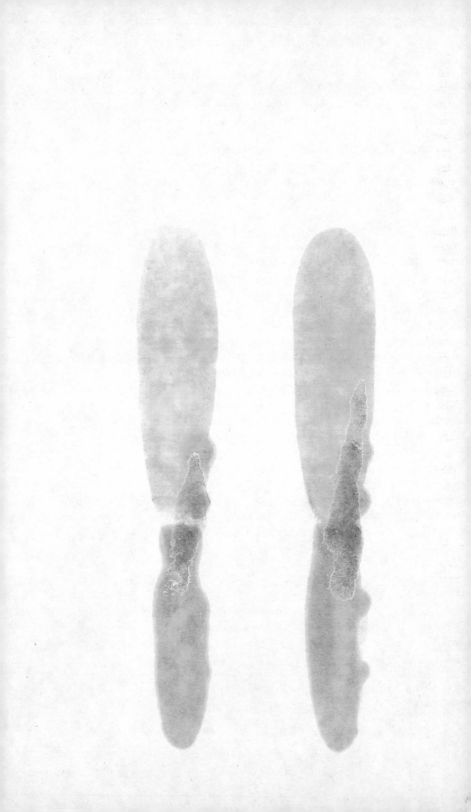